SO-AEH-922

Resistance Training for Special Populations

RESISTANCE TRAINING
FOR SPECIAL POPULATIONS

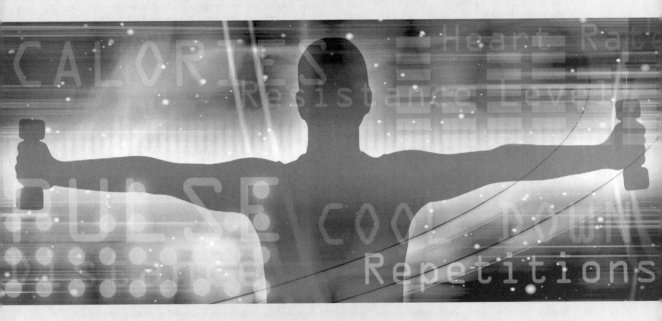

ANN MARIE SWANK, PhD
PATRICK HAGERMAN, Ed.D

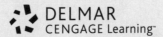

DELMAR
CENGAGE Learning™

Australia • Brazil • Japan • Korea • Mexico • Singapore • Spain • United Kingdom • United States

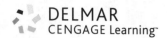

Resistance Training for Special Populations
By Ann Marie Swank and Patrick Hagerman

Vice President, Career and Professional Editorial: Dave Garza

Director of Learning Solutions: Matthew Kane

Acquisitions Editor: Matt Seeley

Managing Editor: Marah Bellegarde

Senior Product Manager: Darcy M. Scelsi

Editorial Assistant: Samantha Zullo

Vice President, Career and Professional Marketing: Jennifer McAvey

Marketing Manager: Kristin McNary

Marketing Coordinator: Erica Ropitsky

Production Director: Carolyn Miller

Content Project Manager: Kenneth McGrath

Art Director: Jack Pendleton

Production Technology Analyst: Mary Colleen Liburdi

For product information and technology assistance, contact us at
Professional & Career Group Customer Support, 1-800-648-7450

For permission to use material from this text or product, submit all requests online at **cengage.com/permissions.**
Further permissions questions can be e-mailed to
permissionrequest@cengage.com.

Library of Congress Control Number: 2008938428

ISBN-13: 978-1-4180-3218-0

ISBN-10: 1-4180-3218-2

Delmar
5 Maxwell Drive
Clifton Park, NY 12065-2919
USA

Cengage Learning products are represented in Canada by Nelson Education, Ltd.

For your lifelong learning solutions, visit **delmar.cengage.com**

Visit our corporate website at **cengage.com.**

Printed in the United States of America
1 2 3 4 5 6 7 12 11 10 09

33090014673646

CONTENTS

DEDICATION

To Carmen, Comehere, Ranger, Jake, Spike, Mookie, Sam, Sebastion, Santino, Puffer, Judy, Sheri, and Ricki for their inspiration, support, and encouragement

FOREWORD

Over the past quarter century, we have found that exercise can benefit every individual, even those with special needs or challenges. The time is right for this new book entitled, *Resistance Training for Special Populations*, in order to gain insights into exercise prescriptions for individuals with chronic disease. This book contains important insights into the modifications and progressions needed to successfully implement an exercise program in these many different populations. Exercise can be a crucial factor for an individual to enhance the quality of life when dealing with chronic disease. More importantly, this book focuses on strength training, which has been found to be one of the most effective modes of exercise for almost every population it has been applied to. During my career I have seen strength training successfully applied to each of the populations covered in this book and people's lives have been improved and the quality of life enhanced. This can only be accomplished if the exercise prescription process is clearly understood as it applies to a specific pathology and more important that the program is individualized. This underscores the importance of individualization of the exercise prescription process within the context of the chronic disease. As Editor, Dr. Ann Swank has put together a highly qualified and talented group of scientists whose insights and work in the various populations covered are exemplary. Unique to this book, after the introduction to the field is a presentation of sample exercise programs or "case studies" designed to enhance muscular strength, power, and endurance presented in a practical, "how to" format. Thus, more than theories, the reader can gain practical insights into the actual programs which have been found successful in their implementation. This format provides a great starting point for understanding the challenges and the implementation of a program. This book will provide the important knowledge base for working with people with such chronic diseases. Ultimately it is the person who we want to help in their struggle to find a better quality of life and survive longer. It is our responsibility to meet this challenge by being fully prepared to give each person our best. This book will help in that preparation and allow us to fulfill the "trust" each person we work with has in our professional ability to meet their needs.

William J. Kraemer
Storrs, CT
August 2008

PREFACE

Resistance Training for Special Populations offers evidence-based strategies for developing resistance training programs for a variety of individuals with various medical conditions. National organizations such as the American College of Sports Medicine (ACSM), National Strength and Conditioning Association (NSCA), American Heart Association (AHA), and the American Association of Cardiovascular and Pulmonary Rehabilitation (AACVPR) support resistance training for all individuals as part of a well rounded fitness program. Most current exercise programming texts for special populations focus on the cardiovascular recommendations. The current text is focused on designing effective resistance training programs with the understanding that a complete health and fitness program should also include cardiovascular and flexibility training.

The textbook is composed of 17 chapters. Chapter 1 presents background information on resistance training program design and the factors such as dosage, rest periods, frequency, etc to consider when developing a program. Chapter 2 presents a "pictorial essay" of each of the different exercises recommended in the subsequent 15 chapters. The remaining 15 chapters each present a special population including: older adults, individuals with osteoporosis, osteoarthritis, low back pain, chronic heart failure, obese adults, youths obesity, individuals with type 1 and type 2 diabetes, coronary heart disease, chronic obstructive pulmonary disease, intellectual disabilities, cancer, stroke, and pregnancy. This list of is by no means an exhaustive one but rather presents special medical conditions for which sufficient evidence exists to support safe and effective resistance training.

Each of the 15 chapters that address a special condition are organized to cover the following topics: prevalence and economic impact; etiology of the condition; specific benefits of resistance training for individuals with particular condition; literature review of relevant resistance training studies (studies that formed the basis of the recommended program); program design considerations; a sample 24-week program and a case study derived from using the 24-week program. The 24-week sample program provides the reader with a starting point for development of their resistance training programs for their own clients/patients. Accompanying the text is a CD which has summaries of the exercise programs developed for each population and space for the student to modify the program as needed. This template offers an evidence-based program as a starting point that can be modified in a variety of ways to fit the needs of individual clients/patients.

As indicated by the author biographies, the contributors for this text are a "who's who" in the strength and conditioning arena. The authors and contributors for the introductory chapters and each of the special populations bring a substantial level of expertise and experience to the table. Each author was able to convey their expertise in a way that students should find helpful as they design programs for their clients and patients.

The audience for whom this text is written is diverse. The text book would be relevant for any undergraduate or graduate programs of strength and conditioning, athletic training, exercise science or exercise physiology, and pre-physical therapy. Each of these graduate and undergraduate programs would have at least one class and possibly several that address principles of exercise training, exercise programming, and strength and conditioning for which this textbook would be appropriate. In addition, this textbook could serve as a reference text for the practicing clinician serving health and wellness clinics, personal training, athletic training, or rehabilitation medicine.

Historically, it was not long ago that resistance training was contraindicated for many medical conditions because of the physiological changes associated with training (increased blood pressure, etc). As research has been done, findings indicate that resistance training is safe, beneficial, and effective for many of these populations. *Resistance Training for Special Populations* presents the relevant research, risks, and benefits and sample programs for a variety of special populations.

Ann M. Swank, Ph.D., FACSM, CSCS

ACKNOWLEDGEMENTS

I would like to thank Patrick Hagerman for agreeing to be a co-editor for this textbook.

I would like to thank all my contributors for their expertise and patience through this entire process.

A special thanks to Dr. William Kraemer for writing the foreword for this textbook and also for contributing.

A final thanks to the University of Louisville administration for providing the time and resources to complete this textbook.

CONTRIBUTORS

Kerry Barnard, MS, CSCS
Southside Regional Medical Center
Petersburg, Virginia
Chapter 12: Resistance-Training Strategies for
Coronary Heart Disease

Sheri Colberg-Ochs, PhD
Old Dominion University
Norfolk, Virginia
Chapter 11: Resistance-Training Strategies for
Individuals with Type 2 Diabetes

Avery Faigenbaum, Ed.D, FACSM, CSCS, FNSCA
The College of New Jersey
Ewing, New Jersey
Chapter 9: Resistance-Training Strategies
for Childhood Obesity

Jeffrey Falkel, PhD, PT, CSCSD
VDP Enterprise
Littleton, Colorado
Chapter 6: Resistance-Training Strategies for
Individuals with Low Back Pain

Bo Fernhall, PhD
University of Illinois
Urbana, Illinois
Chapter 14: Resistance-Training Strategies
for Individuals with Intellectual Disabilities

Daniel E. Forman, MD
Brigham and Women's Hospital
Boston, Massachusetts
Chapter 3: Resistance-Training Strategies
for the Elderly

Karen L. Frost, PhD
University of Louisville
Louisville, Kentucky
Chapter 5: Resistance-Training Strategies for
Individuals with Osteoarthritis

Kara Mohr, PhD, FACSM
Mohr Results, Inc.
Louisville, Kentucky
Chapter 8: Resistance-Training Strategies for
Adult Obesity

Patrick Hagerman, Ed.D, CSCSD, NSCA-CPT
Quest Personal Training
Tulsa, Oklahoma
Kevin Heffernan, Ph.D.
Tufts Medical Center, Boston, Mass
Chapter 16: Resistance-Training Strategies for
Stroke Survivors

Kimberly Clark, MPH
University of Louisville
Louisville, Kentucky
Chapter 15: Resistance-Training Strategies for
Individuals with Cancer

Mark Kaelin, MS, CSCS
Bellarmine University
Louisville, Kentucky
Chapter 13: Resistance-Training Strategies for
Individuals with Asthma and COPD

William Kraemer, PhD, CSCS, FACSM, FNSCA
University of Connecticut
Storrs, Connecticut
Chapter 1: Overview of Training and Progression
Strategies

Steven Keteyian, PhD, FACSM
William Ford Center for Athletic Medicine
Detroit, Michigan
Chapter 7: Resistance-Training Strategies for
Individuals with Chronic Heart Failure

Robert Kipp, MS, CSCS
Louisville Athletic Club
Louisville, Kentucky

Chapter 2: Compendium of Resistance-Training
Exercises
Tom LaFontaine, PhD, FACSM
FitHealth
University of Missouri–Columbia
Columbia, Missouri
Chapter 10: Resistance-Training Strategies for
Individuals with Type 1 Diabetes

Sharon I. Larose, BS
Brigham and Women's Hospital
Boston, Massachusetts
Chapter 3: Resistance-Training Strategies for
the Elderly

John Manire, MS
University of Louisville
Lousiville, Kentucky
Chapter 2: Compendium of Resistance-Training
Exercises

Bonita L. Marks, PhD, FACSM
University of North Carolina at Chapel Hill
Chapel Hill, North Carolina
Chapter 4: Resistance-Training Strategies for
Individuals with Osteoporosis

Chris Mohr, PhD, RD
Mohr Results Inc.
Louisville, Kentucky
Chapter 8: Resistance-Training Strategies for
Adult Obesity

Michelle Mottola, PhD, FACSM
R. Samuel McLaughlin Foundation
University of Western Ontario
London, Ontario, Canada
Chapter 17: Resistance-Training Strategies for
Pregnant Woman

Jennifer Olive, PhD
Chapter 11: Resistance-Training Strategies for
Individuals with Type 2 Diabetes

Matthew J. Peterson, PhD
Durham Department of Veteran Affairs
Medical Center
Durham, North Carolina
Chapter 4: Resistance-Training Strategies for
Individuals with Osteoporosis

Nicholas Ratamess, PhD
The College of New Jersey
Ewing, New Jersey
Chapter 1: Overview of Training and Progression
Strategies

Jeffrey L. Roitman, Ed.D, FACSM
Rockhurst University
Kansas City, Missouri
Chapter 10: Resistance-Training Strategies for
Individuals with Type 1 Diabetes

Paul Salmon, PhD, MS
University of Louisville
Louisville, Kentucky
Chapter 15: Resistance-Training Strategies for
Individuals with Cancer

Kathy M. Shipp, PT, MHS, PhD
Duke University
Durham, North Carolina
Chapter 4: Resistance-Training Strategies for
Individuals with Osteoporosis

Robert Topp, PhD, RN
University of Louisville
Louisville, Kentucky
Chapter 5: Resistance-Training Strategies for
Individuals with Osteoarthritis

Lynn B. Wilson, MA
DePuy Spine, a Johnson & Johnson Company
Raynham, Massachusetts
Chapter 3: Resistance-Training Strategies for the
Elderly

REVIEWERS

Stacey Buser, MS, ATC
The University of Akron
Akron, Ohio

Donald M. Cummings, PhD
East Stroudsburg University
East Stroudsburg, Pennsylvania

L. Jerome Brandon, Phd, FACSM
Georgia State University
Atlanta, Georgia

Shannon Gaul
Lane Community College
Eugene, Oregon

Marla M. Graves, PhD
Arkansas State University
Jonesboro, Arkansas

Misty Hood
Highland Community College
Highland, Kansas

Timothy G. Howell, Ed.D, ATC, CSCS
Alfred University
Alfred, New York

Mark A. Lafferty, BA, BS, MS, MEd, PhD
Delaware Technical and Community College
Wilmington, Delaware

Jennifer Pintar, PhD, MPH
Youngstown State University
Youngstown, Ohio

Steve Rathbone, DA, ATC
Concord University
Athens, West Virginia

Scott C. Swanson, PhD
Ohio Northern University
Ada, Ohio

Adam J. Thompson, PhD, ATC, LAT
Indiana Wesleyan University
Marion, Indiana

Celete M. Weuve, MA, ATC, CSCS, LAT
Nicholls State University
Thibodaux, Louisiana

K. Sean Willeford, MS, ATC, LAT
Texas Christian University
Fort Worth, Texas

ABOUT THE AUTHORS

Ann Marie Swank, PhD, is a Professor of Exercise Physiology at the University of Louisville. She is also Director of the Exercise Physiology Laboratory. She is a Fellow of the American College of Sports Medicine. She is also certified through the National Strength and Conditioning Association as a CSCS and through the American College of Sports Medicine as an Exercise Specialist and Program Director. She has been teaching a wide range of exercise physiology courses and coordinating the internship program at the University of Louisville for 24 years.

Patrick S. Hagerman, Ed.D., CSCS, NSCA-CPT, FNSCA, is the Director of Sport Skill Development for Quest Personal Training Inc. He has been a certified coach for USA Weightlifting and USA Triathlon, a collegiate strength and conditioning coach, university professor, athlete and author. Dr. Hagerman has written five books, chapters in seven textbooks, over 30 professional articles, and is the Assistant Editor-in-Chief of the Strength and Conditioning Journal. He holds both NSCA and ACSM certifications, and is a Fellow of the National Strength and Conditioning Association.

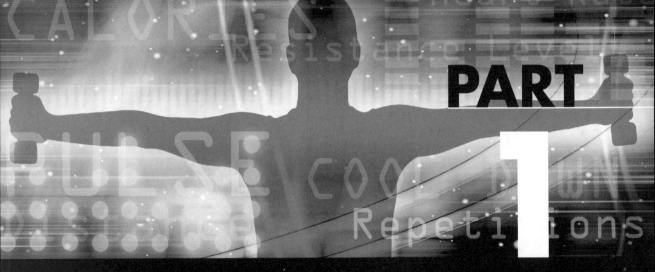

PART 1

OVERVIEW OF TRAINING

Chapter 1 Resistance Training and Progression Strategies for Special Populations

Chapter 2 Compendium of Resistance Training Exercises

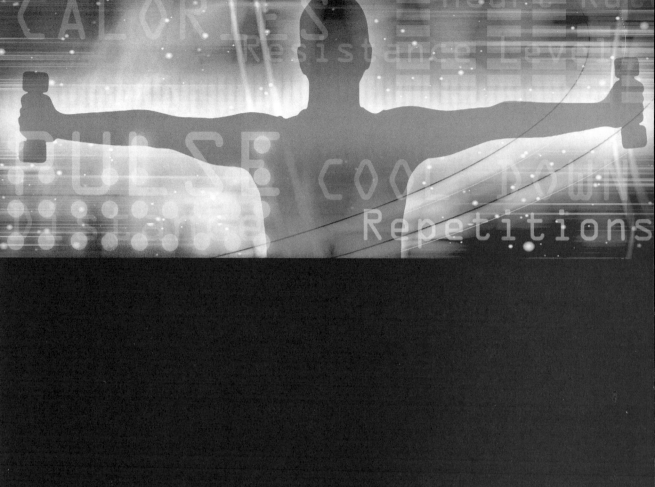

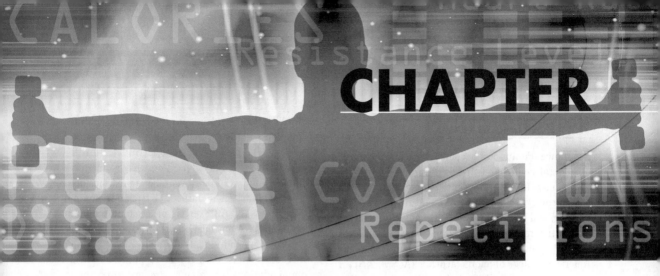

CHAPTER 1

RESISTANCE TRAINING AND PROGRESSION STRATEGIES FOR SPECIAL POPULATIONS

Objectives

Upon completion of this chapter, the reader should be able to:

- ○ Discuss the preplanning that needs to occur prior to designing a resistance-training program
- ○ Discuss the acute program variables and how manipulation of each can be used to target improvements in muscular strength, power, hypertrophy, and local endurance
- ○ Discuss program design for novice, intermediate, and advanced training, with an emphasis on the novice and intermediate classifications with respect to the recommendations provided by the American College of Sports Medicine
- ○ Explain the basic principles of progression for novice, intermediate, and advanced training

INTRODUCTION

Resistance training has become a critical component of general health and fitness programs due to the role it plays in increasing muscular strength, power, hypertrophy, local muscular endurance, speed, balance, and coordination (37). Because of the array of benefits, resistance training has now been recommended by national health organizations such as the American College of Sports Medicine (ACSM; 2, 3) for virtually all individuals, including adolescent, healthy adult, elderly, and clinical populations. Appropriate program design is critical to successful resistance training at any level. Program design entails goal setting, proper exercise instruction (e.g., technique, breathing, correct use of equipment, etc.), methods of evaluation, the correct application of program variables consistent with program goals, and specific methods of progression targeting particular areas of muscular fitness. This chapter discusses the critical components of resistance-training program design as well as progression strategies for those individuals targeting improved levels of fitness.

PLANNING THE RESISTANCE-TRAINING PROGRAM

The first step in program design is to obtain medical clearance. Although an individual may appear healthy, and the risk of serious illness or death via a cardiovascular event during exercise is very low (<6 individuals per 100,000), it is recommended that screening take place to ensure that resistance training is beneficial rather than injurious. The ACSM, the American Heart Association (AHA), and the National Strength and Conditioning Association (NSCA) have published guidelines addressing the procedures used for pre-exercise screening to ensure safe participation in resistance training (4, 48). The ACSM and AHA recommend all exercise facilities screen individuals prior to participation (4), and such screening typically occurs at the time of membership purchase. Screening can identify those individuals at risk and may be accomplished using a medical history questionnaire

(e.g. PAR-Q) or health-appraisal document (4). Information regarding cardiovascular risk factors and musculoskeletal problems can be identified. Health-appraisal documents should be interpreted by qualified facility personnel (4). In the event that a predisposition to injury or illness is identified, physician screening may be necessary. All exercise professionals should adhere to the recommendations of these organizations when screening individuals for resistance training. Failure of a client or member to abide by these recommendations, or to sign a release form, may exclude them from exercise participation (4).

The second step in preplanning involves goal setting via a **needs analysis** that consists of answering relevant questions based upon resistance-training goals. Some common questions that need to be addressed include (38):

○ Are there any health or injury concerns that may limit the exercises performed or the exercise intensiy?

○ What types of equipment (e.g., free weights, machines, bands/tubing, medicine balls, functional, etc.) are available and preferred?

○ What is the targeted training frequency?

○ Are there any time constraints that may affect workout duration?

○ What muscle groups need special attention? All major muscle groups are trained, but some may require prioritization based upon strengths and weaknesses.

○ What are the targeted energy systems (e.g., aerobic or anaerobic)?

○ Are isometric muscle actions needed in addition to concentric and eccentric muscle actions?

○ If the individual is training for a sport or activity, what are the most common sites for injury?

These are general questions addressing program goals. Each of the subsequent chapters addressing special populations will discuss more specific population-based goals. The program goals are subsequently determined from the information gained from these questions. Some common goals include increase in muscle size, strength, power, speed, local muscular endurance, balance and proprioception, coordination, flexibility, reductions in body fat, improvements in general health, and rehabilitation from injury. Most programs aim to collectively improve several of these components as opposed to only focusing on one. Along with goal setting, the magnitude of improvement and the nature of the program need to be established. **Recreational training** involves resistance training for moderate improvements in muscle strength, local muscular endurance, and hypertrophy for general fitness; whereas **competitive training** involves resistance training to maximize muscle hypertrophy, strength, power, and local muscular endurance. **Maintenance training** involves resistance training to maintain the current level of muscular fitness rather than to develop further gains. A benefit of maintenance programs is that in the short term, reductions in training volume, frequency, and intensity may be used without a significant reduction in muscular fitness. These programs are commonly used by athletes during the competitive season and in the general fitness setting. However, it is important to note that long-term maintenance training could result in detraining if the exercise volume, frequency, and intensity do not meet a minimum training threshold.

RESISTANCE-TRAINING PROGRAM DESIGN

The resistance-training program is composed of variables that include 1) specific muscle actions used during an exercise, 2) intensity, 3) mode, 4) sequence of exercises, 5) rest intervals between sets, 6) repetition velocity, and 7) training frequency. Manipulation of these variables affects the training stimulus and leads to goal-specific adaptations. Designing a proper resistance-training program involves manipulation of each variable specific to the targeted goals.

Muscle Actions

Muscle actions refer to the type of contractions performed. Resistance training consists predominantly of dynamic muscle actions, which include both **concentric muscle action (CON)**, or muscle shortening, and **eccentric muscle action (ECC)**, or muscle lengthening. The ACSM recommends inclusion of both regardless of training goals; therefore the role of manipulating muscle actions is minimal at any level of training (3); however, there is a question as to whether **isometric muscle actions (ISOM)**, static actions with minimal change in length, should be included.

When comparing ISOM to dynamic resistance training, ISOM training can increase dynamic strength when multiple-joint angles are trained, and dynamic training can increase ISOM muscle strength. However, the trained muscle action will yield the greatest improvement when that action is specifically tested (5, 45), meaning that ISOM strength shows the greatest improvement after training with ISOM actions. Isometric training is often overlooked and has numerous benefits for all populations. Loaded ISOM contractions are encountered many times during training, such as when gripping the weights, during pauses in between CON and ECC muscle actions, and during failed or nearly failed CON repetitions. Other than the aforementioned scenarios, performing specific ISOM sets appears to be most common in early injury rehabilitation and in advanced resistance-training programs to enhance maximal strength. For example, a popular ISOM training modality is **functional isometrics**, which involve performing isometric actions at specific weak points in a range of motion as a means of increasing strength at that particular point. Functional isometrics have not been extensively investigated in special populations, but they are believed to favor improvements in muscular strength.

Exercise Selection

Exercise selection refers to types of exercises chosen for inclusion in the program. Resistance-training exercises are either single or multiple joint. **Single-joint exercises** stress one joint or major muscle group, whereas **multiple-joint exercises** stress more than one joint or major muscle group. Both types are effective for increasing muscular strength. Single-joint exercises, such as the triceps extension or biceps curl, have been used to target specific muscle groups and are less complex. Multiple-joint exercises—such as the bench press, squat, and power clean—involve a higher degree of coordination, especially the total-body Olympic lifts; and due to the larger muscle-mass involvement and subsequent amount of weight used, these exercises have generally been regarded as the most effective exercises for increasing muscular strength and power (15, 38). Total-body exercises, such as the power snatch and power clean, have been regarded as the most effective exercises for increasing muscle power, because they require fast-force production to successfully complete each repetition (17).

Large muscle mass exercises elicit the greatest acute metabolic responses. For example, exercises such as the squat, leg press, leg extension, and bent-over row have been shown to elicit greater rates of oxygen consumption than the behind-the-neck shoulder press, bench press, upright row, and arm curl (6). In addition, these exercises produce substantial acute hormonal responses in comparison to smaller-mass exercises (39). These results have direct implications for resistance-training programs targeting improvements in local muscle endurance, lean body mass, and reductions in body fat.

Single- and multiple-joint exercises have also been described as closed-chain or opened-chain kinetic exercises. A **closed-chain kinetic exercise** is one where the distal segments are fixed, as in the leg press, squat, and deadlift; **opened-chain kinetic exercise,** such as leg extensions and leg curls, enables the distal segment to freely move against a resistance. Both stress each joint differently, however, the effects on performance are less clear.

The primary consideration in selecting which exercises to include in a training program is the goals of the individual. An argument can be made for the benefits of any given exercise; however, it is the relationship between an exercise and achievement of the overall training goal that is most important.

As a general rule, the exercises chosen should challenge the individual, should be within the individual's capabilities, and should impact the final result in some direct way. In sports, this is often achieved by choosing sport-specific exercises or exercises that mimic some part of the required skills. Among general and special populations, exercises should enhance activities of daily living and improve the individual's ability to interact with the environment, as well as increasing the ability to maintain a healthy lifestyle.

Exercise Sequencing and Structure of Training Routines

Exercise sequencing refers to the order in which exercises are placed within a training session. The sequencing of exercises and the number of muscle groups trained significantly affects the acute expression of muscular strength. Prior to discussing the effects of different sequencing strategies, it is important to identify which muscle groups will be trained. Three training-routine structures common to resistance training determine which muscle groups are trained: 1) total-body routines, 2) upper- and lower-body split routines, and 3) muscle-group split routines. **Total-body routines** involve performance of exercises stressing all major muscle groups and include one or two exercises for each major muscle group. **Upper- and lower-body split routines** involve performance of upper-body exercises during one workout and lower-body exercises during another. **Muscle-group split routines** involve the performance of exercises for specific muscle groups during the same workout (e.g., chest and triceps during one workout, biceps and back during another, and legs and shoulders during a third, separate workout). All three are effective for improving muscular fitness, and it appears that individual goals, time or frequency, and personal preferences often determine which type of structure will be used. The major differences between these structures lies in the magnitude of specialization observed during each training session and the amount of recovery between each session. More exercises for a specific muscle group may be performed during a muscle-group split routine as opposed to fewer exercises per muscle group in a total-body routine.

General recommendations for exercise sequencing can be made depending on whether a person is training for strength, hypertrophy, power, or local muscular endurance. Acute lifting performance and optimal strength increases depend on where an exercise is placed in a workout sequence (59, 61, 62). For instance, an individual will usually be able to perform more repetitions or use heavier weights during multiple-joint exercises when those exercises are performed early in a workout rather than toward the end. In addition, large muscle-mass exercises performed early have a stimulatory effect on small muscle-mass exercises performed later in the workout. Hansen and colleagues (23) reported greater ISOM strength increases in arm musculature when arm training was preceded by lower-body exercises. They also found greater acute elevations in growth hormone and testosterone when large muscle-mass exercises preceded small-mass exercises. Considering that multiple-joint exercises have been shown to increase muscular strength, hypertrophy, and power, maximizing performance of these exercises by including them early in the training session, when fatigue is minimal, may be necessary for optimal gains (3).

Multiple-joint exercises, such as Olympic lifts, have been used extensively for power training. Because they require rapid force production, the inclusion of these exercises is necessary for increased power. These exercises also require additional time for learning proper technique and need to be performed first in the workout, when fatigue is minimal. Performing explosive exercises early on may also enhance performance of basic multiple-joint strength exercises such as squats, when the squat follows the Olympic lift in sequence (62).

The sequencing of exercises for local muscular endurance training may not be as critical in comparison to strength and power training, because fatigue is a necessary component of local muscular endurance training. Therefore other variations, in addition to the aforementioned strategies, may be used for local muscular endurance training. The sequencing strategies for strength, power, and hypertrophy training suggested by the ACSM (3) are presented in Table 1-1. Exceptions to these recommendations do exist, especially if the

Table 1-1 Exercise Sequencing Strategies for Strength and Power Training

Total-Body Routine

- Perform large muscle group exercises before small muscle group exercises.
- Perform multiple-joint exercises before single-joint exercises.
- Perform Olympic lifts before basic strength exercises (i.e., squats, bench presses), and do the most complex exercises first.
- Rotate upper- and lower-body exercises and opposing (agonist–antagonist) exercises.

Upper- and Lower-Body Split Routine

- Perform large muscle group exercises before small muscle group exercises.
- Perform multiple-joint exercises before single-joint exercises.
- Rotate opposing (agonist–antagonist) exercises.

Muscle Group Split Routines

- Perform multiple-joint exercises before single-joint exercises.
- Perform high-intensity exercises (i.e., those having a higher percent of one-repetition maximum [1RM]) before low-intensity exercises.

Source: Kraemer WJ, Ratamess NA. Fundamentals of resistance training: progression and exercise prescription. *Med Sci Sport Exes*. 2004;36:674–688.

individual is training specifically for muscle endurance or, to a certain extent, muscle hypertrophy. In addition, other exceptions may relate to warm-up exercises and weakness prioritization.

Intensity

Intensity describes the amount of weight, or load, lifted and is highly dependent upon other variables such as exercise order, volume, frequency, muscle action, repetition speed, and amount of rest between sets. Altering the training load can significantly affect the acute metabolic, hormonal, neural, and cardiovascular responses to training. The intensity prescribed also depends upon individual training status and goals and is often listed as a percentage of a person's **one-repetition maximum (1RM)**. The term 1RM refers to the maximum amount of weight that can be lifted one time with proper technique. Other terms often used to describe intensity are multiples of 1RM, such as 6RM, which indicates a load that can be lifted a maximum of 6 repetitions with proper technique. Any number placed before the RM designation indicates the maximum number of repetitions possible with that load (e.g., 3RM, 5RM, 10RM, etc.).

In novices—that is, previously untrained individuals—light loads approximately 45 to 50 percent of 1RM or less may increase dynamic muscular strength, because this initial phase of lifting is characterized by improved motor learning and coordination (1, 58). At the novice or beginning level of training, strength increases are a by-product of learning correct form and technique, so heavy weights are not required to increase strength. The ACSM recommends an intensity of approximately

50 to 70 percent of 1RM, depending on the person's goals (3), but heavier loading will be needed to increase maximal strength as the individual moves from novice to intermediate or advanced levels of training (19, 27; see Table 1-2).

Maximizing strength, power, and hypertrophy may only be accomplished when the maximal number of **motor units** are recruited. Heavy loading in trained individuals is needed to recruit the high-threshold motor units that may not be activated during light to moderate lifting. Therefore, the ACSM recommends 70 to 100 percent of 1RM for advanced strength training, for individuals with several years of lifting experience and a firm strength base, and hypertrophy training (3). However, the human body cannot withstand lifting heavy weights on a weekly basis, so the use of heavy weights systematically included in specific training phases using periodization of loading is most critical and produces the best results in advanced lifters (38).

Intensity is also related to the number of repetitions prescribed. There is an inverse relationship between weight lifted and repetitions performed. As the %1RM increases, and the load becomes heavier,

Table 1-2 ACSM Recommendations

Training for Strength, Power, Hypertrophy, and Muscular Endurance

Strength	Power	Hypertrophy	Muscular Endurance
%1RM	50–70% Novice 30–80% 70–100% Intermediate to Advanced	30–60%	70–80%
Rest	2–3 minutes for multiple-joint exercises		1–2 minutes for high-repetition sets
Interval	1–2 minutes for single-joint exercises >3 minutes for advanced lifters		<1 minute for moderate-repetition sets
Frequency	2–3 days per week for novices; 2–4 days per week for intermediate to advanced lifters		

Source: American College of Sports Medicine: Position stand: Progression models in resistance training for healthy adults. *Med Sci Sports Exerc.* 2002;34:364–380.

the number of repetitions per set decreases. As the %1RM decreases, and the load becomes lighter, the number of repetitions per set increases. Research has shown that training with loads corresponding to 80 to 85 percent of 1RM and higher resulted in 1 to 6 repetitions per set and were most effective for increasing maximal dynamic strength (10). This loading range appears to maximally recruit muscle fibers and will specifically increase dynamic 1RM strength. Although strength can increase with lighter loads corresponding to approximately 70 to 80 percent of 1RM, it is believed that this range may not be as effective in increasing maximal strength in advanced resistance-trained individuals compared to heavier loading (>80 percent of 1RM).

The 6RM to 12RM loading range (70 to 80 percent of 1RM) is typically used in programs that target muscular hypertrophy (38). Although heavy loading is effective for increasing muscle size, it has been suggested that the 6RM to 12RM loading range may provide the best combination of load and volume (38). Loads lighter than this (50 to 70 percent of 1RM or 12RM to 15RM and lighter) rarely increase maximal strength but are very effective for increasing absolute local muscular endurance (10). Thus, a continuum exists on the loading-volume axis such that high load and low repetitions are most specific to increasing strength, whereas low load and high repetitions are most specific to endurance (38). The ACSM recommends 30 to 80 percent of 1RM for advanced endurance training, depending on the selected repetition number and rest interval length (3); that is, higher repetitions of 20 to 25 or more are performed with light loads, whereas heavier loads with moderate repetitions of 10 to 15 can be used successfully, especially when combined with short rest intervals (<2 min).

Training to increase muscle power is multifactorial. Given that both force and velocity are relevant components to maximizing power, training to increase muscular power requires two general loading strategies. First, moderate to heavy loads are required to recruit high-threshold, fast-twitch motor units needed for strength enhancement. However, higher loads are accompanied by lower velocities. Thus, the second strategy is to incorporate light to moderate loads performed at an explosive lifting velocity. Depending on the exercise in question, this loading range may encompass 30 to 60 percent of 1RM, as recommended by the ACSM (3).

In addition, **ballistic resistance exercise** can enhance 1RM strength (42). The advantage of ballistic resistance exercise is that the load is maximally accelerated either by jumping, such as in jump squats, or by releasing the weight using specialized equipment such as the Plyo Power System. However, traditional repetitions result in a deceleration phase, which limits power development throughout the complete range of motion. During traditional resistance-training exercises performed at an explosive velocity, a recent study has shown that 40 to 60 percent of 1RM may be most beneficial for bench presses, and 50 to 70 percent may be most beneficial for squats (60), thereby demonstrating that a slightly higher load is necessary for power training when nonballistic repetitions are performed. Thus, training for maximal power requires various loading strategies performed at high velocity.

Although each training zone has its advantages, devoting 100 percent of training to one general RM zone or intensity runs a very high risk of the individual encountering training plateaus or becoming overtrained, so it is not recommended. It is important to note that intensity is exercise dependent. For example, Hoeger and colleagues (25) showed that 80 percent of 1RM corresponded to 10RM for exercises such as the bench press, leg extension, and lat pulldown; however, this intensity corresponded to only 6RM for the leg curl, 7RM to 8RM for the arm curl, and 15RM for the leg press. Therefore, it appears that optimal strength, hypertrophy, and local muscular endurance training requires the systematic use of various loading strategies to target all facets of muscular development.

Once training intensity has been prescribed, three basic methods are used to increase loading during progression: 1) increasing relative load percentage, 2) training within a repetition maximum zone, and 3) increasing absolute amounts. Increasing relative load percentage is common in periodized programs. An individual may train at 70 percent of 1RM for an exercise during one phase and 80 percent in the next phase.

Training within an RM zone requires an increase in repetitions for one workload until a target is reached. For instance, in an 8RM to 12RM zone, an individual selects an 8RM load and then performs 8 repetitions. Within the next few training sessions, the individual increases repetitions with that load until 12 repetitions are performed on consecutive days. Loading is increased and the individual subsequently performs 8 repetitions. So as the individual becomes stronger, more repetitions are possible with the same weight; and when the maximum number of repetitions for that RM zone has been reached, load is increased. An increase in load requires a decrease in repetitions, an inverse relationship, so the individual will train with the new load until they can increase the number of repetitions again.

Increasing load in absolute amounts is common. For example, the individual completes 6 repetitions with 100 kg on the bench press. Subsequently, the individual continues to perform 6 repetitions but with a greater load (e.g., 105 kg). An absolute amount of weight is added to the exercise while the individual attempts to perform a similar number of repetitions. All of these methods have been studied and have been shown to be very effective for resistance training (37, 38). Ultimately, it may be the preference of the exercise professional or the trainee as to which method or combination of methods will be used, because they are all effective.

Volume

Training volume is a summation of the total number of sets and repetitions performed during a workout. It can be manipulated by changing the number of repetitions performed per set, the number of sets performed per exercise, or the number of exercises performed per session. The number of repetitions performed per set is dependent on the weight used, as noted earlier. Although training volume has been studied to varying degrees, the exact number of sets performed per muscle group during a workout still remains unclear.

The comparison of single- and multiple-set resistance-training programs has received considerable attention and has been a topic of much debate since the 1970s.

In most of the studies to date, one set per exercise, performed for 8 to 12 repetitions at an intentionally slow lifting velocity, has been compared to both periodized and nonperiodized multiple-set programs (3, 36, 40). Several studies have been criticized because the number of sets per exercise was not separated from other variables such as intensity, frequency, and repetition velocity, therefore making it difficult to ascertain if the observed differences were the result of the number of sets per exercise or from some other uncontrolled variable (3, 36, 40). However, the purpose of some of these studies was to make general program comparisons in response to the emergence in popularity of single-set programs and the subsequent unsubstantiated marketing claims associated with their efficacy. This concern notwithstanding, comparisons between a single-set training program and various multiple-set programs of various intensities have yielded conflicting results. Some studies have reported similar strength increases between single- and multiple-set programs (3), whereas others pronounced multiple-set programs superior in previously untrained individuals (9, 51). A recent report in untrained older adults showed that 20 weeks of multiple-set training was superior to one set for increasing maximal strength and endurance in most exercises; however, no differences in functional performance were observed among groups (16). Another study in resistance-trained post-menopausal women showed that multiple-set training resulted in a 3 to 6 percent strength increase, whereas single-set training resulted in a 1 to 2 percent *reduction* in strength (34).

In a meta-analysis, Peterson and colleagues (52) reported that performance of approximately 8 sets per muscle group produced the greatest effect size for strength increases. Most studies have used 2 to 6 sets per exercise and have found substantial increases in strength in trained and untrained individuals (38). However, similar strength increases have been found in novice individuals who trained using 2 and 3 sets and 2 and 4 sets (50). Three sets have also been reported as being superior to 1 and 2 (8). Based on these studies, it appears that untrained individuals respond favorably to several multiple-set programs. No study has shown single-set training to be superior to multiple-set training in either trained or untrained individuals.

Accordingly, the ACSM has recommended 1 to 3 sets for novice or beginning training (3). Considering that the early phase of resistance training is characterized by improvements in muscle activation and coordination, it may be that lifting volume is not critical during the initial 6 to 12 weeks. However, long-term resistance training studies have predominantly shown that a higher volume of resistance exercise is necessary to generate a higher rate of progression. Thus, the ACSM has recommended multiple sets for intermediate training—that is, training for several months to a few years—and advanced resistance training (3). Typically, 3 to 6 sets per exercise are most common during resistance training, but more and less have also been used successfully. In resistance-trained individuals, multiple-set programs have been shown to be superior for muscle strength, local muscular endurance, power, and hypertrophy increases (36, 56). Therefore, the number of sets selected per exercise should vary depending on the training goals.

As mentioned earlier, volume is the sum of the number of sets, repetitions, and exercises performed at a given intensity or load. Because intensity and volume are inversely related; increases in training volume with low-repetition, high-intensity programs should be closely monitored and intensity possibly reduced to lower the risk of overtraining.

Traditional resistance training—high load, low repetition, and long rest periods—produces significant hypertrophy; however, the total volume involved with traditional resistance training may not maximize hypertrophy (15, 38). Total volume, in addition to the forces developed, plays a critical role for gains in muscular hypertrophy. This finding has been supported in part by greater hypertrophy associated with high-volume, multiple-set programs compared to low-volume, single-set programs in resistance-trained individuals (36, 40). Muscular endurance and hypertrophy programs using moderate to heavy loads, moderate to high repetitions, multiple sets per exercise, and at least six exercises are generally regarded as high-volume programs.

High-intensity, low-repetition sets (<6 repetitions) appear to be most conducive to enhancing maximal strength and the force component of the power equation; very light to moderate loads performed for multiple sets of high repetitions, characteristic of local muscular endurance training, are considered to be very high in total volume but not optimal for hypertrophy or strength. Multiple-set strength and power training with heavy loads and low repetitions using a moderate to high number of sets is generally considered a low-volume program.

Finally, it is important to point out that not all exercises need to be performed with the same number of sets; emphasis on higher or lower training volume is related to the program priorities as well as to the muscles trained in an exercise movement. Low-volume programs can provide a solid variation during the larger training cycle and therefore have a place when properly incorporated into a conditioning program.

One intensity/volume program design issue is whether or not each set should be performed to muscular exhaustion, or failure. Repetitions are performed with RM loading until another repetition cannot be performed with proper technique without assistance. Some programs consist entirely of performing each set to failure, whereas some programs limit or do not perform sets to failure, such as Olympic-style lifts. The rationale for training to failure is to maximize motor-unit activity and muscular adaptation. Performing each set to failure produces higher levels of fatigue during subsequent sets of the same exercise, resulting in lower volume unless load modifications are made (7). The challenge is to designate the proper proportion of the total sets performed to failure while still minimizing the risk of overtraining and injury. Drinkwater and associates (13) compared equal volume/intensity programs either to failure (4 sets of 6 repetitions) or not to failure (8 sets of 3 repetitions) and found that training to failure resulted in a greater increase in 6RM bench presses (9.5 percent) compared to nonfailure (5 percent). Recent investigations have shown that not performing each set to failure (3 sets of 10 reps) versus performing each set to failure (6 sets of 5 reps) with the same load resulted in similar increases in 1RM bench press, squat, and muscle power. However, muscular endurance was enhanced further via training to failure (31). Thus, it appears that training to failure has a more prominent effect on enhancing muscular endurance. Training to failure or nonfailure are both effective for increasing strength, but caution is needed, because training to failure induces a larger magnitude of neuromuscular fatigue.

Although it is still unclear how to systematically include sets to failure, evidence supports both philosophies for optimal resistance training, and the goal of the exercise may be critical to the decision. Complex exercises that require high force, high velocity, increased power production, and proper technique—such as Olympic lifts, variations, and ballistic exercises—are best performed with minimal fatigue. Consequently, training to failure may be counterproductive. There is evidence showing that fatigue may enhance the resistance-training process for less complex exercises (13). Resistance training with multiple-joint, single-joint, and basic strength exercise to failure at least part of the time may be beneficial. Not every set is performed to failure, but it does appear that at least a few sets, perhaps the last 1 to 2 sets of an exercise, need to be performed to failure to maximally increase muscle strength.

Rest Intervals

Rest intervals refer to the amount of time taken in between sets and exercises. The amount of rest between sets and exercises significantly affects the metabolic, hormonal, and cardiovascular responses to an acute bout of resistance exercise, as well as performance of subsequent sets and training adaptations (38). Rest-interval length is selected based on training intensity, goals, fitness level, and targeted energy system utilization. The metabolic response to resistance exercise depends on the rest-interval length. Strength and power training that utilize heavy loads and 1 to 6 repetitions with long rest intervals, predominantly stress the ATP-PC system, the primary energy system used for high-intensity exercise lasting up to 20 seconds. Hypertrophy and strength training, utilizing moderate-to-heavy loads and 6 to 12 repetitions with moderate to short rest intervals, is supported mostly by energy provided by ATP-PC and glycolysis, an anaerobic energy

system characterized by the breakdown of glucose for energy liberation that often results in increased blood lactate production with only minor contributions from aerobic metabolism. Local muscular endurance training, with high repetitions and short rest intervals, involves a higher contribution of energy from aerobic metabolism. Thus, the rest interval influences the relative contribution of the three energy systems.

Rest-interval length affects subsequent adaptations in 1RM strength. Strength and power performance is highly dependent upon anaerobic energy release, primarily via the phosphagens (ATP-PC), and the majority of phosphagen repletion occurs within 3 minutes. Therefore, performance of maximal lifts requires maximal energy substrate availability prior to the set with minimal or no fatigue. This finding emphasizes the importance of recovery during optimal strength and power training. Studies have shown greater strength increases when long versus short rest periods—2 to 3 minutes versus 30 to 40 seconds—are used. Robinson and colleagues (57) reported a 7 percent versus 2 percent increase in squat performance after 5 weeks of training with 3-minute versus 30-second rest intervals respectively. Pincivero and colleagues (53) reported significantly greater strength gains— 5 to 8 percent—when 160-second rest intervals were used compared to 40-second intervals. Acute force and power production may be compromised with short rest periods lasting a minute or less (46). Repetition number decreased with each successive set when performing 5 sets of 15RM of squats or bench presses when less than 2-minute rest intervals were used between sets (65). In addition, the pattern of decline in performance is comparable between low and moderately high intensities ranging between 50 and 80 percent of 1RM (64). When using a 10-repetition squat protocol, 2 minutes of rest was not sufficient to maintain performance over 6 sets, but it was sufficient for 2 to 3 sets (55). Thus, greater declines in performance are seen as the rest interval becomes shorter. Therefore, the ACSM has recommended at least 2- to 3-minute rest intervals for multiple-joint exercises and 1 to 2 minutes for single-joint exercises for novice to intermediate strength and power training; for advanced strength and power training, more than 3 minutes was recommended (3; see Table 1-2).

Rest-interval length will vary according to the goals of a particular exercise, so not every exercise will use the same rest interval. Muscle strength may be increased using short rest periods but at a slower rate compared to long rest periods, thus demonstrating the need to establish goals for the magnitude of strength improvement sought prior to selecting a rest interval.

Targeting the glycolytic and ATP-PC energy systems may enhance training for hypertrophy in addition to heavy-resistance exercise. For this aspect of hypertrophy training, such as bodybuilding programs, less than 2 minutes of rest between sets appears to be effective. These rest intervals appear to be a potent anabolic hormone stimulator, stimulating local blood flow and resulting in significant lactate production. Studies that have restricted blood flow and used light loading during resistance exercise, thereby increasing the concentrations of metabolites and the anaerobic nature of the exercise stimulus, have shown prominent increases in muscle hypertrophy comparable to heavier loading, thus demonstrating the utility of blood flow and/or metabolite accumulation during resistance training (63). This finding may be one explanation for the efficacy of bodybuilding programs that use moderate loading and high volume with short rest intervals for increasing muscle hypertrophy. However, it appears that maximal hypertrophy may be attained through the combination of strength and hypertrophy training, using variation in rest-interval length depending on the loading, to maximize the mechanical and metabolic responses, which is why the ACSM has recommended 2 to 3 minutes of rest between heavy exercises and 1 to 2 minutes for other exercises for advanced hypertrophy training (3).

Rest intervals also have a substantial impact on local muscular endurance. Local muscular endurance improves during resistance training with greater effects observed with **absolute muscular endurance,** the maximal number of repetitions performed with a specific pretraining load (29), and only limited effects in **relative local muscular endurance,** endurance assessed at a specific relative intensity, or percent of 1RM (41). Training to increase local muscular endurance requires that the individual

1) perform high repetitions in long-duration sets and/ or 2) minimize recovery between sets. Minimizing recovery between sets is an important stimulus with regard to the adaptations within skeletal muscle necessary to improve local muscular endurance (e.g., to increase mitochondrial and capillary number, fiber-type transitions, and buffer capacity). The ACSM has recommended 1- to 2-minute rest intervals in conjunction with high-repetition sets and less than 1-minute rest intervals for moderate repetition ranges (3). Another consideration when selecting rest intervals between sets is the number of exercises performed per muscle group during a workout. As a muscle is worked repeatedly with different exercises, fatigue will build. Therefore rest intervals will vary for each exercise in a workout, and fatigue associated with previous exercises must be considered when performing exercises later in the workout.

Repetition Velocity

Repetition velocity refers to the time it takes to perform a single repetition, and it is usually divided into the CON and ECC portions of the movement. **Dynamic constant external resistance** training poses different stresses when examining lifting velocity. Since force equals mass times acceleration, application of high levels of force leads to greater acceleration of the weight. Likewise, significant reductions in force production are observed when the intent is to perform the repetition slowly. However, it is important to note that two types of low-velocity contractions exist, *unintentional* and *intentional*. Unintentional low velocities are used during high-intensity repetitions in which either loading and/or fatigue are responsible for the low velocity. Mookerjee and Ratamess (44) have shown that during a 5RM bench press, the concentric phase for the first 3 repetitions was approximately 1.2 to 1.6 seconds in duration, whereas the last 2 repetitions were approximately 2.5 and 3.3 seconds respectively due to fatigue. These data demonstrate the impact of loading and fatigue on repetition velocity in individuals performing each repetition with maximal effort.

Intentional low velocities are used with submaximal weights where the individual has greater control of the velocity. CON force production is substantially lower for an intentionally slow speed of lifting (5-second CON, 5-second ECC), compared to a traditional moderate velocity (1- to 2-second CON, 1- to 2-second ECC) with a corresponding lower neural activation (35). This finding indicates that motor-unit activity may be limited when intentionally lifting a weight slowly. Although intentionally slow repetitions may provide some benefit for local muscular endurance and hypertrophy training, the lighter loads may not provide an optimal stimulus for improving 1RM strength in resistance-trained individuals. When performing a set of 10 repetitions using a very low velocity (10-second CON, 5-second ECC) compared to a low velocity (2-second CON, 4-second ECC), a 30 percent reduction in training weight resulted, leading to significantly less strength gains in most of the exercises tested after 10 weeks of training (33). Compared to low velocities, moderate velocities (1- to 2-second CON, 1- to 2-second ECC) and high velocities (<1-second CON, 1-second ECC) proved more effective for enhanced muscular performance, increasing the number of repetitions performed and increasing work, power output, volume, and the rate of strength gains (38).

Critical to resistance training is the intent to move the weight as quickly as possible to optimize neural activation and force output. Recent studies have shown **intentional high velocities** to be more effective for advanced training than traditionally lower velocities with similar loading. Jones and colleagues (32) found that if bar velocity was maximized, 1RM squats increased by 11.5 percent after 10 weeks of resistance training with a light load, 40 to 60 percent of 1RM, that would typically produce minimal strength gains. This technique, called **compensatory acceleration,** requires the individual to accelerate the load maximally throughout the range of motion during the CON action to maximize bar velocity. A major advantage is that this technique can be used with heavy loads, and it is considered especially effective for multiple-joint exercises.

Lifting velocity is critical for power training. Power production is greatest when the optimal combination

of force and velocity are attained. Neuromuscular contributions to maximal power development include 1) maximal rate of force development; 2) muscular strength at low and high repetition velocities; 3) stretch-shortening cycle performance; and 4) coordination of movement pattern and skill. To maximize power training, heavy resistance training needs to be accompanied by explosive exercises.

A limitation to performing high-velocity repetitions with free weights is the **deceleration phase,** which occurs near the end of the CON range of motion, where bar velocity decreases prior to completion of the repetition to bring the bar to a stop and to prevent injury. The length of this phase depends on the weight lifted and the initial velocity, because the load is decelerated for a considerable proportion, 24 to 40 percent, of the CON movement (14, 49). The length of the deceleration phase increases to 52 percent of the CON movement when performing the lift with a lower percentage (81 percent) of 1RM (14). Thus, power improvements may be most specific only to the initial segment of the range of motion.

Ballistic resistance exercise—that is, explosive movements that enable acceleration throughout the full range of motion (e.g., loaded jump squat, bench throw, and shoulder throw)—has been shown to limit this problem. Loaded jump squats at 30 percent of 1RM have been shown to increase vertical jump performance more than traditional back squats, plyometrics, and jump squats performed at 80 percent of 1RM (42, 66). Research indicates that peak power was significantly greater for the shoulder throw than the shoulder press at both 30 and 40 percent of 1RM (11). These studies indicate the importance of minimizing the deceleration phase when maximal power is the training goal (11, 42, 46).

Many recent investigations have examined the effects of power training in older adults (22, 43, 54). Typically, light to moderate loading is lifted at high velocities during the CON phase. Part of the reason stems from the fact that power is a variable more closely related to balance, fall prevention, and performance of activities of daily living, and it is lost to a greater extent than maximal strength.

These studies have shown that power training may be more effective than traditional resistance training for improving functional capacity in older adults. Studies have shown that muscle strength, walking capacity, rising from a chair, reaching ability, and balance are significantly enhanced following power training (24, 28). In fact, lifting velocity with a light load, 40 percent of 1RM, has been shown to correlate with improvements in balance (46). Power appears to increase similarly when different loads are lifted at high velocities; however, muscle strength and endurance are increased to a greater extent with heavy loading, i.e. 80 > 50 > 20% of 1RM (12). And it has also been shown that power training in the elderly is safe (24).

Training for local muscular endurance, and in some respects hypertrophy, may require a spectrum of velocities with various loading strategies (3). High, moderate, and low velocities are effective for improving local muscular endurance during dynamic constant external resistance training, depending on the number of repetitions performed. The critical component to local muscular endurance training is to prolong the duration of the set. Two effective strategies used to prolong set duration are 1) moderate repetition using an intentionally low velocity and 2) high repetition using moderate to high velocities. Training with intentionally low velocity and light loads places steady tension on the muscles for an extended period and may be more metabolically demanding than moderate and high velocities when the same number of repetitions are performed. However, it is difficult to perform a high number of repetitions using intentionally low velocities. Training strategies that employ both low velocity with moderate repetitions and moderate to high velocities with high repetitions increase the glycolytic and oxidative demands of the stimulus, thereby serving as an effective means of increasing local muscular endurance.

Frequency

Frequency refers to the number of times certain exercises or muscle groups are trained per week. It is dependent on several factors, including volume and intensity, exercise selection, level of conditioning and/or training status, recovery ability, nutritional intake, and training goals. The number of training sessions performed during a specific period, such as one week, may affect subsequent resistance-training adaptations. Training with heavy loads increases the recovery time needed prior to subsequent sessions, especially for multiple-joint exercises involving similar muscle groups. The use of extremely heavy loads may require 72 hours of recovery, whereas large and moderate loads may require less recovery time. Untrained women of various ages may only recover approximately 94 percent of their strength 2 days following a lower-body workout consisting of 5 sets of 10 repetitions with a 10 RM load (21). Numerous resistance-training studies have used frequencies of 2 to 3 alternating days per week in previously untrained individuals. This frequency has been shown to be an effective initial frequency, whereas 1 to 2 days per week appears to be an effective maintenance frequency for those individuals already engaged in a resistance-training program. In a few studies, training 4 to 5 days per week was superior to training 3 days per week, which was superior to training 1 and 2 days per week; and training 2 days per week was superior to training for 1 day for increasing maximal strength (18, 30). A recent study in older women demonstrated that strength increased similarly when training 1, 2, or 3 days per week; however, 3 days was superior to 1 and 2 for improving coordination, balance, and muscular endurance (47). The ACSM recommends 2 to 3 days per week as the optimal frequency in novices (3; see Table 1-2). An increase in training experience does not require a change in frequency but may coincide with alterations in other acute variables, such as exercise selection, volume, and intensity. Increasing training frequency may enable greater specialization, such as greater exercise selection and volume per muscle group, in accordance with more specific goals. Performing upper- and lower-body split routines or muscle-group split routines during a workout are common at this level of training in addition to total-body workouts to accommodate higher frequency. Hence, training 2 to 4 days per week is recommended (3).

Advanced training frequency varies considerably. Football players with varied training backgrounds who trained 4 to 5 days per week achieved better results than those who trained either 3 or 6 days per week (26, 27). Advanced weight lifters and bodybuilders use high frequency training four to six times per week. The frequency for elite weight lifters and bodybuilders may be even greater. Double-split routines—that is, two training sessions per day with emphasis on different muscle groups—are common during training and can result in the completion of 8 to 12 training sessions per week. Training frequencies as high as 18 sessions per week may occur for Olympic weight lifters. The rationale for this high-frequency training is that frequent short sessions followed by periods of recovery, supplementation, and food intake allow for high-intensity training via maximal energy utilization and reduced fatigue during exercise performance. One study reported greater increases in muscle cross-sectional area and strength when training volume was divided into two sessions per day rather than one (20). Elite power lifters typically train 4 to 6 days per week. In accordance, the ACSM has recommended 4 to 6 days per week for advanced training (3), although elite athletes may train with higher frequency. Note that not all muscle groups are trained specifically at every workout using a high frequency. Rather, each major muscle group may be trained two to three times per week despite the large number of workouts.

BASIC PRINCIPLES OF PROGRESSION

Lifting weights does not ensure optimal gains in muscular fitness. Effort and systematic structuring of the training stimulus ultimately determine the level of adaptation. The most successful resistance-training programs are those that are individualized to meet specific goals. Each individual will respond differently to resistance training.

Progression may be defined as "the act of moving forward or advancing toward a specific goal." The primary goal of resistance training is to improve some component of fitness or health until a certain level has been attained. For improvements to occur, the program used must be systematically altered so that the body is forced to adapt to the changing stimuli. Although continuing to improve at the same rate over long-term training, the proper manipulation of

program variables can limit training plateaus. Three general principles of progression are 1) progressive overload, 2) variation, and 3) specificity. Figure 1-1 depicts the principles of progression.

Any resistance-training program can be successful as long as certain principles are adhered to. *Progressive overload* entails increasing the stress placed on the body. *Variation* refers to consistently altering the stimuli. *Specificity* refers to adaptations that take place that are specific to the variables listed. Although some degree of transfer is evident, successful programs are designed specifically to goals.

The rate of progression during resistance training depends on several factors, including the training status of the individual. The largest rates of strength improvement occur in untrained individuals, because the window of adaptation is greatest at this point. Because neural adaptations predominate initially, it is difficult to differentiate the efficacy of various training programs. Several low-intensity, low-volume programs have yielded results similar to higher-intensity, higher-volume programs (38). However, many of these programs yielded inferior results in individuals with greater levels of strength and experience. Resistance-trained individuals show a slower rate of progression such that beginners have shown over 100 percent increases in strength, whereas elite athletes may improve only 1 to 2 percent over the course of a year (3). These results show that the rate and magnitude of progression decrease with higher levels of conditioning. Simple or basic programs can be very effective initially and are recommended. However, resistance-training program design must incorporate progressive overload, specificity, and variation to a greater degree to progress to a higher level. Therefore, the higher the level of conditioning, the more specific and scientific the program design needs to be. As long as the principles of progressive overload, variation, and specificity are adhered to, any resistance-training program can be successful.

Progressive overload entails increasing the stress placed on the body. Figure 1-1 discusses ways in which progressive overload can be introduced in a resistance-training program. **Variation** refers to

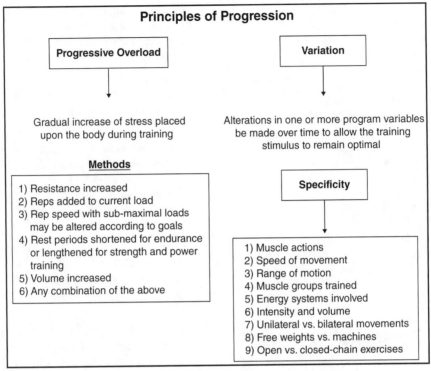

Figure 1-1 Principles of progression.
© Delmar/Cengage Learning.

consistently altering the stimuli. Because the human body can adapt to a workout within a couple of weeks, variation ensures that adaptations continue beyond the initial training period. **Specificity** refers to adaptations that are specific to the variables listed. Although some degree of transfer is evident, successful programs are designed specifically to goals.

Summary

Specific needs and goals should be addressed prior to resistance training. The resistance-training program should be basic initially for untrained individuals but should become more specific with greater variation in acute program variables during progression. Manipulation of the program variables may be performed in numerous ways. Progression may be maximized by the incorporation of progressive overload, specificity, and training variation in the program.

Key Terms

Absolute muscular endurance
Ballistic resistance exercise
Closed-chain kinetic exercise
Compensatory acceleration
Competitive training
Concentric muscle action (CON)
Deceleration phase
Dynamic constant external resistance
Eccentric muscle action (ECC)
Exercise selection
Exercise sequencing
Frequency
Functional isometrics
Intensity
Intentional high velocities
Intentional low velocities
Isometric muscle action (ISOM)
Maintenance training

Motor unit
Multiple-joint exercise
Muscle actions
Muscle-group split routine
Needs analysis
One-repetition maximum (1RM)
Opened-chain kinetic exercise
Progression
Progressive overload
Recreational training
Relative local muscular endurance
Repetition velocity
Rest intervals
Single-joint exercises
Specificity
Total-body routine
Training volume
Unintentional low velocities
Upper- and lower-body split routine
Variation

Study Questions

1. What type of exercises, loading, speeds, and rest intervals are needed for optimal power training?

2. Explain the factors that affect the number of sets performed in each workout.

3. What are the most critical concepts to resistance-training progression?

4. Using light weights for high repetitions at a moderate to low velocity is an effective way to increase what aspect of performance?

5. Provide an example of a single-joint exercise, a closed-chain kinetic exercise, and an opened-chain kinetic exercise.

References

1. Anderson T, Kearney JT. Effects of three resistance training programs on muscular strength and absolute and relative endurance. *Res Q.* 1982;53:1–7.

2. American College of Sports Medicine. Position stand: The recommended quantity and quality of exercise for developing and maintaining cardiorespiratory and muscular fitness and flexibility in healthy adults. *Med Sci Sports Exerc.* 1998;30:975–991.

3. American College of Sports Medicine: Position stand: Progression models in resistance training for healthy adults. *Med Sci Sports Exerc.* 2002;34:364–380.

4. American College of Sports Medicine and American Heart Association. Joint position stand: Recommendations for cardiovascular screening, staffing, and emergency policies at health/fitness facilities. *Med Sci Sports Exerc.* 1998;30:1009–1018.

5. Baker D, Wilson G, Carlyon R. Generality versus specificity: A comparison of dynamic and isometric measures of strength and speed-strength. *Eur J Appl Physiol.* 1994; 68:350–355.

6. Ballor DL, Becque MD, Katch VL. Metabolic responses during hydraulic resistance exercise. *Med Sci Sports Exerc.* 1987;19:363–367.

7. Benson C, Docherty D, Brandenburg J. Acute neuromuscular responses to resistance training performed at different loads. *J Sci Med Sport.* 2006;9:135–142.

8. Berger RA. Comparison of the effect of various weight training loads on strength. *Res Q.* 1963;36:141–146.

9. Borst SE, Dehoyos DV, Garzarella L, et al. Effects of resistance training on insulin-like growth factor-1 and IGF binding proteins. *Med Sci Sports Exerc.* 2001;33:648–653.

10. Campos GER, Luecke TJ, Wendeln HK, et al. Muscular adaptations in response to three different resistance-training regimens: Specificity of repetition maximum training zones. *Eur J Appl Physiol.* 2002;88:50–60.

11. Dalziel WM, Neal RJ, Watts MC. A comparison of peak power in the shoulder press and shoulder throw. *J Sci Med Sport.* 2005;5:229–235.

12. De Vos NJ, Singh NA, Ross DA, Stavrinos TM, Orr R, Fiatarone-Singh MA. Optimal load for

increasing muscle power during explosive resistance training in older adults. *J Gerontol A Biol Sci Med Sci.* 2005;60:638–647.

13. Drinkwater EJ, Lawton TW, Lindsell RP, Pyne DB, Hunt PH, McKenna MJ. Training leading to repetition failure enhances bench press strength gains in elite junior athletes. *J Strength Cond Res.* 2005;19:382–388.

14. Elliott BC, Wilson GJ, Kerr GK. A biomechanical analysis of the sticking region in the bench press. *Med Sci Sports Exerc.* 1989;21:450–462.

15. Fleck SJ, Kraemer WJ. *Designing Resistance Training Programs.* 3rd ed. Champaign, IL: Human Kinetics. 2003:151–186.

16. Galvao DA, Taaffe DR. Resistance exercise dosage in older adults: Single-versus multiset effects on physical performance and body composition. *J Am Geriatr Soc.* 2005;53:2090–2097.

17. Garhammer J. A comparison of maximal power outputs between elite male and female weight lifters in competition. *Int J Sports Biomech.* 1991;7:3–11.

18. Graves JE, Pollock ML, Leggett SH, Braith RW, Carpenter DM, Bishop LE. Effect of reduced training frequency on muscular strength. *Int J Sports Med.* 1988;9:316–319.

19. Häkkinen K, Alen M, Komi PV. Changes in isometric force and relaxation time, electromyographic and muscle fibre characteristics of human skeletal muscle during strength training and detraining. *Acta Physiol Scand.* 1985;125:573–585.

20. Häkkinen K, Kallinen M. Distribution of strength training volume into one or two daily sessions and neuromuscular adaptations in female athletes. *Electromyogr Clin Neurophysiol.* 1994;34:117–124.

21. Häkkinen K. Neuromuscular fatigue and recovery in women at different ages during heavy resistance loading. *Electromyogr Clin Neurophysiol.* 1995;35:403–413.

22. Häkkinen K, Kraemer WJ, Newton RU, Alen M. Changes in electromyographic activity, muscle fibre and force production characteristics during heavy resistance/power strength training in middle-aged and older men and women. *Acta Physiol Scand.* 2001;171:51–62.

23. Hansen S, Kvorning T, Kjaer M, SjØgaard G. The effect of short-term strength training on human skeletal muscle: The importance of physiologically elevated hormone levels. *Scand J Med Sci Sports.* 2001;11:347–354.

24. Henwood TR, Taaffe DR. Improved physical performance in older adults undertaking a short-term programme of high-velocity resistance training. *Gerontology.* 2005;51:108–115.

25. Hoeger WW, Barette SL, Hale DF, Hopkins DR. Relationship between repetitions and selected percentages of one-repetition maximum. *J Appl Sport Sci Res.* 1987;1:11–13.

26. Hoffman JR, Kraemer WJ, Fry AC, Deschenes M, Kemp DM. The effect of self-selection for frequency of training in a winter conditioning program for football. *J Appl Sport Sci Res.* 1990;3:76–82.

27. Hoffman JR, Kang J. Strength changes during an in-season resistance-training program for football. *J Strength Cond Res.* 2003;17:109–114.

28. Holviala JH, Sallinen JM, Kraemer WJ, Alen MJ, Häkkinen K. Effects of strength training on muscle strength characteristics, functional capabilities, and balance in middle-aged and older women. *J Strength Cond Res.* 2006;20:336–344.

29. Huczel HA, Clarke DH. A comparison of strength and muscle endurance in strength-trained and untrained women. *Eur J Appl Physiol.* 1992;64:467–470.

30. Hunter GR. Changes in body composition, body build, and performance associated with different weight training frequencies in males and females. *NSCA Journal.* 1985;7:26–28.

31. Izquierdo M, Ibanez J, Gonzalez-Badillo JJ, et al. Differential effects of strength training leading to failure versus not to failure on hormonal responses, strength, and muscle power gains. *J Appl Physiol.* 2006;100:1647–1656.

32. Jones K, Bishop P, Hunter G, Fleissig G. The effects of varying resistance-training loads on intermediate- and high-velocity-specific adaptations. *J Strength Cond Res.* 2001;15:349–356.

33. Keeler LK, Finkelstein LH, Miller W, Fernhall B. Early-phase adaptations to traditional-speed vs. superslow resistance training on strength and aerobic capacity in sedentary individuals. *J Strength Cond Res.* 2001;15:309–314.

34. Kemmler WK, Lauber D, Engelke K, Weineck J. Effects of single- vs. multiple-set resistance training on maximum strength and body composition in trained postmenopausal women. *J Strength Cond Res.* 2004;18:689–694.

35. Keogh JWL, Wilson GJ, and Weatherby RP. A cross-sectional comparison of different resistance training techniques in the bench press. *J Strength Cond Res.* 1999;13:247–258.

36. Kraemer WJ. A series of studies – The physiological basis for strength training in American football: Fact over philosophy. *J Strength Cond Res.* 1997;11:131–142.

37. Kraemer WJ, Ratamess NA. Physiology of resistance training: Current issues. *Orthop Phys Therapy Clin North Am Exerc Tech.* Philadelphia, PA: W.B. Saunders; 2000;9(4):467–513.

38. Kraemer WJ, Ratamess NA. Fundamentals of resistance training: Progression and exercise prescription. *Med Sci Sports Exerc.* 2004;36:674–688.

39. Kraemer WJ, Ratamess NA. Hormonal responses and adaptations to resistance exercise and training. *Sports Med.* 2005; 35:339–361.

40. Marx JO, Ratamess NA, Nindl BC, et al. The effects of single-set vs. periodized multiple-set resistance training on muscular performance and hormonal concentrations in women. *Med Sci Sports Exerc.* 2001;33:635–643.

41. Mazzetti SA, Kraemer WJ, Volek JS, et al. The influence of direct supervision of resistance training on strength performance. *Med Sci Sports Exerc.* 2000;32:1175–1184.

42. McBride JM, Triplett-McBride T, Davie A, Newton RU. The effect of heavy- vs. light-load jump squats on the development of strength, power, and speed. *J Strength Cond Res.* 2002;16:75–82.

43. Miszko TA, Cress ME, Slade JM, Covey CJ, Agrawal SK, Doerr CE. Effect of strength and power training on physical function in community-dwelling older adults. *J Gerontol A Biol Sci Med Sci.* 2003;58:171–175.

44. Mookerjee S, Ratamess NA. Comparison of strength differences and joint action durations between full and partial range-of-motion bench press exercise. *J Strength Cond Res.* 1999;13:76–81.

45. Morrissey MC, Harman EC, Johnson MJ. Resistance training modes: Specificity and effectiveness. *Med Sci Sports Exerc.* 1995;27:648–660.

46. Orr R, De Vos NJ, Singh NA, Ross DA, Stavrinos TM, Fiatarone-Singh MA. Power training improves balance in healthy older adults. *J Gerontol A Biol Sci Med Sci.* 2006;61:78–85.

47. Nakamura Y, Tanaka K, Yabushita N, Sakai T, Shigematsu R. Effects of exercise frequency on functional fitness in older adult women. *Arch Gerontol Geriatr.* 2007;44(2):163–173.

48. National Strength and Conditioning Association. Strength and conditioning professional standards and guidelines. May 2001.

49. Newton RU, Kraemer WJ, Häkkinen K, Humphries BJ, Murphy AJ. Kinematics, kinetics, and muscle activation during explosive upper-body movements. *J Appl Biomech.* 1996;12:31–43.

50. Ostrowski KJ, Wilson GJ, Weatherby R, Murphy PW, Lyttle AD. The effect of weight training volume on hormonal output and muscular size and function. *J Strength Cond Res.* 1997;11:148–154.

51. Paulsen G, Myklestad D, Raastad T. The influence of volume of exercise on early adaptations to strength training. *J Strength Cond Res.* 2003;17:113–118.

52. Peterson MD, Rhea MR, Alvar BA. Maximizing strength development in athletes: A meta-analysis to determine the dose–response relationship. *J Strength Cond Res.* 2004;18:377–382.

53. Pincivero DM, Lephart SM, Karunakara RG. Effects of rest interval on isokinetic strength and functional performance after short-term high-intensity training. *Br J Sports Med.* 1997;31:229–234.

54. Porter MM. Power training for older adults. *Appl Physiol Nutr Metabol.* 2006;31:87–94.

55. Ratamess NA, Kraemer WJ, Volek JS, et al. Kinetic characteristics of a back-squat protocol in resistance-trained men. *National Strength and Conditioning Association National Conference.* 2004.

56. Rhea MR, Alvar BA, Ball SD, Burkett LN. Three sets of weight training superior to 1 set with equal intensity for eliciting strength. *J Strength Cond Res.* 2002;16:525–529.

57. Robinson JM, Stone MH, Johnson RL, Penland CM, Warren BJ, Lewis RD. Effects of different weight training exercise/rest intervals on strength, power, and high intensity exercise endurance. *J Strength Cond Res.* 1995;9:216–221.

58. Rutherford OM, Jones DA. The role of learning and coordination in strength training. *Eur J Appl Physiol.* 1986;55:100–105.

59. Sforzo GA, Touey PR. Manipulating exercise order affects muscular performance during a resistance exercise training session. *J Strength Cond Res.* 1996;10:20–24.

60. Siegel JA, Gilders RM, Staron RS, Hagerman FC. Human muscle power output during upper- and lower-body exercises. *J. Strength Cond Res.* 2002;16:173–178.

61. Simao R, Farinatti PTV, Polito MD, Maior AS, Fleck SJ. Influence of exercise order on the number of repetitions performed and perceived exertion during resistance exercises. *J Strength Cond Res.* 2005;19:152–156.

62. Spreuwenberg LP, Kraemer WJ, Spiering BA, et al. Influence of exercise order in a resistance-training exercise session. *J Strength Cond Res.* 2006;20:141–144.

63. Takarada Y, Takazawa H, Sato Y, Takebayashi S, Tanaka Y, Ishii N. Effects of resistance exercise combined with moderate vascular occlusion on muscular function in humans. *J Appl Physiol.* 2006;88:2097–2106.

64. Willardson JM, Burkett LN. The effect of rest interval length on bench press performance with heavy vs. light loads. *J Strength Cond Res.* 2006a;20:396–399.

65. Willardson JM, Burkett LN. The effect of rest interval length on the sustainability of squat and bench press repetitions. *J Strength Cond Res.* 2006b;20:400–403.

66. Wilson GJ, Newton RU, Murphy AJ, Humphries BJ. The optimal training load for the development of dynamic athletic performance. *Med Sci Sports Exerc.* 1993;25:1279–1286.

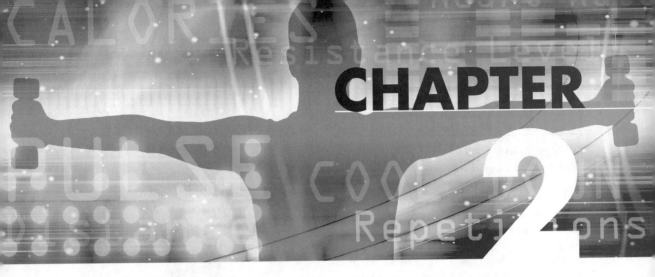

CHAPTER 2

COMPENDIUM OF RESISTANCE-TRAINING STRATEGIES

Objectives

Upon completion of this chapter, the reader should be able to:

- ○ Select appropriate resistance-training exercises for an individual in a variety of resistance-training modes
- ○ Correctly and safely demonstrate all resistance-training exercises in this chapter
- ○ Identify resistance-training exercise variations to individualize exercise prescriptions
- ○ Safely progress a resistance-training program exercise prescription
- ○ Learn proper spotting techniques for resistance-training exercises in this chapter

INTRODUCTION

Throughout this text, specific examples of recommended exercises are provided for each of the populations addressed. While the recommended exercises are by no means a complete list of possible exercises, they provide an evidence-based starting point from which the exercise professional can provide an appropriate resistance-training program. This chapter is a compendium of all of the recommended exercises listed in Chapters 3 through 17. Exercises are organized into groups according to the type of equipment being used. These include selectorized and plate-loaded machines, resistance bands or tubing, dumbbells and barbells, cable/pulley systems, and body-weight exercises. Body-weight exercises include the use of ankle weights, stability balls, and medicine balls. Instructions are provided covering the recommended technique for each exercise, but these may need to be modified according to the needs and abilities of the individual (1).

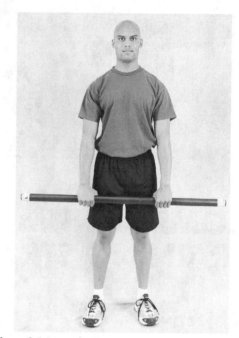

Figure 2-1 Pronated grip.

Courtesy of Patrick Hagerman, Ed.D. Quest Personal Training, Inc.

GRIPS

There are various grips involved in resistance training. The appropriate grip and any possible grip variations for each exercise are provided in the exercise description. Figures 2-1 through 2-4 illustrate the **pronated, supinated,** and **alternating grips** that may be used on the barbell or dumbbell, as well as the **neutral grip** for dumbbells.

In addition to the appropriate grip when using a barbell, correct placement of the hands on the bar is important. A **normal grip** is defined as the shoulder-width distance of the individual, so it will differ according to the size of the individual performing the exercise. A **narrow grip** is any grip smaller than shoulder width, and a **wide grip** is any grip larger than shoulder width. Figures 2-5 through 2-7 illustrate normal, narrow, and wide grips on the barbell.

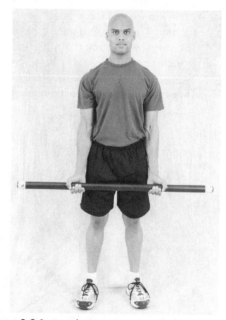

Figure 2-2 Supinated grip.

Courtesy of Patrick Hagerman, Ed.D. Quest Personal Training, Inc.

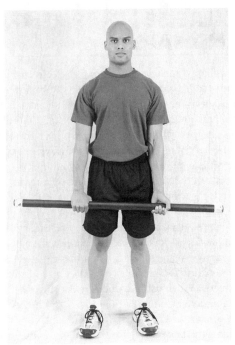

Figure 2-3 Alternating grip.
Courtesy of Patrick Hagerman, Ed.D. Quest Personal Training, Inc.

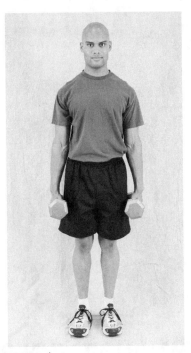

Figure 2-4 Neutral grip.
Courtesy of Patrick Hagerman, Ed.D. Quest Personal Training, Inc.

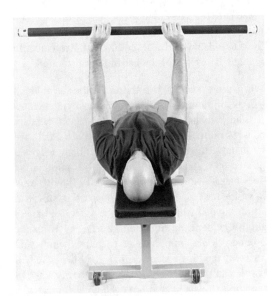

Figure 2-5 Normal grip width.
Courtesy of Patrick Hagerman, Ed.D. Quest Personal Training, Inc.

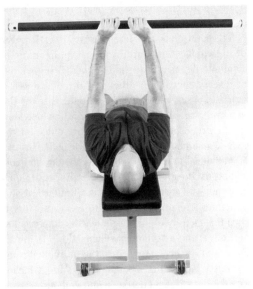

Figure 2-6 Narrow grip width.
Courtesy of Patrick Hagerman, Ed.D. Quest Personal Training, Inc.

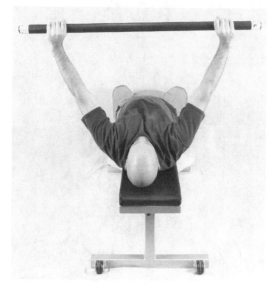

Figure 2-7 Wide grip width.
Courtesy of Patrick Hagerman, Ed.D. Quest Personal Training, Inc.

BREATHING TECHNIQUE

Proper breathing is important for effective and safe resistance training. Improper technique can result in discomfort and excessive heart rate and blood pressure responses (2, 3). For the healthy individual, such responses may not pose a serious risk. However, for individuals with cardiovascular, pulmonary, or metabolic disease, or for individuals at higher risk for disease, elevated heart rate and blood pressure responses to resistance training may increase the risk for a cardiovascular event (3). Generally, the individual should exhale during the concentric phase of the exercise and inhale during the eccentric phase. Instruct the individual to exhale during exertion and to avoid holding the breath throughout the entire set. Holding the breath with a closed epiglottis is called the **Valsalva maneuver**. The only exception to breath holding is when the intensity of the weight reaches 80 percent or more of the one-repetition maximum (1RM). To initiate movement at these intensities, the individual must generate a higher intra-abdominal pressure, which is accomplished by holding the breath without a closed glottis. After the movement has begun, the individual should exhale and relieve the pressure.

EXERCISE EQUIPMENT AND SAFETY

This chapter includes exercises for selectorized and plate-loaded machines, dumbbells and barbells, resistance tubing, and body-weight exercises using medicine balls, ankle weights, and stability balls. An often overlooked area in exercise training is the safety of the equipment. Always examine the equipment before using it to avoid injuring the client or others in the exercise area. Examine the exercise machine for worn or missing pads, frayed or nicked cables, and broken handles, weight pins, or clamps. Likewise, do not use any resistance tube that shows obvious areas of weakness. Dumbbells are rarely damaged, but if using magnetic weights on the dumbbell, make sure they are attached correctly. When using barbells make sure the rack is properly anchored and the individual hooks are not broken or cracked. Lift the weight plates by flexing the knees, grabbing with both hands, and lifting with the legs, not the back. The weight plates should face inward on the bar and must be secured in place with a lock collar. Two common errors are improperly balanced weight or incorrect weight. Make sure the same amount of weight is placed on both sides of the bar, and check that the weight on the bar adds up to the desired weight. Remember to include the weight of the bar in the calculation.

When using a **stability ball**, the proper size and inflation affects both exercise safety and intensity. Puncture-resistant balls are preferred over non–puncture-resistant balls. Stability balls are sold in various sizes and vary by manufacturer. The correct size for body height is printed on the packaging; however, this information does not take into account leg length. The best way to ensure the proper ball size is to have the individual sit on the ball with an upright torso, feet and knees slightly wider than hip width, and feet flat on the ground. Viewed from the side, examine the hips and knees. If the hips are lower than the knees the ball is too small. Conversely, if the hips are higher than the knees, the ball is too large. Figure 2-8 illustrates different size stability balls. Related to proper stability, ball size is dependent on the degree of inflation.

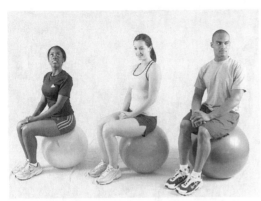

Figure 2-8 Different sizes of stability balls for different leg lengths.
Courtesy of Patrick Hagerman, Ed.D. Quest Personal Training, Inc.

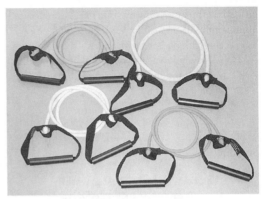

Figure 2-9 Different sizes of resistance tubing.
Courtesy of Patrick Hagerman, Ed.D. Quest Personal Training, Inc.

Inflation should be checked periodically and should result in a 1- to 2-inch depression when pressed with the thumb. A new stability ball will be stiffer than an older one. Underinflation increases the risk of improper body alignment, whereas overinflation increases both the risk of rupture and the ability to balance while seated or lying on the stability ball.

EXERCISE PROGRESSION

The most common way to progress exercise intensity is to increase the resistance by adding more weight to the machine, dumbbell, or barbell. When using a resistance tube, resistance can be increased by using a thicker tube (Figure 2-9). Tube color often indicates the degree of resistance and is specific to the manufacturer (e.g., yellow, green, red, blue, and black range from easiest to hardest). In some instances using the next hardest tube may be too difficult for the client. In those instances combining two easier tubes, or folding one easier tube in half, can create an intermediate level.

Stability ball exercise progression is dependent on the client's position on the ball. In any position the easiest level is for the feet and knees to be wider apart. Moving the feet and knees closer together increases the difficulty by decreasing the stability of the position. Likewise, performing exercises with both legs is easier than with one leg. In either the prone, supine, or side-lying positions, the angle of incline of the torso to the ground can be changed to affect exercise intensity. The easiest level of difficulty is when the torso is inclined approximately 80 degrees relative to the ground. Decreasing the incline increases the difficulty, so the most difficult level would be reached when the torso is parallel to the floor.

SPOTTING

Spotting is required during exercises in which a weight is held above the head or chest. The spotter's primary responsibility is to keep the individual safe during the exercise by ensuring that the equipment, usually a barbell or dumbbell, does not fall on the person lifting it. However, the ability to effectively spot a client may be used to enhance training, and the spotter may assist the client through the last few repetitions of a set. This action is referred to as **assisting** rather than *spotting*. To ensure the safety of the individual and the spotter, the spotter must be positioned to have the most leverage possible in case the individual loses control of the weight. Spotting is performed in kneeling, standing, or sitting positions as outlined below.

Kneeling

- ◯ Stand with feet shoulder width apart.
- ◯ Slowly lower the body until one knee and the other foot sits firmly on the floor.
- ◯ Keep the spine in a neutral position.

Standing

- ◯ Stand with feet shoulder width apart and knees slightly flexed.
- ◯ Keep the spine in a neutral position.

Sitting

- ◯ Sit on a stool or bench with feet flat on the floor, shoulder width apart.
- ◯ Keep the spine in a neutral position.

SELECTORIZED AND PLATE-LOADED MACHINE EXERCISES

The exercises in this section utilize either a selectorized or plate-loaded machine. A **selectorized machine** utilizes a stack of weights into which the user inserts a pin to select the desired resistance. A **plate-loaded machine** requires the user to add free-weight style plates to the machine for resistance. Both machine types provide a fixed-movement pattern that is specific to the machine, and a different machine is usually employed for each exercise.

Leg Press

Starting Position: Sit in the leg-press machine and place both feet on the platform, spaced slightly wider than shoulder width, with the toes turned slightly out. Be sure to keep the feet completely on the platform; do not let them hang over the edge. Adjust the seat forward

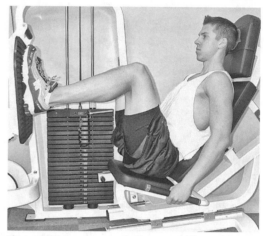

Figure 2-10 Leg press start/finish position.
Courtesy of Patrick Hagerman, Ed.D. Quest Personal Training, Inc.

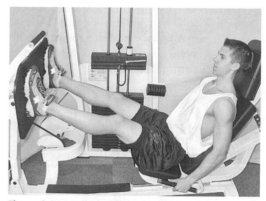

Figure 2-11 Leg press midpoint.
Courtesy of Patrick Hagerman, Ed.D. Quest Personal Training, Inc.

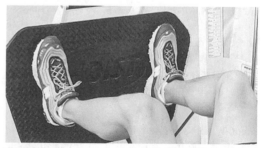

Figure 2-12 Proper foot position for the leg press: shoulder width apart, toes slightly turned out.
Courtesy of Patrick Hagerman, Ed.D. Quest Personal Training, Inc.

or back until the knees are bent just under 90 degrees. Some machines allow adjustment of the angle of the backrest, which allows changes to the starting angle of hip flexion. Adjust this angle so that the thighs are not in contact with the chest and the stomach is not pressed into the legs. Select the appropriate weight, making sure the selector pin is pushed all the way in. In this position, the hips, buttocks, and shoulders should all be in contact with the seat.

Movement: Push against the platform with both feet at the same time, putting equal pressure on the heels and balls of the feet; do not allow the focus to be on the toes, which will make this movement a calf exercise. Push until the legs are almost completely straight without locking them out. Slowly bend the legs, letting the platform move back to the starting position. When the weights almost touch the stack, start another repetition until the set is complete.

Seated Calf Raises

Starting Position: Place the appropriate weight on the machine. Sit in the seat, place both feet on the footplate, and slide the knees under the knee pads. Only the toes and the balls of the feet will be on the footplate, the rest of the foot will be hanging over

the edge. Adjust the knee pads so that they are snug against the knees; any space between the knees and the knee pads prevents the correction execution of this exercise. Most machines have handgrips on top of the knee pads. Place the hands either on these handgrips or on top of the legs. If using the handgrips, do not pull on the knee pad; this would be using the arms instead of the calf muscles.

Movement: Push on the balls of the feet to raise the heels as high as possible. On the first repetition, the bar that supports the machine and weight will move out of the way. Lower the heels as far as possible, to the "down" position; then push up on the balls of the feet again, raising the heels as far as possible to the "up" position. Repeat, lowering and raising the heels until the set is complete. On the last repetition, when the heels are at the highest point, move the bar that supports the machine and weight back into place, and slowly lower the heels back to the starting point.

Precaution: Do not try to get out of the machine until the support bar is back in place; it holds the weight that was added. Sliding the knees out of the machine without using the support bar may cause injury or damage the machine.

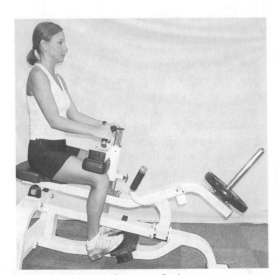

Figure 2-13 Seated calf raise start/finish position.
Courtesy of Patrick Hagerman, Ed.D. Quest Personal Training, Inc.

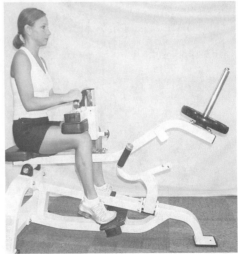

Figure 2-14 Seated calf raise midpoint.
Courtesy of Patrick Hagerman, Ed.D. Quest Personal Training, Inc.

Leg Extension or Knee Extension

Starting Position: Sit down in the machine and adjust the seat back so that the knees line up with the machine's pivot point. This point will always be evident and is usually at the edge of the seat, or it can be found on the machine's instruction card. If the knees are too far forward, there will be too much strain on the knees at the beginning of the exercise. Place both feet behind the footpad. Adjust the height of the pad so that it rests just above the feet on the shins, so that it does not push down on the top of the foot. Some machines automatically adjust themselves by means of a pivoting footpad. Select the appropriate weight, making sure the selector pin is pushed all the way in.

Movement: Hold onto the handles and straighten out both legs simultaneously as far as possible. Slowly lower the legs back down to the starting position, but do not let the weight stack come to rest. Just before the weights touch the stack, start another repetition until the set is complete.

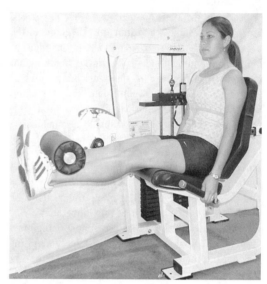

Figure 2-16 Leg extension/knee extension midpoint.
Courtesy of Patrick Hagerman, Ed.D. Quest Personal Training, Inc.

Precaution: This exercise should be done slowly and with control. Moving too fast and "kicking" the footpad up in the air and off the shins could cause injury or damage the equipment.

Lying Leg Curls

Starting Position: Determine the location of the knee pivot point on the machine. Commonly, this point is at the edge of the padding. Stand at the end of the bench, knees against the padding, and lie down; this should align the knees with the machine pivot point. If not, adjust forward or backward until the correct position is found. The kneecaps should always hang off the end of the bench. Some machines have pads for the elbows to rest on, and some machines have a flat bench with handles underneath. Either way, lie down flat and place the elbows and hands in the proper position. The Achilles tendon should be underneath the footpad. Some machines adjust this pad automatically; if yours does not, adjust the pad so that it is not pushing down on the heel or foot. Select the appropriate weight, making sure the selector pin is pushed all the way in. If the machine uses plates for resistance, add the weight before lying down.

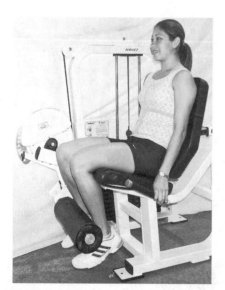

Figure 2-15 Leg extension/knee extension start/finish position.
Courtesy of Patrick Hagerman, Ed.D. Quest Personal Training, Inc.

Movement: Bend the knees and try to bring the footpad all the way up to touch the buttocks. Slowly let the footpad back down until the weights almost touch the stack. Start another repetition until the set is complete.

Precaution: As the weights increase and the intensity rises, the hips may lift up during the movement. This body movement is a normal reaction to the mechanics of the exercise, but it decreases the effectiveness of the exercise. Prevent this movement by pushing the hips down into the pad during the movement.

Seated Leg Curl

Starting position: Sit on the machine and adjust the seat back so that the knees line up with the machine's pivot point. The seat is usually quite short on these machines and may stop about halfway to the knees, so be sure to identify the proper pivot point. Place the feet and legs on top of the leg pad.

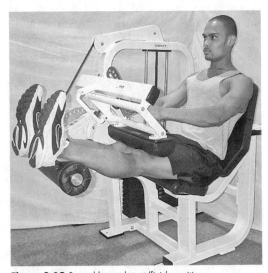

Figure 2-19 Seated leg curl start/finish position.
Courtesy of Patrick Hagerman, Ed.D. Quest Personal Training, Inc.

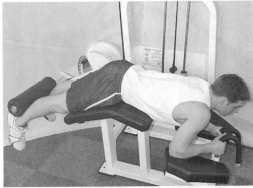

Figure 2-17 Lying leg curl start/finish position.
Courtesy of Patrick Hagerman, Ed.D. Quest Personal Training, Inc.

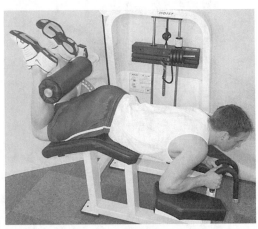

Figure 2-18 Lying leg curl midpoint.
Courtesy of Patrick Hagerman, Ed.D. Quest Personal Training, Inc.

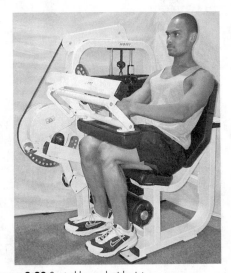

Figure 2-20 Seated leg curl midpoint.
Courtesy of Patrick Hagerman, Ed.D. Quest Personal Training, Inc.

Adjust the leg pad so that it is in contact with the Achilles tendon and not pushing on the foot. Adjust the thigh pad until it is snug against the top of both legs. Select the appropriate weight, making sure the selector pin is pushed all the way in.

Movement: Hold on to the hand grips, and bend both knees to pull the leg pad down and under the seat as far as possible. Slowly straighten the legs until the weights almost touch the stack. Then begin another repetition until the set is complete.

Chest Press

Starting position: Adjust the seat up or down so that the handles are at chest height when the individual is sitting upright. Most chest-press machines have a horizontal and a vertical set of handles. Grasp the horizontal handles and lift the elbows up so they are at the same height as the hands and shoulders. Sit up straight in the chair so the back is flat against the pad and both feet are flat on the ground. Select the appropriate

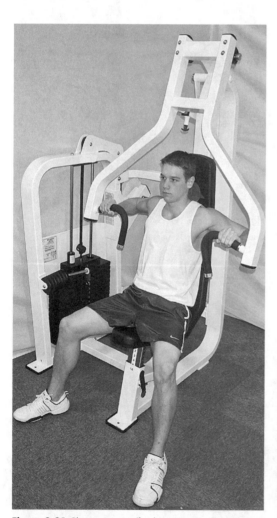

Figure 2-21 Chest press start/finish position.
Courtesy of Patrick Hagerman, Ed.D. Quest Personal Training, Inc.

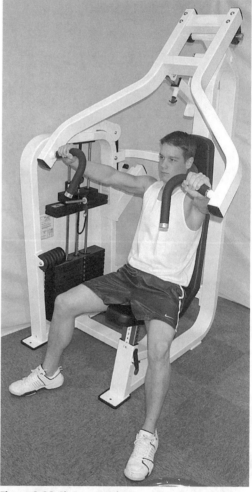

Figure 2-22 Chest press midpoint.
Courtesy of Patrick Hagerman, Ed.D. Quest Personal Training, Inc.

weight, making sure the selector pin is pushed all the way in.

Movement: Push the handles out until both arms are completely straight. Keep the back and shoulders against the seat and do not lean forward. Slowly bend at the elbows to let the handles come back toward the starting position until the weights almost touch the stack, then begin another repetition until the set is complete.

Chest Fly

Starting position: Adjust the seat up or down so that while holding both handles out to the sides, the hands and shoulders are at the same level. Next, adjust the range of motion of the machine arms so that the hands are resting just behind the shoulders.

Select the appropriate weight, making sure the selector pin is pushed all the way in.

Movement: Maintain a slight bend in the elbows as the hands are brought forward together in front of the body. When the hands meet, slowly return the weight to the starting position until the weights almost touch the stack, and then begin another repetition until the set is complete.

Precaution: While a greater range of motion may be possible by setting the machine arms to begin farther behind the shoulders, this positioning may compromise shoulder integrity and cause injury. Also, do not lean forward during this exercise. Keep the back flat against the pad and the head out of the way of the arms of the machine.

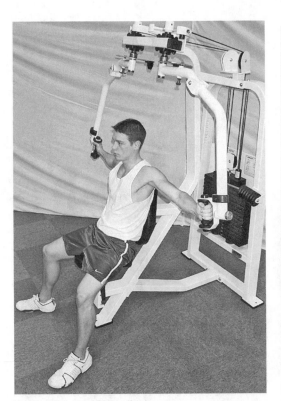

Figure 2-23 Chest fly start/finish position.
Courtesy of Patrick Hagerman, Ed.D. Quest Personal Training, Inc.

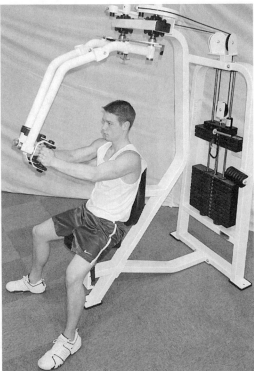

Figure 2-24 Chest fly midpoint.
Courtesy of Patrick Hagerman, Ed.D. Quest Personal Training, Inc.

Seated Row

Starting position: Adjust the seat height up or down so that the arms are horizontal, not angled up or down, while holding the handles of the machine. Most seated row machines have both horizontal and vertical handles; grasp the horizontal set. Hold the elbows up so that they are at the same level as the hands and shoulders. Sit upright so that the chest is against the chest pad. Select the appropriate weight, making sure the selector pin is pushed all the way in. The feet may be placed on the floor or on the footpad, if the machine is so equipped.

Movement: Pull back on both handles simultaneously, moving the elbows behind the body as far as possible while keeping them at shoulder height. Slowly straighten the arms back to the starting position. Just before the weights touch, begin another repetition until the set is complete.

Variation: Grasp the vertical set of handles and allow the elbows to move down along the sides of the body during the movement.

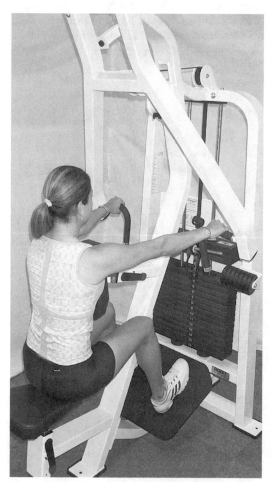

Figure 2-25 Seated row start/finish position.
Courtesy of Patrick Hagerman, Ed.D. Quest Personal Training, Inc.

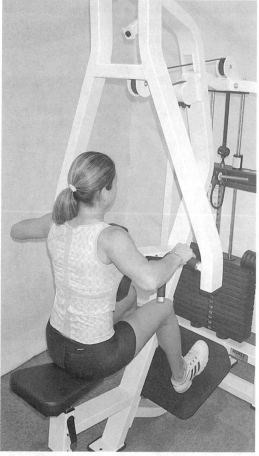

Figure 2-26 Seated row midpoint.
Courtesy of Patrick Hagerman, Ed.D. Quest Personal Training, Inc.

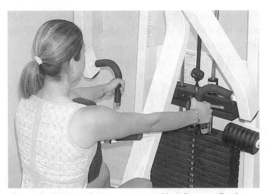

Figure 2-27 Seated row using vertical handles start/finish position.
Courtesy of Patrick Hagerman, Ed.D. Quest Personal Training, Inc.

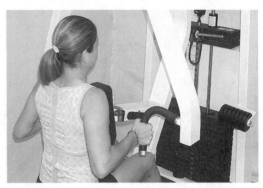

Figure 2-28 Seated row using vertical handles midpoint.
Courtesy of Patrick Hagerman, Ed.D. Quest Personal Training, Inc.

Shoulder Press

Starting position: Sit down and adjust the seat up or down so that the handles are at the same height as the shoulders. If the seat is too high, it will be difficult to grip the handles and perform the movement. If the seat is too low, range of motion will be decreased. There are usually two sets of handles, one set pointing toward the head and one set pointing away from the machine. Use whichever set is most comfortable; the movement is essentially the same. Select the appropriate weight, making sure the selector pin is pushed all the way in. Sit up straight in the seat, keeping the back as flat as possible during the movement. Place both feet flat on the floor with a wide stance for good balance.

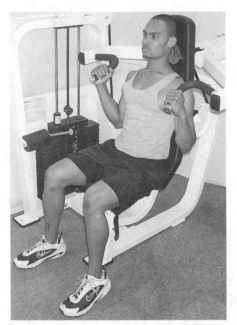

Figure 2-29 Shoulder press start/finish position.
Courtesy of Patrick Hagerman, Ed.D. Quest Personal Training, Inc.

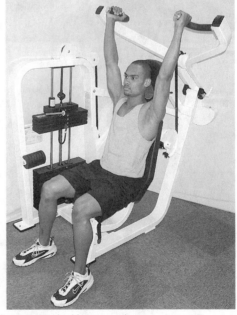

Figure 2-30 Shoulder press midpoint.
Courtesy of Patrick Hagerman, Ed.D. Quest Personal Training, Inc.

Movement: Push both arms toward the ceiling until they are completely straight. Slowly let the arms back down until the weight stack almost touches, then push back up to complete another repetition until the set is complete.

Precaution: If the back arches during the movement, lower the weight. Arching the back hyper-extends the vertebrae, a position that can lead to low back pain.

Biceps Curl

Starting position: Sit in the machine and adjust the height of the seat or arm pad, depending on the model of bench. The goal is to sit comfortably with the upper arm flat against the padding. If the elbows are the only part of the arm touching the pad, then the seat is too high. If the elbows do not touch the pad at all, but the top of the arm near the armpit touches it, the seat is too low. Select the appropriate weight, making sure the selector pin is pushed all the way in. Grasp the handle with a normal and supinated grip, palms facing up. Adjust where the elbows rest on the padding so that they line up with the machine pivot point, the hinge or axis where the handle is attached to the machine.

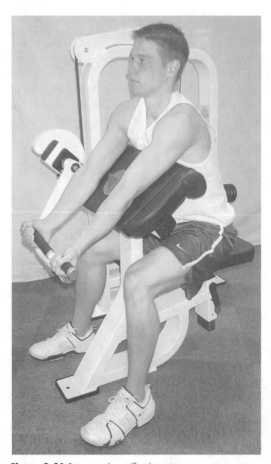

Figure 2-31 Biceps curl start/finish position.
Courtesy of Patrick Hagerman, Ed.D. Quest Personal Training, Inc.

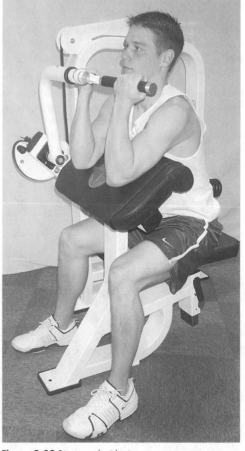

Figure 2-32 Biceps curl midpoint.
Courtesy of Patrick Hagerman, Ed.D. Quest Personal Training, Inc.

Movement: Keep the elbows aligned with the pivot point, pulling the bar up toward the shoulders just under the chin. Slowly lower the handle back down, making sure to straighten the arms completely before starting the next repetition. If the weight stack touches before the arms are completely straight, adjust either the seat or the alignment of the elbows.

Precaution: Do not "bounce" the weight at the bottom of the repetition as a means of using momentum to begin the next repetition. Bouncing the weight can strain the elbow tendons or sprain the elbow ligaments.

Triceps Extension

Starting position: Sit down and adjust the height of the seat so that the elbows and a large portion of the upper arms are touching the pad. If only the elbows are touching the pad, the seat is too high. If the elbows are not touching the pad, the seat is too low. Select the appropriate weight, making sure the selector pin is pushed all the way in. Grasp the handles, one in each hand, and pivot the handle arm back toward you. Slide forward or back in the seat until the elbows line up with the pivot point of the machine; the pivot point is where the handles

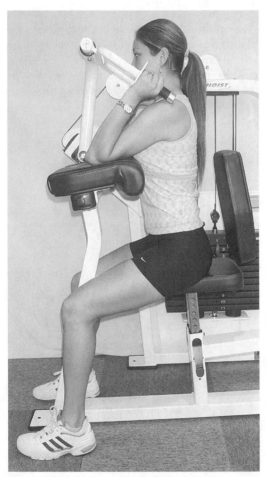

Figure 2-33 Triceps extension start/finish position.
Courtesy of Patrick Hagerman, Ed.D. Quest Personal Training, Inc.

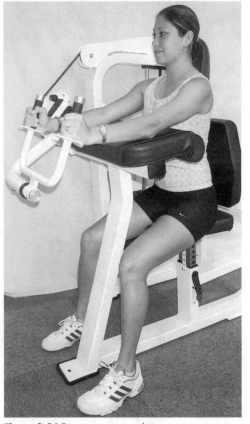

Figure 2-34 Triceps extension midpoint.
Courtesy of Patrick Hagerman, Ed.D. Quest Personal Training, Inc.

are attached to the axis of the machine. The back-support pad can be used to help maintain an upright seated position, so adjust it to touch the back.

Movement: Push against the handles until both arms are completely straight. Slowly bend at the elbows to return the handles to the starting position, making sure the elbows stay planted against the pad.

Precaution: Keep your head upright and facing the handles. Leaning forward may cause the handles to hit the head.

Trunk Flexion, or Abdominal Curl

Starting position: There are two main variations of the abdominal machine: one places a padded bar across the chest to push against, and the other uses padded elbow rests to push against. Sit down

and adjust the seat height so that the hips line up with the machine pivot point. Select the appropriate weight, making sure the selector pin is pushed all the way in. If the machine uses a padded bar across the chest, grab hold of the handles on the bar or simply "hug" the bar. If the machine has elbow pads, it will also have handles to hold. Place the elbows on the pads, and hold the handles.

Movement: Bend at the waist, and push against the chest bar or elbow pads, depending on the equipment. Bend the body as far forward as possible, moving the head toward the knees. Slowly return to the starting position. Repeat until the set is complete.

Precautions: If the machine has foot straps or a bar to anchor the feet, do not use them; these attachments allow the body to use the hip flexor muscles instead of the abdominals. Place the feet flat on the floor or on the platform provided.

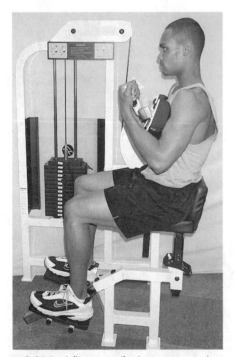

Figure 2-35 Trunk flexion start/finish position on machine with padded chest bar.

Courtesy of Patrick Hagerman, Ed.D. Quest Personal Training, Inc.

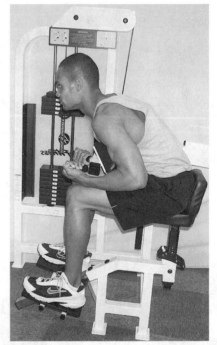

Figure 2-36 Trunk flexion midpoint on machine with padded chest bar.

Courtesy of Patrick Hagerman, Ed.D. Quest Personal Training, Inc.

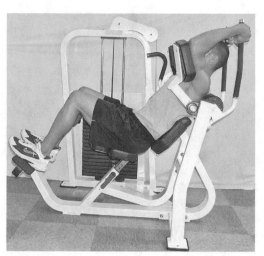

Figure 2-37 Trunk flexion start/finish position on machine with elbow pads.

Courtesy of Patrick Hagerman, Ed.D. Quest Personal Training, Inc.

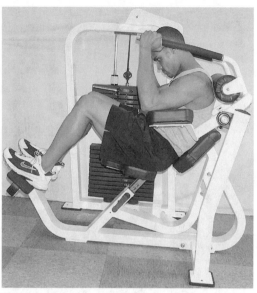

Figure 2-38 Trunk flexion midpoint on machine with elbow pads.

Courtesy of Patrick Hagerman, Ed.D. Quest Personal Training, Inc.

Assisted Dips

Starting position: Select an appropriate weight, making sure the selector pin is all the way in. On an assisted-dip machine, more weight makes the exercise easier, because this particular machine acts as a counterweight to the individual's body weight. Climb onto the machine using the steps provided. If using a Gravitron machine, place both knees on the knee pads in the areas indicated. If using another brand of assisted-dip machine, stand on a plate rather than kneeling. Hold on to the machine's arms, one hand on each side, using a neutral grip, palms facing toward the body. Begin with the arms completely straight.

Movement: Keeping the torso straight, slowly bend both arms to lower the body toward the floor. Stop when the elbows and shoulders are at the same height, or when the upper arms are parallel with the floor. Push on both hands to straighten the arms until you reach the starting position. Repeat to complete the set.

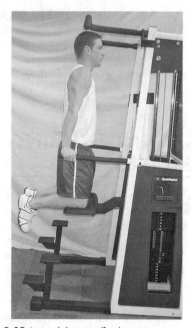

Figure 2-39 Assisted dips start/finish position.

Courtesy of Patrick Hagerman, Ed.D. Quest Personal Training, Inc.

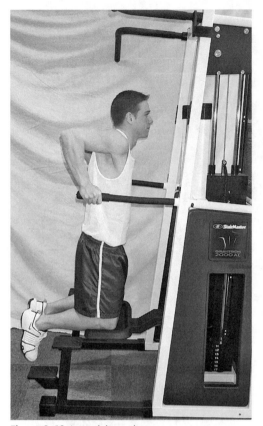

Figure 2-40 Assisted dips midpoint.
Courtesy of Patrick Hagerman, Ed.D. Quest Personal Training, Inc.

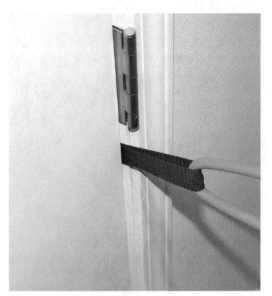

Figure 2-41 Resistance tubing door anchor.
Courtesy of Patrick Hagerman, Ed.D. Quest Personal Training, Inc.

anchor, or placed under one foot so that body weight holds the tubing in place.

Tubing Biceps Curls

Starting position: Stand with the feet about a foot apart, one foot in front of the other. Hold the ends of the tubing in each hand using a supinated grip, palms facing up. Keep the arms relaxed and down at the sides of the body. To anchor the tubing, place the center of the tubing under the arch of the front foot, and place most of the body weight on that foot.

Movement: To work both arms at the same time, keep the elbows at the sides of the body and bend the arms to curl the tubing up to the shoulders. Slowly let the tubing back down by straightening at the elbows until the arms are again relaxed at the sides of the body. To work one arm at a time, keep one arm at the side of the body while the other arm completes a repetition. Alternate left and right repetitions, or complete an entire set on one arm, followed by the other. When isolating one arm, keep holding the tubing in the other hand for support and balance.

RESISTANCE-TUBING EXERCISES

Resistance tubing can be used to mimic virtually any exercise machine available. The compact size and versatility of resistance tubing make it a good choice for individuals who train at home or while traveling. Resistance tubing must be anchored at one or both ends, depending on the exercise, to provide a solid foundation from which the tubing can be pulled. In some cases, the tubing may be wrapped around a pole or exercise machine, attached to a doorway by means of a tubing–door

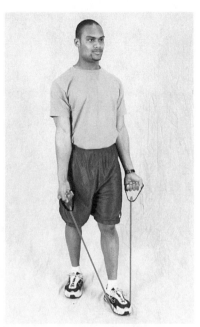

Figure 2-42 Tubing biceps curl start/finish position.
Courtesy of Patrick Hagerman, Ed.D. Quest Personal Training, Inc.

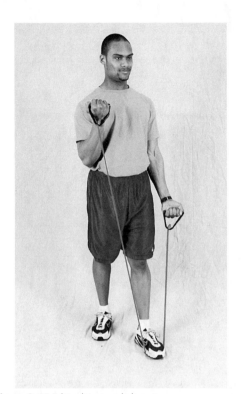

Figure 2-44 Tubing biceps curl alternating arms.
Courtesy of Patrick Hagerman, Ed.D. Quest Personal Training, Inc.

Tubing Triceps Pushdown

Starting position: Attach the tubing to the top of a doorway or loop it over the top of a tall machine in the gym. Make sure that each side is hanging down at an equal length. Grasp one end of the tubing in each hand using a pronated grip, palms facing down. Stand as close to the tubing as possible without standing underneath it. Keep the feet apart, one foot in front of the other. Place the elbows at the sides of the body, and bend them so that the hands are as close to the shoulders as possible. The tubing should have some stretch in it at this point. If the tubing is too long, it can be wrapped around the hands or the top of the machine to take out some slack; wrapping will also increase the resistance of the tubing. If wrapping causes the tubing to be too tight, take the slack out by kneeling on the floor instead of standing.

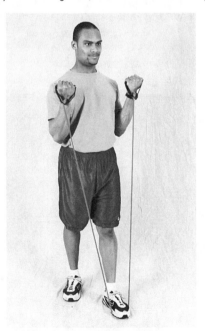

Figure 2-43 Tubing biceps curl midpoint.
Courtesy of Patrick Hagerman, Ed.D. Quest Personal Training, Inc.

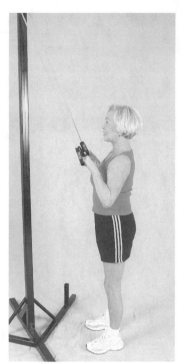

Figure 2-45 Tubing triceps pushdown start/finish position.
Courtesy of Patrick Hagerman, Ed.D. Quest Personal Training, Inc.

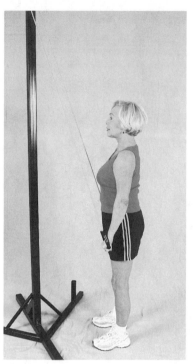

Figure 2-46 Tubing triceps pushdown midpoint.
Courtesy of Patrick Hagerman, Ed.D. Quest Personal Training, Inc.

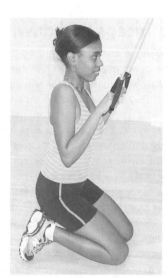

Figure 2-47 Tubing triceps pushdown kneeling start/finish
position.
Courtesy of Patrick Hagerman, Ed.D. Quest Personal Training, Inc.

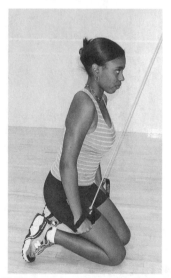

Figure 2-48 Tubing triceps pushdown kneeling midpoint.
Courtesy of Patrick Hagerman, Ed.D. Quest Personal Training, Inc.

Movement: Keep the elbows at the sides of the body, pressing the hands down until the arms are completely straight. Slowly allow both hands to return to their starting position near the shoulders.

Seated Row with Tubing

Starting position: Wrap the tubing around a pole or through the tubing–door anchor about a foot off the ground. Sit on the floor facing the tubing; hold one handle in each hand with the arms straight out in front of the body at shoulder height. Shift back until there is some stretch in the tubing. Bend the knees slightly so that the heels are in contact with the floor and can provide some support, and sit up straight.

Movement: Pull the handles to the stomach, allowing the elbows to move down to the sides and back

behind the body. Slowly allow the arms to return to the starting position.

Variation: Keep the elbows held at shoulder level as the tubing is pulled back. During this movement, the elbows will move out away from and behind the body instead of staying low and close to the body.

Standing Row with Tubing

Starting position: Wrap the tubing around a pole, or through a tubing–door anchor, at about chest height. Hold one handle in each hand with the arms out in front of the body at shoulder height. Step back until the tubing stretches a little. Stand upright, and keep the back straight and still. Place one foot in front of the other for a good base of support.

Movement: Hold the elbows up at shoulder level, pulling back on both handles. Pull back as far as possible, or until the hands reach the shoulders. Slowly allow the tubing to return to the starting position.

Variation: Keep the elbows down at the sides of the body while pulling the hands back to the chest.

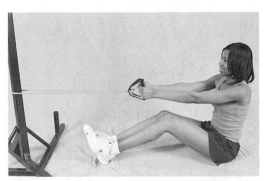

Figure 2-49 Tubing seated row start/finish position.
Courtesy of Patrick Hagerman, Ed.D. Quest Personal Training, Inc.

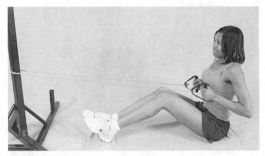

Figure 2-50 Tubing seated row midpoint.
Courtesy of Patrick Hagerman, Ed.D. Quest Personal Training, Inc.

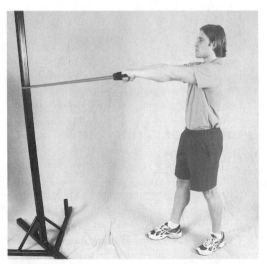

Figure 2-51 Tubing standing row start/finish position.
Courtesy of Patrick Hagerman, Ed.D. Quest Personal Training, Inc.

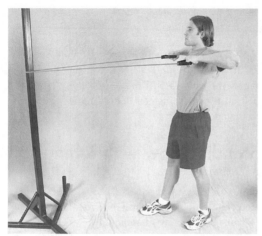

Figure 2-52 Tubing standing row midpoint.
Courtesy of Patrick Hagerman, Ed.D. Quest Personal Training, Inc.

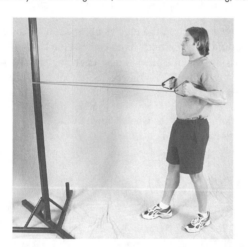

Figure 2-53 Tubing standing row variation midpoint.
Courtesy of Patrick Hagerman, Ed.D. Quest Personal Training, Inc.

Seated Hamstring Curl with Tubing

Starting position: Wrap the tubing around a pole or through a tubing–door anchor at ground level. Place the toe of each foot through a handle, and wrap the tubing around the shins a couple of times to keep it in place; if the tubing is not wrapped around the shins, it will slip off halfway through the exercise. Sit on the edge of a chair facing the anchor. Straighten both legs, and place the heels on

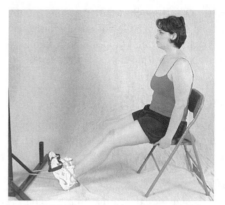

Figure 2-54 Tubing seated leg curl start/finish position.
Courtesy of Patrick Hagerman, Ed.D. Quest Personal Training, Inc.

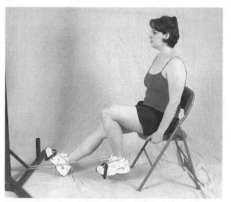

Figure 2-55 Tubing seated leg curl midpoint.
Courtesy of Patrick Hagerman, Ed.D. Quest Personal Training, Inc.

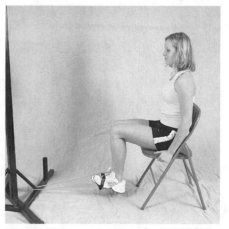

Figure 2-56 Tubing seated leg curl variation midpoint.
Courtesy of Patrick Hagerman, Ed.D. Quest Personal Training, Inc.

the floor, toes pointed toward the ceiling. Move the chair back until the tubing has a little stretch to it. Hold on to the sides of the chair.

Movement: Pull one foot towards the body and under the chair as far as possible; the other foot remains on the floor for support. Slowly let the foot back out. Alternate repetitions on the left and right leg, or complete a set with one leg and then the other.

Variation: Work both legs at the same time. This variation is more difficult, because the tubing will tend to pull back quickly, so hold on to the back of the chair.

Chest Press with Tubing

Starting position: Wrap the tubing around a pole, or through a tubing–door anchor, at chest height. Hold one end of the tubing in each hand, and face away from the anchor. Hold the elbows up in the air behind the body at shoulder height with the hands just under the shoulders. Place one foot in front of the other to create a solid base.

Movement: Push forward with both hands until the arms are straight out in front of the body. Slowly bend at the elbows, and bring the hands back to their starting position near the shoulders. The tubing will tend to pull back quickly, so control the return to starting position.

Variations: Instead of moving both arms at the same time, alternate repetitions on the left and right sides. Hold the tubing in place as you normally would, but keep one hand at the shoulder as the other hand presses out. The resistance can also be increased by placing both handles in one hand and completing a set of single-arm presses.

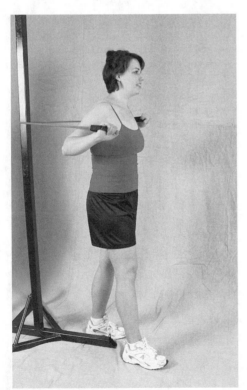

Figure 2-57 Tubing chest press start/finish position.
Courtesy of Patrick Hagerman, Ed.D. Quest Personal Training, Inc.

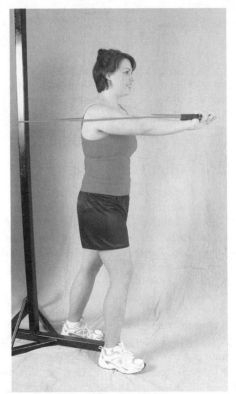

Figure 2-58 Tubing chest press midpoint.
Courtesy of Patrick Hagerman, Ed.D. Quest Personal Training, Inc.

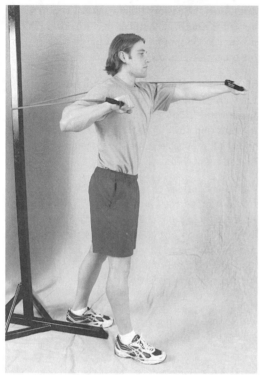

Figure 2-59 Tubing chest press variation midpoint.
Courtesy of Patrick Hagerman, Ed.D. Quest Personal Training, Inc.

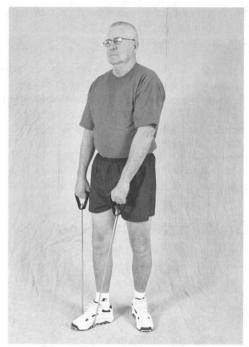

Figure 2-60 Tubing front raise start/finish position.
Courtesy of Patrick Hagerman, Ed.D. Quest Personal Training, Inc.

Front Raise with Tubing

Starting position: Hold one end of the tubing in each hand with arms held down in front of the body. Stand with one foot slightly in front of the other, and place the middle of the tubing under the front foot to anchor it. If there is slack in the tubing, either wrap it around the hands or the foot to tighten it.

Movement: Keeping the arms straight, lift both hands up in front of the body until they are at shoulder level. Slowly lower both arms back to the starting position. If lifting both arms at the same time is too difficult, keep one arm down and only lift one arm at a time, alternating left and right repetitions.

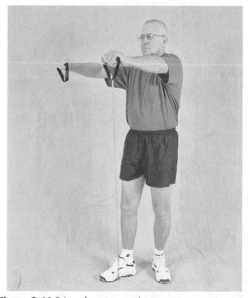

Figure 2-61 Tubing front raise midpoint.
Courtesy of Patrick Hagerman, Ed.D. Quest Personal Training, Inc.

Standing Hamstring Curl with Tubing

Starting position: Wrap the tubing around a pole, or through a tubing–door anchor, at ground level. Place the toe of each foot through a handle, and wrap the tubing around the shins a couple of times to keep it in place; if the tubing is not wrapped around the shins, it will slip off during the exercise. Stand facing the door or pole that anchors the tubing and hold on to it for support. Step back until there is no slack in the tubing.

Movement: Shift all the body weight to one foot, and lift the other foot about an inch off the floor. Bend that knee to lift the foot up and behind the body as far as possible, attempting to touch the heel to the buttocks. While the foot is moving, keep the knees close together so that the hip does not move. Slowly return the foot to the floor. Alternate left and right, or complete a set on one leg then the other.

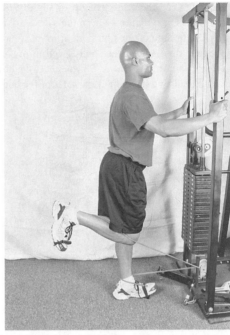

Figure 2-63 Tubing standing leg curl midpoint.
Courtesy of Patrick Hagerman, Ed.D. Quest Personal Training, Inc.

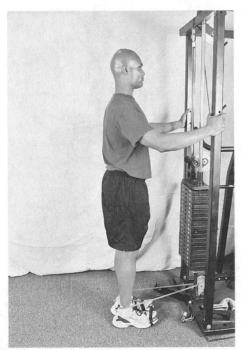

Figure 2-62 Tubing standing leg curl start/finish position.
Courtesy of Patrick Hagerman, Ed.D. Quest Personal Training, Inc.

DUMBBELL AND BARBELL EXERCISES

Dumbbells and barbells are two of the most basic tools of resistance exercise. A **dumbbell** (DB) is made of a short bar with weights on each end, and it is meant to be held in one hand. A **barbell** (BB) is made of a longer bar with weights on each end, and it is meant to be held in both hands. Barbells come in 4-foot and 6-foot lengths, along with a variation called the **EZ-curl barbell** that is bent or "wavy" to accommodate a more comfortable grip.

Dumbbell Lateral Raise

Starting position: Stand with the feet apart, one foot slightly behind the other for balance. Hold a dumbbell in each hand against the outside of the thighs with a neutral grip, palms facing the legs.

Movement: Keep the arms straight or slightly bent at the elbow. Lift both arms out to the sides until the dumbbells are shoulder height. Both arms must move at the same time and at the same speed to prevent unnecessary strain to the back. Slowly lower the arms back to the starting position at the sides of the body.

Dumbbell Front Raise

Starting position: Stand with the feet slightly apart, one foot in front of the other. Hold a dumbbell in each hand, arms straight down in front of the body, using a pronated grip, palms facing the legs.

Movement: Slowly lift one arm straight out in front of the body until it reaches shoulder level. Keep the arm as straight as possible. Slowly lower the dumbbell back down to the leg and repeat with the other arm, alternating left and right arms until the set is complete.

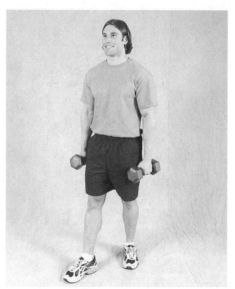

Figure 2-64 DB lateral raise start/finish position.
Courtesy of Patrick Hagerman, Ed.D. Quest Personal Training, Inc.

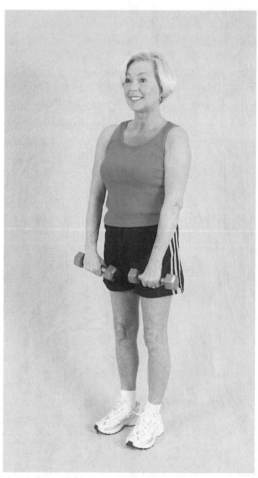

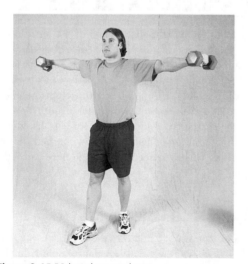

Figure 2-65 DB lateral raise midpoint.
Courtesy of Patrick Hagerman, Ed.D. Quest Personal Training, Inc.

Figure 2-66 DB front raise start/finish position.
Courtesy of Patrick Hagerman, Ed.D. Quest Personal Training, Inc.

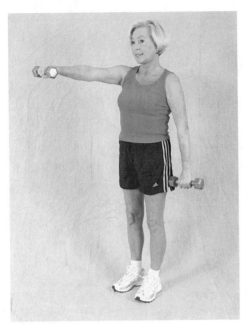

Figure 2-67 DB front raise midpoint.
Courtesy of Patrick Hagerman, Ed.D. Quest Personal Training, Inc.

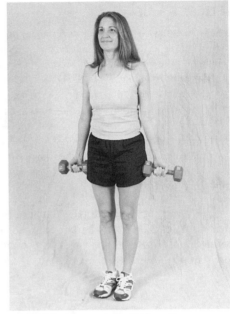

Figure 2-68 DB biceps curl start/finish position.
Courtesy of Patrick Hagerman, Ed.D. Quest Personal Training, Inc.

Dumbbell Biceps Curl

Starting position: Stand with the feet apart and a dumbbell in each hand in a supinated grip, palms facing away from you. Hold the arms at the sides of the body, and allow the dumbbells to rest against the outside of the thighs.

Movement: To prevent leaning back, perform the curl with one arm at a time. Keep the elbow at the side of the body, do not let it move forward at all, and smoothly pull the dumbbell up by bending at the elbow as far as possible, or until the dumbbell reaches the shoulder. Once at the top of the curl, slowly lower the dumbbell back down to rest beside the leg. Alternate arms, allowing one arm to rest while the other is working.

Variation: To perform the curl with both arms at the same time, stand so that one foot is in front of the other. This positioning provides a wide base of support to prevent any leaning back during the curl. Pull both arms up at the same time, and slowly lower them back down.

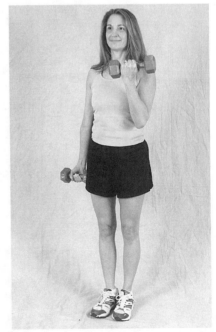

Figure 2-69 DB biceps curl midpoint.
Courtesy of Patrick Hagerman, Ed.D. Quest Personal Training, Inc.

Preacher Curl

Starting position: On a preacher-curl bench, begin by adjusting the height of the seat or the arm pad, depending on the model of bench, so that the upper arm is flat on the padding. If the elbows are the only part of the arm touching the pad, then the seat is too high. If the elbows cannot touch the pad, but the top of the arm near the armpit touches it, the seat is too low. Hold an EZ-curl barbell using a normal and supinated grip. Depending on the design of the bar, a narrow grip may have to be used instead of a normal grip.

Movement: Curl the bar up to the shoulders, just under the chin. Slowly let the bar back down, lowering it until the arms are completely straight before starting the next repetition.

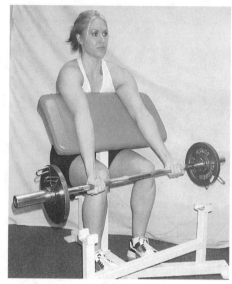

Figure 2-70 Preacher curl start/finish position.
Courtesy of Patrick Hagerman, Ed.D. Quest Personal Training, Inc.

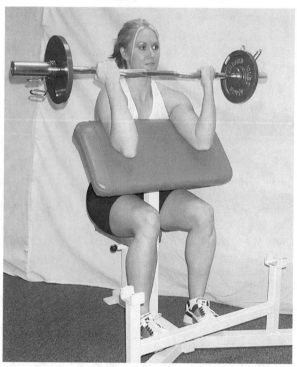

Figure 2-71 Preacher curl midpoint.
Courtesy of Patrick Hagerman, Ed.D. Quest Personal Training, Inc.

Barbell Biceps Curl

Starting position: Stand with the feet apart, one foot slightly behind the other. Hold a barbell in both hands using a normal and supinated grip, palms facing away from the body. Make sure the hands are evenly spaced from the center or ends of the bar. Let the barbell rest against the front of the thighs.

Movement: While keeping the body still and the elbows at the sides of the body, bend at both elbows to curl the barbell up to the shoulders. Both sides of the barbell should reach the shoulders at the same time, so curl with a steady, balanced movement. Slowly lower the barbell down to the thighs, allowing the arms to reach a straight position before starting another repetition.

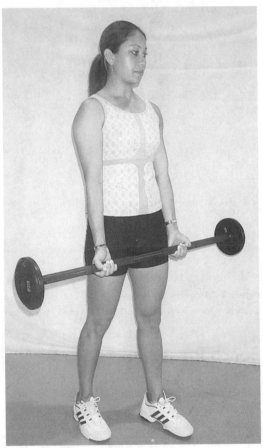

Figure 2-72 BB biceps curl start/finish position.
Courtesy of Patrick Hagerman, Ed.D. Quest Personal Training, Inc.

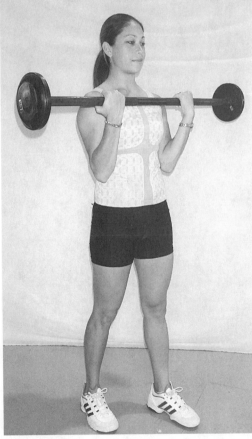

Figure 2-73 BB biceps curl midpoint.
Courtesy of Patrick Hagerman, Ed.D. Quest Personal Training, Inc.

Hammer Curl

Starting position: Stand with the feet apart. Hold a dumbbell in each hand, resting against the outsides of the thighs in a neutral grip, palms facing the legs. Keep the arms relaxed at the sides of the body.

Movement: Keep one arm at rest while pulling the other dumbbell up to the shoulder by bending at the elbow. The elbow should remain at the side of the body while lifting the dumbbell, and only the forearm and hand should move. Slowly lower the dumbbell back down, and repeat with the other arm.

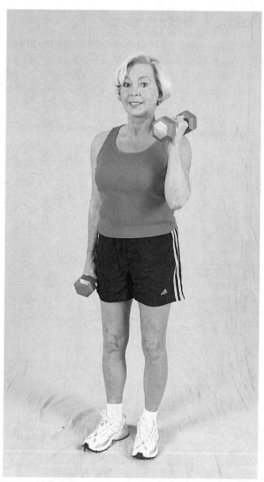

Figure 2-75 Hammer curl midpoint.
Courtesy of Patrick Hagerman, Ed.D. Quest Personal Training, Inc.

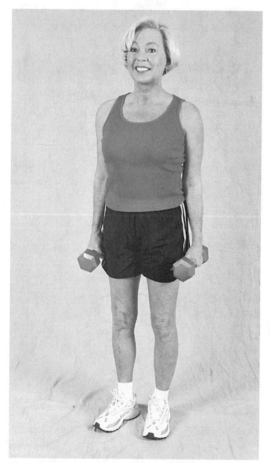

Figure 2-74 Hammer curl start/finish position.
Courtesy of Patrick Hagerman, Ed.D. Quest Personal Training, Inc.

Bench Press

Starting position: Using a flat bench, lie down in a supine position, face up, placing the feet flat on the floor. Grasp the bar using a normal, pronated grip. Be sure the hands are an equal distance from the middle of the bar. Lift the bar off its resting hooks, and hold it over the chest. Do not let the bar move over the head or stomach. Find the point at which the arms are perfectly vertical, and the bar will feel relatively light.

Movement: Slowly lower the bar down to within an inch of the chest; the bar should never touch the chest. As the bar is moving down, the elbows should move out away from the sides of the body. Push the bar back up until the arms are straight, again moving the bar in a straight line. If the bar moves more toward the head or stomach, make adjustments to keep it positioned over the chest.

Precautions: Do not perform this exercise without a spotter. Do not "bounce" the bar off the chest.

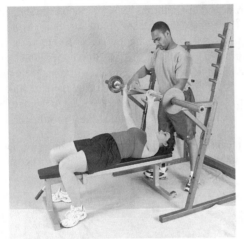

Figure 2-76 Bench press start/finish position.
Courtesy of Patrick Hagerman, Ed.D. Quest Personal Training, Inc.

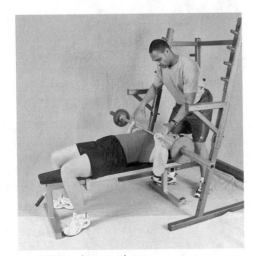

Figure 2-77 Bench press midpoint.
Courtesy of Patrick Hagerman, Ed.D. Quest Personal Training, Inc.

Barbell Incline Press

Starting position: Using an inclined bench, lie down in a supine position, face up. The incline of most benches is approximately 45 degrees, but this incline can vary slightly without any significant difference in results. Grasp the bar with a normal, pronated grip. Lift the bar off the rack, and hold it straight up in the air over the chest and head. Find the point at which the arms are perfectly vertical, and the bar will feel relatively light.

Movement: Slowly lower the bar to within an inch of the chest. As the bar is lowered, the elbows should move out away from the sides of the body. Do not let it come down over the head or stomach; keep it over the chest. Push the bar back up until the arms are completely straight.

Precautions: Do not perform this exercise without a spotter, and do not "bounce" the bar off the chest.

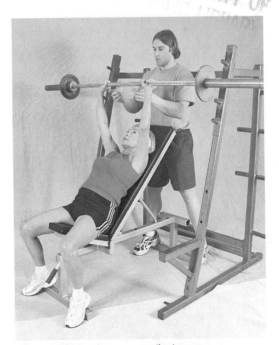

Figure 2-78 BB incline press start/finish position.
Courtesy of Patrick Hagerman, Ed.D. Quest Personal Training, Inc.

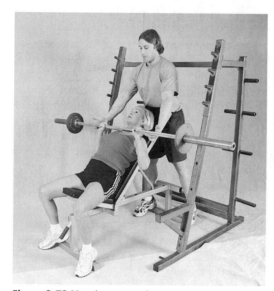

Figure 2-79 BB incline press midpoint.
Courtesy of Patrick Hagerman, Ed.D. Quest Personal Training, Inc.

Dumbbell Chest Press

Starting position: Hold a dumbbell in each hand, using a pronated grip. Lie down on a flat bench in a supine position (face up, on the back), placing the feet flat on the floor. Hold the dumbbells directly above each shoulder, and move the elbows away from the sides of the body until they are in line with the shoulders.

Movement: Press the dumbbells straight up in the air over the chest until the arms are completely straight. Do not allow the dumbbells to hover over the head or stomach; they should always be directly over the chest and shoulders. Slowly lower the dumbbells back down to the starting position. While the dumbbells are moving up and down, they should follow a straight, smooth path. If they move out to the sides in a circular path to the top, bring them back in line.

Precautions: Do not perform this exercise without a spotter.

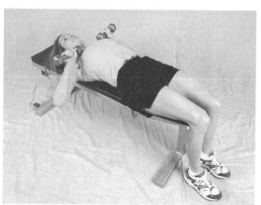

Figure 2-80 DB chest press start/finish position. This exercise should be performed with a spotter, however to focus on the technique, the spotter was not included in the photo.
Courtesy of Patrick Hagerman, Ed.D. Quest Personal Training, Inc.

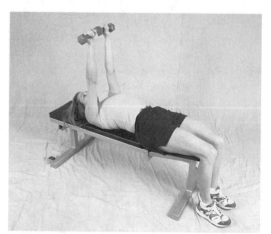

Figure 2-81 DB chest press midpoint This exercise should be performed with a spotter, however to focus on the technique, the spotter was not included in the photo.
Courtesy of Patrick Hagerman, Ed.D. Quest Personal Training, Inc.

Dumbbell Incline Press

Starting position: Using an inclined bench, lie down in a supine position (face up, on the back). The incline of most benches is approximately 45 degrees, but this can vary slightly without any significant difference in results. Hold a dumbbell in each hand using a pronated grip. Hold the dumbbells directly above each shoulder, and move the elbows away from the sides of the body until they are in line with the shoulders.

Movement: Press the dumbbells straight up in the air over the chest until the arms are completely straight. Do not allow the dumbbells to hover over the head or stomach; they should always be directly over the chest and shoulders. Slowly lower the dumbbells back down to the starting position. While the dumbbells are moving up and down, they should follow a straight, smooth path. If they move out to the sides in a circular path to the top, bring them back in line.

Precautions: Do not perform this exercise without a spotter.

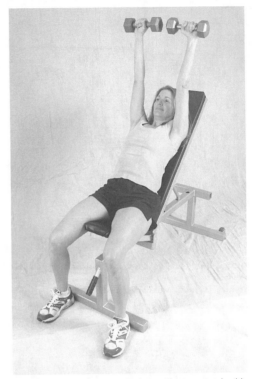

Figure 2-83 DB incline press midpoint. This exercise should be performed with a spotter, however to focus on the technique, the spotter was not included in the photo.
Courtesy of Patrick Hagerman, Ed.D. Quest Personal Training, Inc.

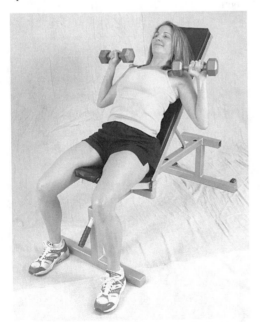

Figure 2-82 DB incline press start/finish position This exercise should be performed with a spotter, however to focus on the technique, the spotter was not included in the photo.
Courtesy of Patrick Hagerman, Ed.D. Quest Personal Training, Inc.

Dumbbell Shoulder Press

Starting position: Sit on a stability ball or on the edge of a bench. Use a bench or chair with a back rest to keep the back straight. Using a pronated grip, hold a dumbbell in each hand and lift them to shoulder level, placing them either in front of the shoulders or to the sides of the shoulders, whichever is more comfortable.

Movement: Press both dumbbells up and over the head at the same time until the arms are completely straight. The dumbbells should naturally move closer together and may even touch at the top. Slowly lower the dumbbells back to the shoulders.

Precautions: Do not perform this exercise without a spotter.

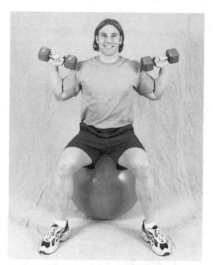

Figure 2-84 DB shoulder press start/finish position. This exercise should be performed with a spotter, however to focus on the technique, the spotter was not included in the photo.

Courtesy of Patrick Hagerman, Ed.D. Quest Personal Training, Inc.

Military Press

Starting position: Using either a military-press bench or an upright seat with a backrest, sit with the back flat against the seat and feet flat on the floor. Grasp the barbell with a normal, pronated grip. Hold the bar directly overhead with the arms fully extended.

Movement: Slowly lower the bar down in front of the head until it reaches chin or shoulder level. As the bar is coming down, the elbows should move down to the sides of the body. Push the bar back over the head, keeping the elbows out away from the sides of the body.

Variation: Perform the military press standing up. Stand with the feet apart, holding the barbell at the shoulders to begin. Press the bar over the head until the arms are straight, then slowly lower it back to the shoulders.

Precautions: Do not perform this exercise without a spotter.

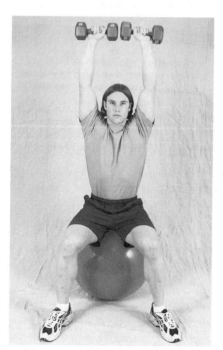

Figure 2-85 DB shoulder press midpoint. This exercise should be performed with a spotter, however to focus on the technique, the spotter was not included in the photo.

Courtesy of Patrick Hagerman, Ed.D. Quest Personal Training, Inc.

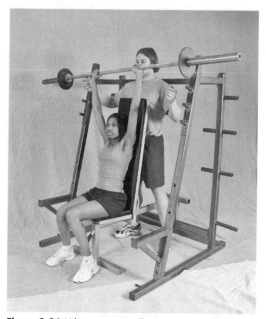

Figure 2-86 Military press start/finish position.

Courtesy of Patrick Hagerman, Ed.D. Quest Personal Training, Inc.

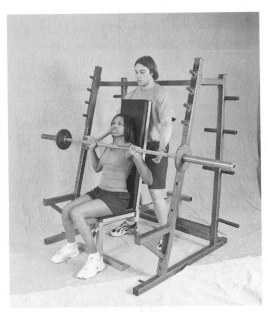

Figure 2-87 Military press midpoint.

Courtesy of Patrick Hagerman, Ed.D. Quest Personal Training, Inc.

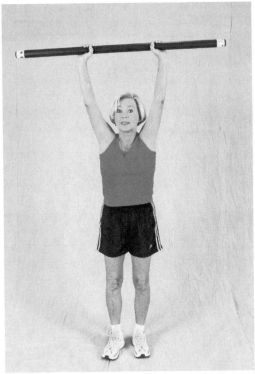

Figure 2-89 Military press standing variation midpoint. This exercise should be performed with a spotter, however to focus on the technique, the spotter was not included in the photo.

Courtesy of Patrick Hagerman, Ed.D. Quest Personal Training, Inc.

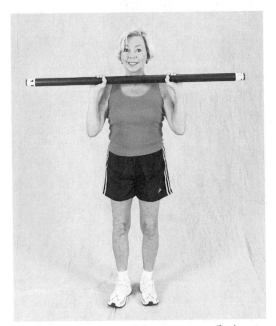

Figure 2-88 Military press standing variation start/finish position. This exercise should be performed with a spotter, however to focus on the technique, the spotter was not included in the photo.

Courtesy of Patrick Hagerman, Ed.D. Quest Personal Training, Inc.

Dumbbell Fly

Starting position: Hold a dumbbell in each hand, and lie down on a flat bench in a supine position (face up, on the back), placing the feet flat on the floor. Using a neutral grip, press the dumbbells up directly over the chest until the arms are straight. Hold the dumbbells together at this point.

Movement: Slightly bend at the elbows, and let the dumbbells move apart and toward the floor in a large arc. Do not bend the elbows any more as the weight goes down, and try to keep the dumbbells as far away from the body as possible at all times. Lower the dumbbells until they are level with the shoulders. Pull the dumbbells back up to their starting position above the chest. This movement should resemble an arc, not a straight-line press. Make sure the dumbbells move at the same speed so one side is not finished before the other.

Precautions: Do not perform this exercise without a spotter.

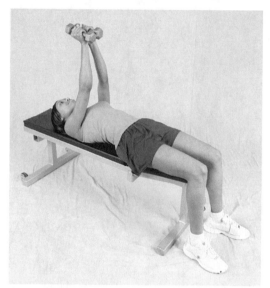

Figure 2-90 DB Fly start/finish position. This exercise should be performed with a spotter, however to focus on the technique, the spotter was not included in the photo.

Courtesy of Patrick Hagerman, Ed.D. Quest Personal Training, Inc.

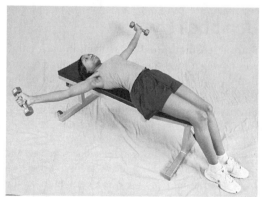

Figure 2-91 DB Fly midpoint. This exercise should be performed with a spotter, however to focus on the technique, the spotter was not included in the photo.

Courtesy of Patrick Hagerman, Ed.D. Quest Personal Training, Inc.

Dumbbell Prone Fly

Starting position: Lie in a prone position, face down, over a stability ball, positioning the ball directly under the middle of the chest just below the chin. Straighten the legs so that the only part of the body touching the floor is the toes. Hold a dumbbell in each hand using a neutral grip. Allow the arms to hang down at the sides of the ball, with a slight bend at the elbows.

Movement: Keeping a slight bend at the elbows, lift both arms out to the sides until the hands are at shoulder height. Slowly lower the arms back to the starting position.

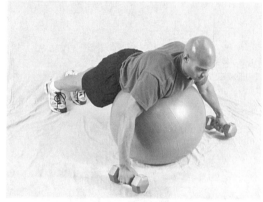

Figure 2-92 Prone fly start/finish position.

Courtesy of Patrick Hagerman, Ed.D. Quest Personal Training, Inc.

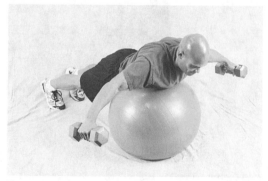

Figure 2-93 Prone fly midpoint.

Courtesy of Patrick Hagerman, Ed.D. Quest Personal Training, Inc.

Dumbbell Incline Fly

Starting position: Hold a dumbbell in each hand, and lie back on an inclined bench in a supine position (face up, on the back), placing both feet flat on the floor. Using a neutral grip, press the dumbbells up directly over the chest until the arms are straight. Hold the dumbbells together at this point.

Movement: Slightly bend at the elbows, and let the dumbbells move apart and toward the floor in a large arc. Do not bend the elbows any more as the weight goes down. Try to keep the dumbbells as far away from the body as possible at all times. Lower the dumbbells until they are level with the shoulders. Pull the dumbbells back up to their starting position above the chest. This movement should resemble an arc, not a straight-line press. Make sure the dumbbells move at the same speed so one side is not finished before the other.

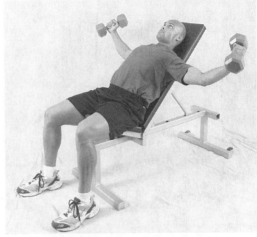

Figure 2-95 DB incline fly midpoint. This exercise should be performed with a spotter, however to focus on the technique, the spotter was not included in the photo.

Courtesy of Patrick Hagerman, Ed.D. Quest Personal Training, Inc.

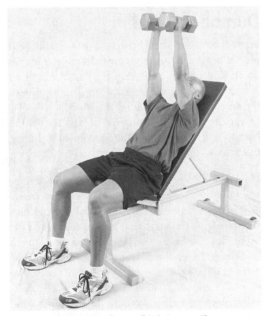

Figure 2-94 DB incline fly start/finish position. This exercise should be performed with a spotter, however to focus on the technique, the spotter was not included in the photo.

Courtesy of Patrick Hagerman, Ed.D. Quest Personal Training, Inc.

Precautions: Do not perform this exercise without a spotter.

Deadlift

Starting position: Stand behind a barbell placed on the floor, feet shoulder width apart. Kneel down and grasp the barbell using a wide and alternating grip. Raise the shoulders and head until the arms are straight, but do not lift the bar. Lower the hips as if sitting down, and flatten the back as much as possible. The feet should be flat on the floor.

Movement: Face forward while lifting the bar off the floor by extending the hips, knees, and ankles simultaneously. The shoulders and hips should rise at the same time and at the same rate. If the hips rise before the shoulders, the movement is incorrect. Keep the bar within an inch of the body, and keep the back completely flat at all times. Rise to a full standing position. Slowly lower the bar back to the floor while keeping the back flat. Bend the knees, hips, and ankles simultaneously again to return to the starting position.

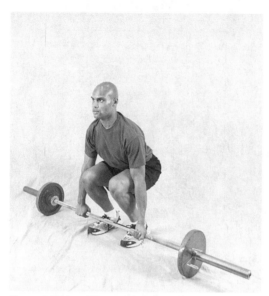

Figure 2-96 Deadlift start position.
Courtesy of Patrick Hagerman, Ed.D. Quest Personal Training, Inc.

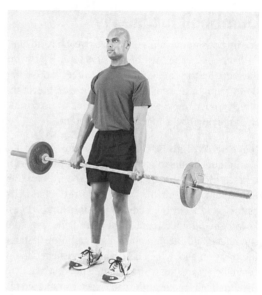

Figure 2-98 Deadlift finish position.
Courtesy of Patrick Hagerman, Ed.D. Quest Personal Training, Inc.

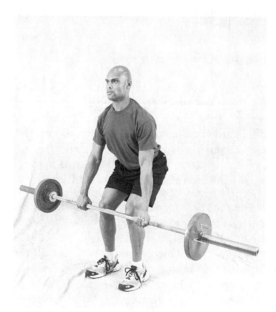

Figure 2-97 Deadlift midpoint position.
Courtesy of Patrick Hagerman, Ed.D. Quest Personal Training, Inc.

Dumbbell Deadlift

Starting position: Stand between a pair of dumbbells placed on the floor, feet approximately 6 inches apart. Kneel down and grasp the dumbbells using a neutral grip. Raise the shoulders and head until the arms are straight, but do not lift the dumbbells. Lower the hips as if sitting down, and flatten the back as much as possible. The feet should be flat on the floor.

Movement: Face forward while lifting the dumbbells off the floor by extending the hips, knees, and ankles simultaneously. The shoulders and hips should rise at the same time and at the same rate. If the hips rise before the shoulders, the movement is incorrect. Keep the dumbbells at the sides of the body, and the back completely flat at all times. Rise to a full standing position. Slowly lower the dumbbells back to the floor, keeping the back flat. Bend the knees, hips, and ankles simultaneously to return to the starting position.

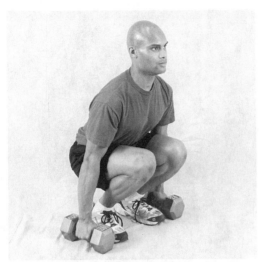

Figure 2-99 DB deadlift start position.
Courtesy of Patrick Hagerman, Ed.D. Quest Personal Training, Inc.

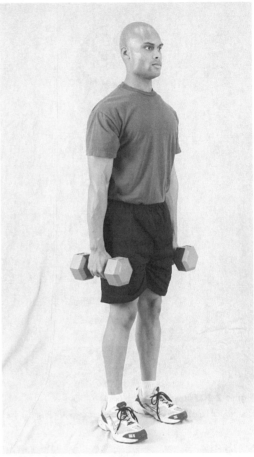

Figure 2-101 DB deadlift finish position.
Courtesy of Patrick Hagerman, Ed.D. Quest Personal Training, Inc.

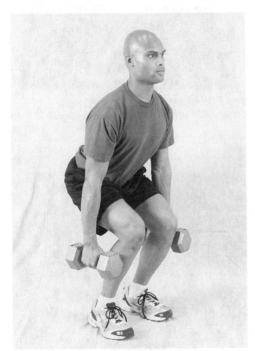

Figure 2-100 DB deadlift midpoint position.
Courtesy of Patrick Hagerman, Ed.D. Quest Personal Training, Inc.

Barbell Squat

Starting position: The barbell squat should always be performed inside of a "squat cage," which has two upright bars that hold the barbell in place as weight is added. With the help of a spotter, add weight to each side of the barbell at the same time, and use locking collars to secure the weights in place. Adjust the catch bars of the squat cage so that they are slightly below the level the barbell will reach at full

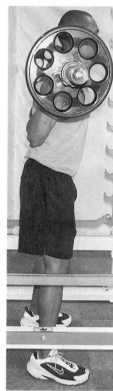

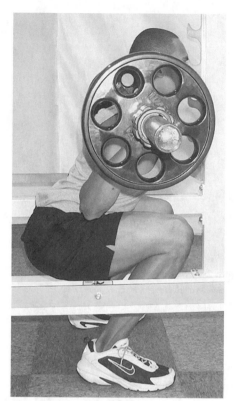

Figure 2-102 Squat start/finish position: side view.
Courtesy of Patrick Hagerman, Ed.D. Quest Personal Training, Inc.

Figure 2-104 Squat midpoint: side view.
Courtesy of Patrick Hagerman, Ed.D. Quest Personal Training, Inc.

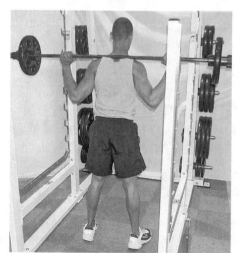

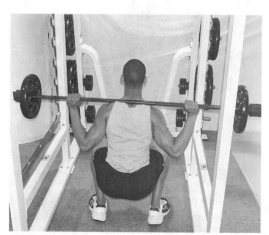

Figure 2-103 Squat start/finish position: rear view.
Courtesy of Patrick Hagerman, Ed.D. Quest Personal Training, Inc.

Figure 2-105 Squat midpoint: rear view.
Courtesy of Patrick Hagerman, Ed.D. Quest Personal Training, Inc.

squat depth. Determine this level by performing an unweighted squat and noting how low the shoulders go: Place the catch bars just below this point. These bars will catch the weighted bar if a repetition cannot be completed. With the barbell resting on the cage, step under the barbell and position it to rest across the top of the shoulders just below the neck. If the bar feels uncomfortable, wrap it with a towel for extra padding. Stand up with the barbell, take a small step back, and position your feet shoulder width apart, toes slightly turned out.

Movement: Keeping your back as straight as possible, bend your knees and hips simultaneously and begin squatting toward the ground. Allow the hips to move behind the body, and allow the shoulders to move forward. Keep the barbell directly over the feet during the entire movement, and squat down until the thighs are parallel with the floor. Stand back up, lifting the hips and shoulders at the same time.

Precautions: If a squat cage equipped with catch bars is not available, the squat can be performed with two spotters, one on each side of the bar to catch it.

Dumbbell Squat

Starting position: Stand with the feet about 6 inches apart, toes slightly turned out. Hold a dumbbell in each hand with a neutral grip. Keep the arms held straight down at the sides of the bo dy during the entire movement.

Movement: Keeping the back straight and head up, slowly bend at both the knees and hips, lowering the body toward the floor. The hips should move out behind the body, and the shoulders should lean forward. Squat until the thighs are parallel with the floor. The dumbbells should move straight down next to the feet but should not touch the floor. Stand back up to the starting position, raising the hips and shoulders at the same time and at the same rate. If the hips rise before the shoulders, the movement is incorrect.

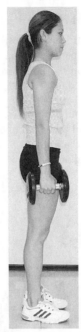

Figure 2-106 DB squat start/finish position.
Courtesy of Patrick Hagerman, Ed.D. Quest Personal Training, Inc.

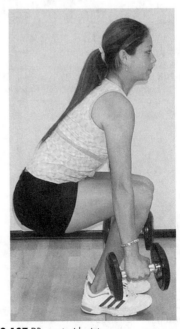

Figure 2-107 DB squat midpoint.
Courtesy of Patrick Hagerman, Ed.D. Quest Personal Training, Inc.

Dumbbell Triceps Press

Starting position: Hold a dumbbell in each hand and lie down on a flat bench in a supine position, placing the feet flat on the floor. Hold the dumbbells over the chest and shoulders using a neutral grip.

Movement: Bend at both elbows, and slowly lower the dumbbells until they are beside the head at ear level. Straighten the arms to push the dumbbells back to the starting position.

Precaution: Do not attempt this exercise without a spotter.

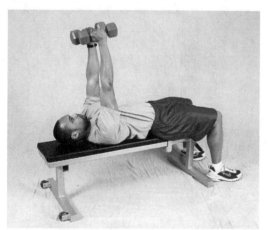

Figure 2-108 DB triceps press start/finish position. This exercise should be performed with a spotter, however to focus on the technique, the spotter was not included in the photo.

Courtesy of Patrick Hagerman, Ed.D. Quest Personal Training, Inc.

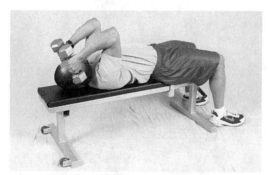

Figure 2-109 DB triceps press midpoint. This exercise should be performed with a spotter, however to focus on the technique, the spotter was not included in the photo.

Courtesy of Patrick Hagerman, Ed.D. Quest Personal Training, Inc.

Dumbbell Triceps Extension

Starting position: Sit on an exercise bench or on top of a stability ball. Hold a dumbbell in one hand, straight up in the air over the head, using a neutral grip. Place the other hand on the knee for support. Keep the back straight at all times.

Movement: Bend at the elbow to lower the dumbbell behind the head. Keep the elbow stationary and pointed up in the air at all times. Lower the dumbbell as far as the elbow will bend. Straighten the arm to lift the dumbbell back overhead.

Precaution: Do not attempt this exercise without a spotter.

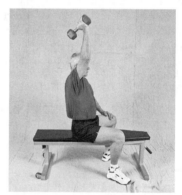

Figure 2-110 DB triceps extension start/finish position. This exercise should be performed with a spotter, however to focus on the technique, the spotter was not included in the photo.

Courtesy of Patrick Hagerman, Ed.D. Quest Personal Training, Inc.

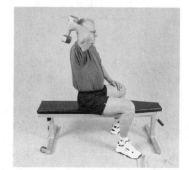

Figure 2-111 DB triceps extension midpoint. This exercise should be performed with a spotter, however to focus on the technique, the spotter was not included in the photo.

Courtesy of Patrick Hagerman, Ed.D. Quest Personal Training, Inc.

Kickbacks

Starting position: To work the left arm, place the right hand and knee on an exercise bench. Hold a dumbbell in the left hand using a neutral grip. The left foot should be on the floor. Keep the back flat and shoulders parallel to the floor. Lift the left elbow up until the upper arm is parallel to the floor and the elbow and shoulder are at the same height.

Movement: Extend the arm behind the body until it is completely straight and the dumbbell is by the

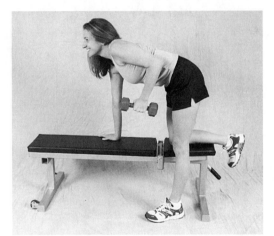

Figure 2-112 Kickbacks start/finish position.
Courtesy of Patrick Hagerman, Ed.D. Quest Personal Training, Inc.

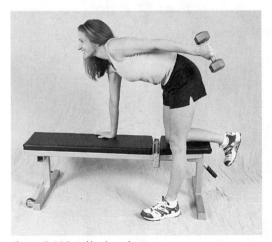

Figure 2-113 Kickbacks midpoint.
Courtesy of Patrick Hagerman, Ed.D. Quest Personal Training, Inc.

hips. Slowly lower the dumbbell back to the starting point. Do not let the dumbbell swing back down or pass the starting point. After completing a set on the left side, turn around, place the left hand and knee on the bench, hold the dumbbell in the right hand, and complete a set for the right arm.

Dumbbell Row, or Bent-Over Row

Starting point: Hold a dumbbell in each hand using a neutral grip, and stand with the feet about 6 inches apart. Bend forward at the waist, keeping the back straight, until the upper body is at a 45-degree angle, or until the back will no longer remain straight. Let the arms hang straight down.

Movement: Keeping the elbows close to the body, pull the dumbbells up to the stomach. Slowly let the arms straighten.

Variation: Work one side at a time by completing a full set with one arm and then the other. When one arm is working, the other arm should be hanging straight down.

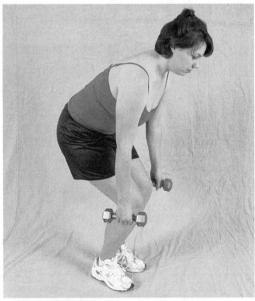

Figure 2-114 DB row or bent-over row start/finish position.
Courtesy of Patrick Hagerman, Ed.D. Quest Personal Training, Inc.

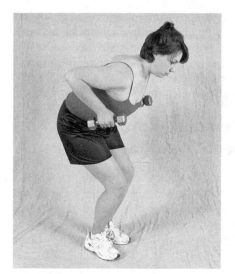

Figure 2-115 DB row or bent-over row midpoint.
Courtesy of Patrick Hagerman, Ed.D. Quest Personal Training, Inc.

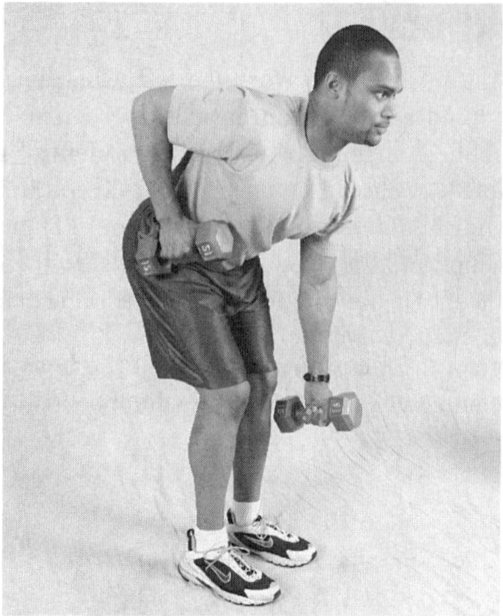

Figure 2-116 DB row or bent-over row variation midpoint.
Courtesy of Patrick Hagerman, Ed.D. Quest Personal Training, Inc.

Dumbbell Upright Row

Starting position: Hold a dumbbell in each hand using a pronated grip, palms facing your legs, arms directly in front of the body against the legs. Stand with the feet slightly apart.

Movement: Lift the elbows straight up in the air, keeping the dumbbells together and in front of the body. Bring the dumbbells right up under the chin. At the highest point, the elbows should be higher than the wrists. Slowly lower the dumbbells back down to the starting point.

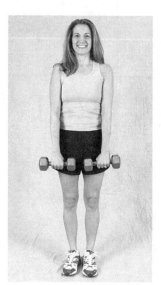

Figure 2-117 DB upright row start/finish position.
Courtesy of Patrick Hagerman, Ed.D. Quest Personal Training, Inc.

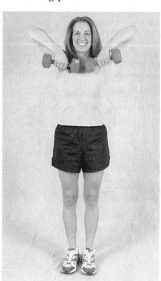

Figure 2-118 DB upright row midpoint.
Courtesy of Patrick Hagerman, Ed.D. Quest Personal Training, Inc.

Dumbbell Shrug

Starting position: Hold a dumbbell in each hand using a neutral grip with arms at the sides of the body. Stand with the feet slightly apart, back straight. Allow arms and shoulders to relax so that the shoulders are pulled down into a depressed position.

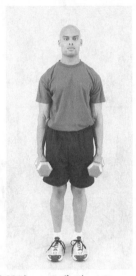

Figure 2-119 DB shrug start/finish position.
Courtesy of Patrick Hagerman, Ed.D. Quest Personal Training, Inc.

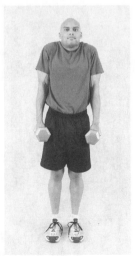

Figure 2-120 DB shrug midpoint.
Courtesy of Patrick Hagerman, Ed.D. Quest Personal Training, Inc.

Movement: Lift both shoulders upward, attempting to touch the shoulders to the ears. As you lift the shoulders, keep the arms completely straight. Slowly lower the shoulders back down until they are completely relaxed.

CABLE/PULLEY-SYSTEM EXERCISES

A **cable/pulley system** uses a stack of weights into which the user must insert a pin to select the desired resistance and a cable to which the user may attach a variety of handles, depending on the exercise. Cable/pulley systems have the advantage of not having a fixed movement, which allows the individual to perform a variety of exercises and movements with a single piece of equipment. The majority of cable/pulley-system exercises employ either a low-pulley or high-pulley setup. The **low-pulley setup** allows the individual to pull the handle up from the floor or from below knee level. The **high-pulley setup** allows the individual to pull the handle down from above the head or from shoulder level.

Lat Pulldown

Starting position: Sit down in the seat facing the weight stack, knees under the pad; the pad provides some leverage to help pull the bar down. Select the appropriate weight, making sure the selector pin is pushed all the way in. Grasp the bar using a normal, pronated grip, palms facing away from the body. No matter how wide the bar is, only use a normal grip; a wide grip prevents a full range of motion.

Movement: Start with both arms completely straight, then pull the bar down in front of the face until it reaches the chin. Slowly let the bar back up, making sure both arms are fully extended before the next repetition. Repeat until the set is complete.

Variations: A normal, supinated grip, as well as a narrow and neutral grip, may be used during this exercise. The movement remains the same.

Precaution: Never pull the bar down behind the head. This movement is a very common mistake that limits the range of motion and may result in shoulder injury.

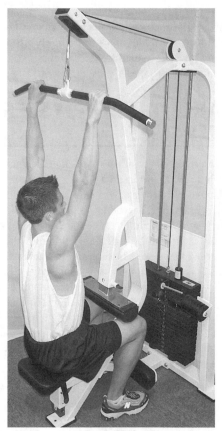

Figure 2-121 Lat pulldown start/finish position.
Courtesy of Patrick Hagerman, Ed.D. Quest Personal Training, Inc.

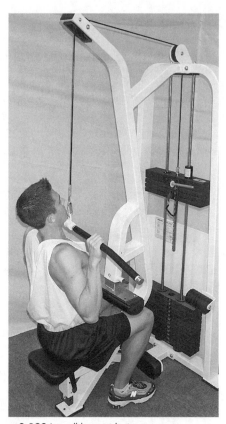

Figure 2-122 Lat pulldown midpoint.
Courtesy of Patrick Hagerman, Ed.D. Quest Personal Training, Inc.

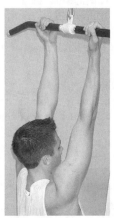

Figure 2-123 Lat pulldown with normal and supinated grip.
Courtesy of Patrick Hagerman, Ed.D. Quest Personal Training, Inc.

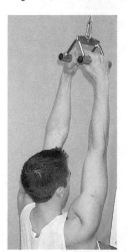

Figure 2-124 Lat pulldown with narrow and neutral grip.
Courtesy of Patrick Hagerman, Ed.D. Quest Personal Training, Inc.

Cable Triceps Pushdown

Starting position: Attach a straight handle or a triceps v-handle to a high pulley. Grasp the handle, one hand on each side of the cable and evenly spaced from the middle, using a pronated grip. Stand as close to the cable as possible without being under it. If the handle swings away from the body during the exercise, move back. Stand with feet apart, one foot in front of the other. Bend at the elbows so that the hands come as close to the shoulders as possible.

Movement: Keep the elbows at the sides of the body, pushing down until both arms are straight. Slowly allow the elbows to bend, and bring the handle back to the starting position.

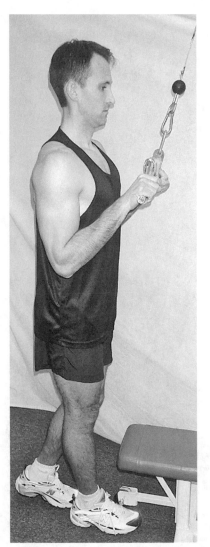

Figure 2-125 Cable triceps pushdown start/finish position.
Courtesy of Patrick Hagerman, Ed.D. Quest Personal Training, Inc.

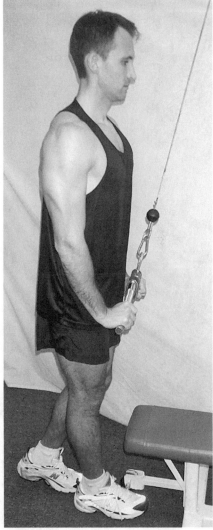

Figure 2-126 Cable triceps pushdown midpoint.
Courtesy of Patrick Hagerman, Ed.D. Quest Personal Training, Inc.

Cable Biceps Curl

Starting position: Attach a straight-handle bar to the low pulley. Grasp the handle with a supinated grip, palms up. Hand placement depends on handle width, so use a grip that allows the hands to be at least 6 inches apart but never wider than the shoulders. Let the arms relax so the bar is hanging in front of the body. Step back about 2 feet from the low pulley, and stand with the feet apart, one foot in front of the other.

Movement: Keep the elbows at the sides of the body, and bend at the elbows to curl the bar up to the shoulders. The elbows should remain stationary at the sides and should not move forward or backward. Slowly lower the bar until the arms are straight.

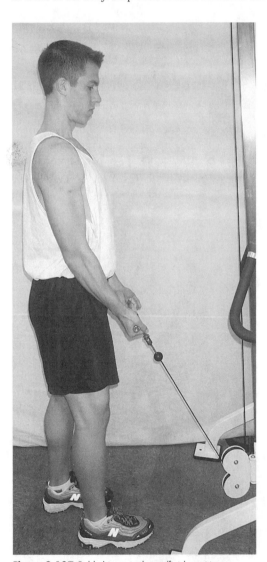

Figure 2-127 Cable biceps curl start/finish position.
Courtesy of Patrick Hagerman, Ed.D. Quest Personal Training, Inc.

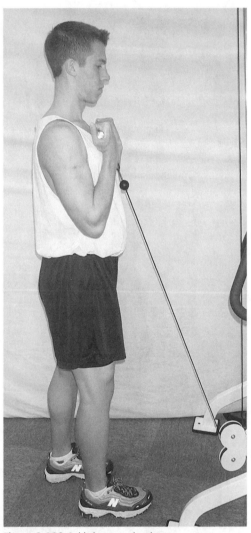

Figure 2-128 Cable biceps curl midpoint.
Courtesy of Patrick Hagerman, Ed.D. Quest Personal Training, Inc.

Cable Leg Curl

Starting position: Attach an ankle strap to a low pulley. Hook the ankle strap to the shin of the right leg. Stand facing the machine, and step back until the cable is tight. Hold on to the machine for support, and keep the back upright and straight at all times. Transfer all the body weight onto the left leg, and hold the right leg about an inch off the ground.

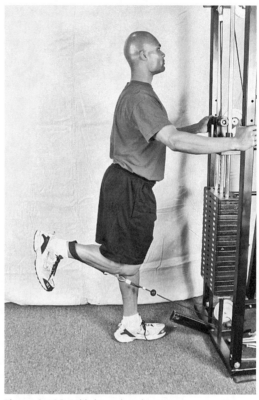

Figure 2-130 Cable leg curls midpoint.
Courtesy of Patrick Hagerman, Ed.D. Quest Personal Training, Inc.

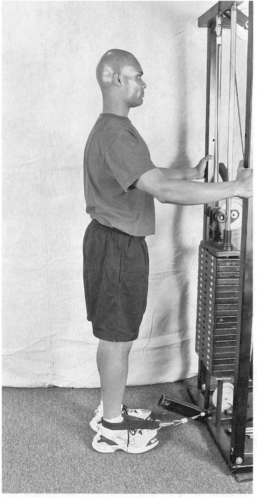

Figure 2-129 Cable leg curls start/finish position.
Courtesy of Patrick Hagerman, Ed.D. Quest Personal Training, Inc.

Movement: Keep the knees together, pulling the right foot up and behind the body. Attempt to touch the right foot to the buttocks. Slowly lower the foot back to the starting position, and complete all repetitions for the set. Switch the ankle strap to the left leg, and complete another set.

Cable Lateral Leg Lift

Starting position: Attach an ankle strap to the low pulley then to one leg. Stand so that the leg being trained first, the one attached to the cable, is farthest away from the machine. Transfer the body weight to the other leg, and hold on to the machine with one hand for support. Place the other hand on your hip.

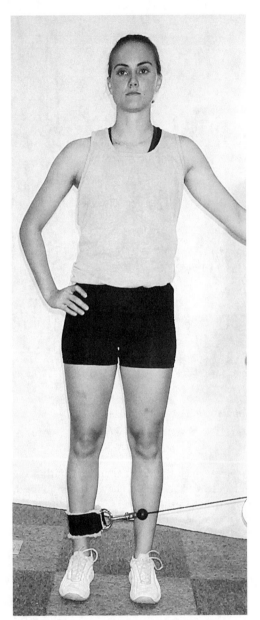

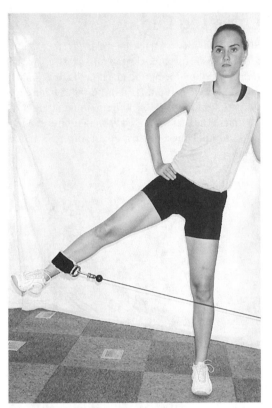

Figure 2-132 Cable lateral leg lift midpoint.
Courtesy of Patrick Hagerman, Ed.D. Quest Personal Training, Inc.

Cable Hip Adduction

Starting position: Attach an ankle strap to the low pulley then to one leg. Stand so that the leg being trained first, the one attached to the cable, is closest to the machine. Step out from the machine until the training leg is held out to approximately a 45-degree angle. Transfer the body weight to the leg farthest away from the machine, holding on to either the machine or a chair with one hand for support; place the other hand on your hip.

Movement: Keep the body upright, and the training leg straight, while pulling it across and in front of the body as far as possible. Slowly let the leg return to the starting position, and complete all the repetitions for that set before switching legs.

Figure 2-131 Cable lateral leg lift start/finish position.
Courtesy of Patrick Hagerman, Ed.D. Quest Personal Training, Inc.

Movement: Keep the body as straight as possible, lifting the leg out to the side as far as possible. Slowly bring the leg back to the starting position; repeat until the set is finished, then switch legs.

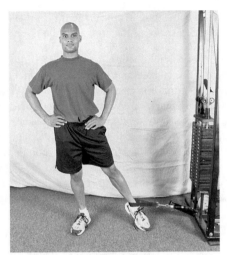

Figure 2-133 Cable hip adduction start/finish position.
Courtesy of Patrick Hagerman, Ed.D. Quest Personal Training, Inc.

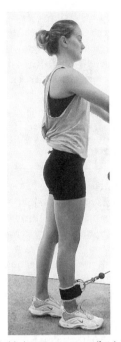

Figure 2-135 Cable hip extension start/finish position.
Courtesy of Patrick Hagerman, Ed.D. Quest Personal Training, Inc.

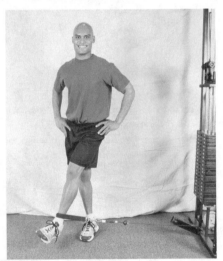

Figure 2-134 Cable hip adduction midpoint.
Courtesy of Patrick Hagerman, Ed.D. Quest Personal Training, Inc.

Cable Hip Extension

Starting position: Attach an ankle strap to a low pulley and then to one leg. Stand facing the machine, holding on to it with both hands for support, and step back until the cable is tight. Transfer all body weight to the leg not being trained, and hold the training leg about an inch off the floor.

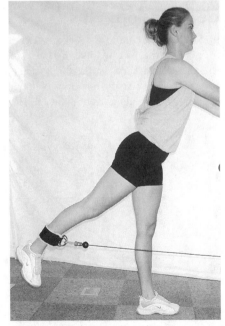

Figure 2-136 Cable hip extension midpoint.
Courtesy of Patrick Hagerman, Ed.D. Quest Personal Training, Inc.

Movement: Keep the training leg straight, pushing it back behind the body as far as possible. Slowly bring the leg back under the body, and repeat until the set is complete. Transfer the ankle strap to the other leg, and complete another set.

BODY-WEIGHT EXERCISES

Our own body weight provides a form of resistance. The main benefit of body-weight exercises is that they usually require no additional equipment. Body-weight exercises are very versatile and always simulate activities of daily living. In some instances, body weight does not provide enough resistance or is too stable to provide the intensity required to stimulate a muscle to work harder than normal. In these instances, **ankle weights,** small weights that are strapped to the ankle; **medicine balls,** balls of varying weights; and stability balls are employed to increase the intensity or difficulty of the exercise.

Back Extension

Starting position: Stand at a 45-degree extension bench, placing the feet against the heel stop or between the heel pads. Adjust the thigh pad so that it is just below the waist and does not interfere with the stomach when bending over the bench. The legs

should remain straight with the toes turned slightly out to the sides. Cross the arms over the chest.

Movement: Slowly bend over the bench until the body is fully relaxed and the head is in the lowest position. Starting with the lower back, roll up slowly, allowing the back to come up one vertebrae at a time. If the back is straight and moving as a single unit, the movement is coming from the hips instead of the spine, which is incorrect. The shoulder and head should be the last part of the body to lift up. Unroll until the body is in a straight line; do not hyperextend the spine.

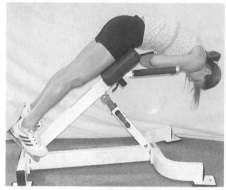

Figure 2-138 Back extension midpoint position.
Courtesy of Patrick Hagerman, Ed.D. Quest Personal Training, Inc.

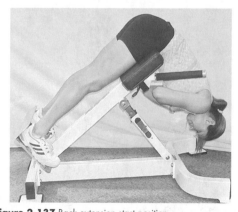

Figure 2-137 Back extension start position.
Courtesy of Patrick Hagerman, Ed.D. Quest Personal Training, Inc.

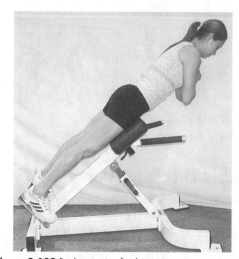

Figure 2-139 Back extension finish position.
Courtesy of Patrick Hagerman, Ed.D. Quest Personal Training, Inc.

Standing Trunk Extension

Starting position: Stand with the head, shoulders, and hips against a wall with feet about a foot in front of the body. Place the hands on top of the thighs. During the exercise, the arms are not used, but do allow the hands to slide up and down the thighs.

Movement: Keep the hips against the wall, tucking the chin to the chest, and slowly roll each vertebrae off the wall, one at a time. Imagine being peeled off the wall from the top down. When the back is entirely off the wall and only the hips remain, slowly rise back to the starting position by rolling the back against the wall one vertebrae at a time, starting at the hips and working up. Concentrate on moving slowly and "unrolling" the body until it is straight again. Once the entire back is against the wall, raise the head up until it rests against the wall; try to stretch up toward the ceiling to extend the back as much as possible.

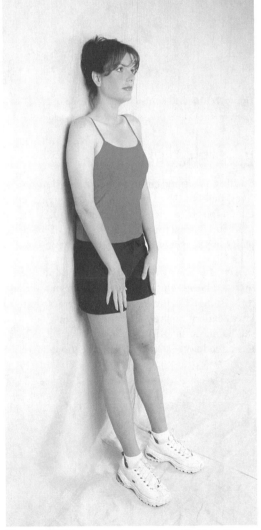

Figure 2-140 Standing trunk extension start/finish position.
Courtesy of Patrick Hagerman, Ed.D. Quest Personal Training, Inc.

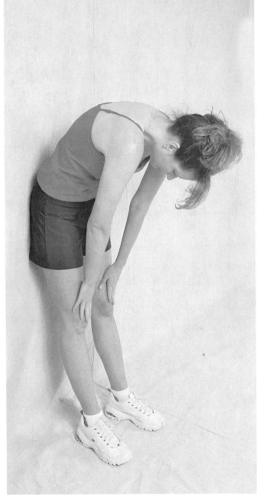

Figure 2-141 Standing trunk extension midpoint.
Courtesy of Patrick Hagerman, Ed.D. Quest Personal Training, Inc.

Kneeling Trunk Extension

Starting position: Kneel down on the floor so that the knees are together and the buttocks are resting on the ankles. Bend forward at the waist as much as possible without lifting the hips. Attempt to touch the forehead to the floor. Allow the arms to relax, and let them lie on the floor beside the body.

Movement: Slowly rise by unrolling the back and lifting one vertebrae at a time until the back is fully upright. Slowly return to the kneeling position to complete another repetition.

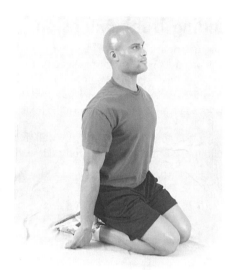

Figure 2-144 Kneeling trunk extension finish position.
Courtesy of Patrick Hagerman, Ed.D. Quest Personal Training, Inc.

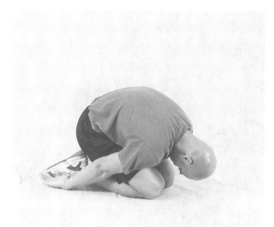

Figure 2-142 Kneeling trunk extension start position.
Courtesy of Patrick Hagerman, Ed.D. Quest Personal Training, Inc.

Back Bridges

Starting position: Lie in a supine position on the floor. Bend at the knees until the feet are no more than a foot from the buttocks, and keep feet flat on the floor. Place both hands at the sides of the body, palms pressing down against the floor.

Movement: Slowly lift the hips up and into the air until the knees, hips, and shoulders are in a straight line. Do not lift the hips up to the point that the knees cannot be seen. Push against the floor with the hands to help lift the hips if needed. Slowly relax and lower the hips back to the ground.

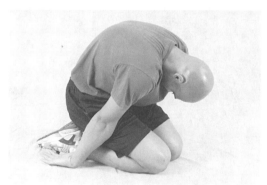

Figure 2-143 Kneeling trunk extension midpoint position.
Courtesy of Patrick Hagerman, Ed.D. Quest Personal Training, Inc.

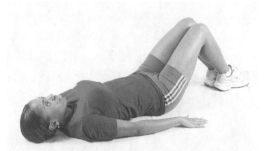

Figure 2-145 Back bridges start/finish position.
Courtesy of Patrick Hagerman, Ed.D. Quest Personal Training, Inc.

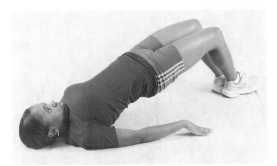

Figure 2-146 Back bridges midpoint.
Courtesy of Patrick Hagerman, Ed.D. Quest Personal Training, Inc.

Horizontal Side Supports

Starting position: Lie on the floor on one side, one leg on top of the other. Prop yourself up on one elbow. Keep the elbow directly under the shoulder, and keep the forearm and hand flat against the ground. At this point none of the upper body should be touching the floor except for the arm. Extend the other arm out and over the head.

Movement: Lift the hips up and off the ground until the body is in a straight line from the feet to the shoulders. Relax back to the floor; repeat until the set is complete, then roll over to the other side and complete another set.

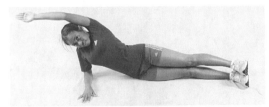

Figure 2-147 Horizontal side supports start/finish position.
Courtesy of Patrick Hagerman, Ed.D. Quest Personal Training, Inc.

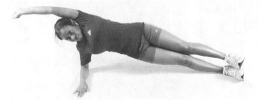

Figure 2-148 Horizontal side supports midpoint.
Courtesy of Patrick Hagerman, Ed.D. Quest Personal Training, Inc.

Erector Lifts

Starting position: Lie in a prone position on the floor. Stretch the arms over the head, point the toes, and allow the body to relax.

Movement: Slowly lift the head, arms, and shoulders up and off the floor as far as possible. Do not push against the floor with the hands. Rise as high as possible, and then slowly relax back to the floor before starting another repetition.

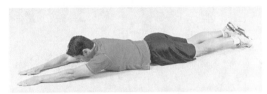

Figure 2-149 Erector lifts start/finish position.
Courtesy of Patrick Hagerman, Ed.D. Quest Personal Training, Inc.

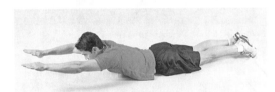

Figure 2-150 Erector lifts midpoint.
Courtesy of Patrick Hagerman, Ed.D. Quest Personal Training, Inc.

Wall Squats

Starting position: Place a stability ball against a wall, then lean back against the ball so the ball is in the curve of the lower back. Position the feet about a foot in front of the body, shoulder width apart and toes turned slightly out. Place the hands on the hips.

Movement: Keep the back and torso upright and straight, slowly bending at the knees and hips to squat down until the thighs are parallel with the floor. While squatting, the ball will roll up toward the shoulders, but the ball should never pass the shoulder blades. If it does, start with the ball placed a little lower on the back. As the ball moves up, concentrate on keeping the back straight, and do not let the hips roll back under the ball. Push back up to the starting position.

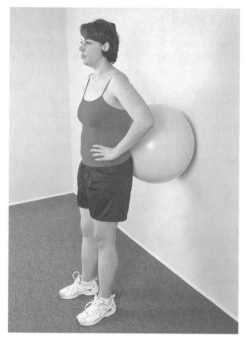

Figure 2-151 Wall squat start/finish position.
Courtesy of Patrick Hagerman, Ed.D. Quest Personal Training, Inc.

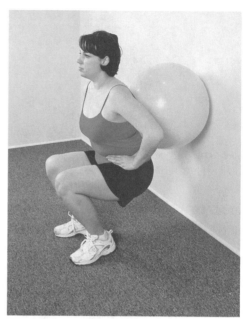

Figure 2-152 Wall squat midpoint.
Courtesy of Patrick Hagerman, Ed.D. Quest Personal Training, Inc.

Lunge

Starting position: Stand with the feet a few inches apart, hands on the hips.

Movement: Starting with either foot, take a step that is approximately two to three times larger than normal. Allow both knees to bend and absorb the impact; the back knee will move toward the floor but should not touch it. Stop when the front thigh is parallel to the floor, and push with the front foot to return to the starting position. If the foot drags back, or if it requires more than one step to return to the starting position, push off with more power initially. Alternate left and right stepping movements to complete the set.

Variations: To increase the intensity, hold a dumbbell in each hand with arms held down at the sides of the body.

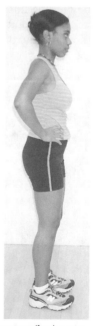

Figure 2-153 Lunge start/finish position.
Courtesy of Patrick Hagerman, Ed.D. Quest Personal Training, Inc.

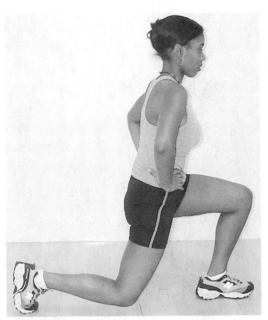

Figure 2-154 Lunge midpoint.
Courtesy of Patrick Hagerman, Ed.D. Quest Personal Training, Inc.

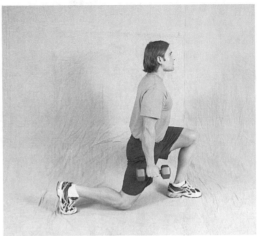

Figure 2-155 Lunge variation with dumbbells.
Courtesy of Patrick Hagerman, Ed.D. Quest Personal Training, Inc.

Step-Ups

Starting position: Stand about 6 to 12 inches from a step or chair that is approximately knee height. Place hands on the hips, and put the left foot on top of the step, completely flat. Do not allow the heel to hang off the edge.

Movement: Shift all the body weight forward and onto the left foot, and push up with the left leg until standing straight on top of the step. Do not push off the floor with the right foot; step down with the left foot first. Try and land on the toes first to absorb the impact, and then bring the right leg down. Now put the right leg on the step, push up with that leg, and then step down on the right leg. Alternate stepping up and down with the left leg and right leg until the set is complete.

Variation: Increase the intensity by holding a dumbbell in each hand with arms held down at the sides of the body.

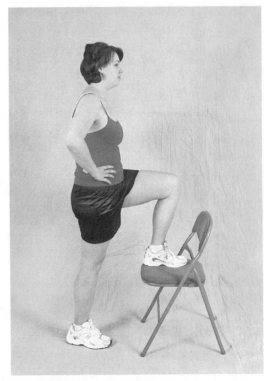

Figure 2-156 Step-up start position.
Courtesy of Patrick Hagerman, Ed.D. Quest Personal Training, Inc.

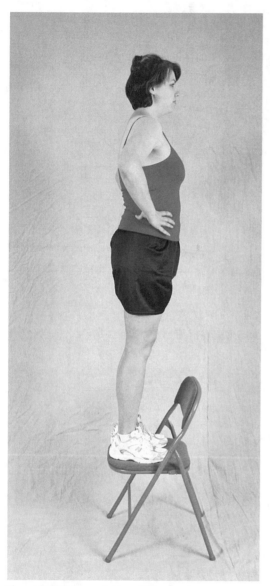

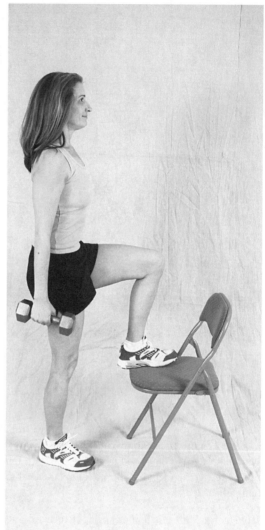

Figure 2-158 Step-up variation with dumbbells.

Courtesy of Patrick Hagerman, Ed.D. Quest Personal Training, Inc.

Figure 2-157 Step-up finish position.

Courtesy of Patrick Hagerman, Ed.D. Quest Personal Training, Inc.

Chair Stands or Sit-to Stands

Starting position: Sit on the edge of a chair, feet in front of the body about 6 inches apart. Either push up by using the arms of the chair, or fold the arms across the chest for a higher intensity exercise.

Movement: Attempt to stand from the chair without using the arms to help push. If pushing with the arms, limit the amount of help provided as much as possible. Stand completely upright, and bend at the knees and hips to sit back down without using the arms.

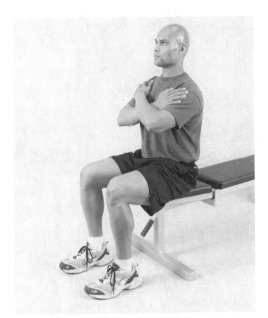

Figure 2-159 Chair stands start/finish position.
Courtesy of Patrick Hagerman, Ed.D. Quest Personal Training, Inc.

Sit-Back Squat, or Body Squat

Starting position: Stand with the feet slightly wider than shoulder width apart, toes turned out slightly. Hold the arms straight out in front of the body: the arms will serve to help with balance during the deepest part of the squat.

Movement: Keep the back flat, eyes focused straight ahead. Bend at the knees and hips to begin squatting. The hips will move behind the body, and the upper body will lean forward. Continue holding the arms straight out in front of the body, and squat down until the thighs are parallel with the floor. Stand back up to resume the starting position.

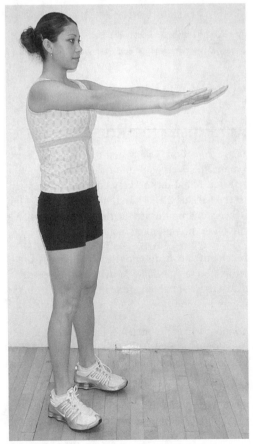

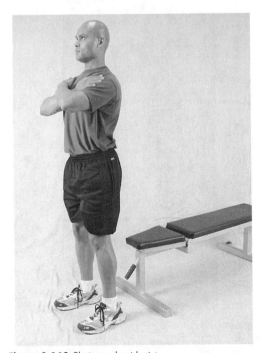

Figure 2-160 Chair stands midpoint.
Courtesy of Patrick Hagerman, Ed.D. Quest Personal Training, Inc.

Figure 2-161 Sit-back squat start/finish position.
Courtesy of Patrick Hagerman, Ed.D. Quest Personal Training, Inc.

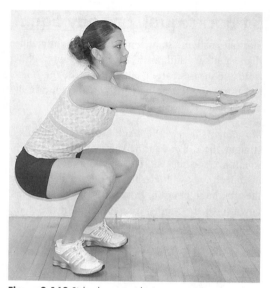

Figure 2-162 Sit-back squat midpoint.
Courtesy of Patrick Hagerman, Ed.D. Quest Personal Training, Inc.

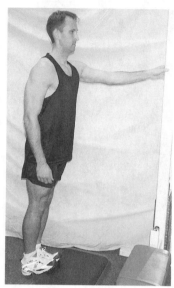

Figure 2-163 Calf raise start/finish position.
Courtesy of Patrick Hagerman, Ed.D. Quest Personal Training, Inc.

Calf Raise (Toe Raise)

Starting position: Use a step that is high enough to allow the heels to drop down without touching the floor. Stand on the very edge of the step with just the balls of the feet and toes on the step. Allow the heels to drop toward the floor as far as possible. Hold on to the wall to maintain balance.

Movement: Push up equally on the balls of the feet as high as possible. Slowly let the heels back down toward the floor, stretching the calves before another repetition.

Variation: For more intensity, use only one leg at a time. Cross one foot behind the other to put all of the body weight on one leg, thus making the calf muscles work twice as hard.

Precaution: During the calf raise, the feet may shift off the edge of the bench. Stop occasionally and reposition the feet.

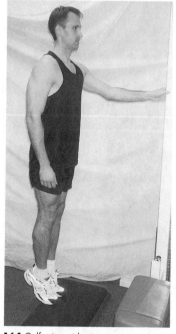

Figure 2-164 Calf raise midpoint.
Courtesy of Patrick Hagerman, Ed.D. Quest Personal Training, Inc.

Sit-Ups

Starting position: Lie down on the floor in a supine position. Cross the arms over the chest, touching the fingers to the shoulders. Bend at the knees so that the feet are about 12 to 18 inches from the buttocks. Either anchor the feet under something heavy, or have a partner hold them down.

Movement: Tuck the chin to the chest, and slowly roll the head and shoulders up and off the floor. When the shoulders are up, continue to lift the entire upper body off the floor until the elbows touch the knees. Slowly lower yourself back to the floor.

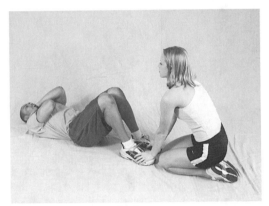

Figure 2-165 Sit-up start/finish position.
Courtesy of Patrick Hagerman, Ed.D. Quest Personal Training, Inc.

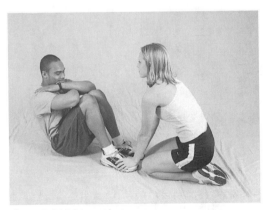

Figure 2-166 Sit-up midpoint.
Courtesy of Patrick Hagerman, Ed.D. Quest Personal Training, Inc.

Side-Lying Sit-Ups

Starting position: Lie down on the floor in a supine position. Hold the hands against the sides of the head, elbows pointing away from the body. Bend at the knees so that the feet are about 12 to 18 inches from the buttocks. Rotate the hips so that the legs fall to the ground on one side of the body. Keep the knees and feet together.

Movement: Tuck the chin to the chest, and slowly roll the head and shoulders up and off the floor. When the shoulders are up, continue to lift the entire upper body off the floor as far as possible. Slowly return to the floor, and complete repetitions until the set is complete, then rotate the hips to the other side of the body to complete the next set.

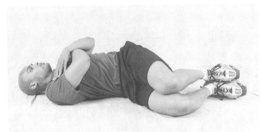

Figure 2-167 Side-lying sit-up start/finish position.
Courtesy of Patrick Hagerman, Ed.D. Quest Personal Training, Inc.

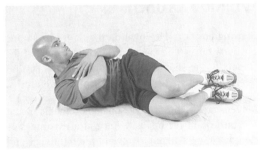

Figure 2-168 Side-lying sit-up midpoint.
Courtesy of Patrick Hagerman, Ed.D. Quest Personal Training, Inc.

Crunch

Starting position: Lie down on the floor in a supine position. Cross the arms over the chest, touching the fingers to the shoulders. Bend at the knees so that the feet are about 12 to 18 inches from the buttocks.

Movement: Tuck the chin to the chest, and roll the head and shoulders up and off the floor. Stop when the shoulder blades leave the floor. Slowly return to the floor by unrolling the shoulders and head.

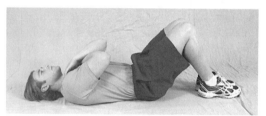

Figure 2-169 Crunch start/finish position.

Courtesy of Patrick Hagerman, Ed.D. Quest Personal Training, Inc.

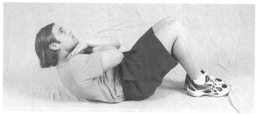

Figure 2-170 Crunch midpoint.

Courtesy of Patrick Hagerman, Ed.D. Quest Personal Training, Inc.

Oblique Crunch

Starting position: Lie down on the floor in a supine position. Cross the arms over the chest, touching the fingers to the shoulders. Bend at the knees so that the feet are about 12 to 18 inches from the buttocks.

Movement: Lift one shoulder up and off the floor, and roll up toward the opposite knee in a twisting motion. Lift the left shoulder toward the right knee and vice versa. Twist and roll up until the shoulder that is still on the floor starts to rise also. Slowly relax and return to the starting position, then repeat the motion to the other side, alternating left and right.

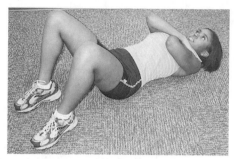

Figure 2-171 Oblique crunch start/finish position.

Courtesy of Patrick Hagerman, Ed.D. Quest Personal Training, Inc.

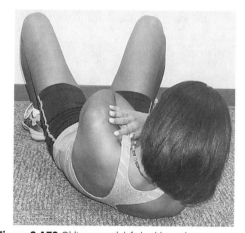

Figure 2-172 Oblique crunch left-shoulder midpoint.

Courtesy of Patrick Hagerman, Ed.D. Quest Personal Training, Inc.

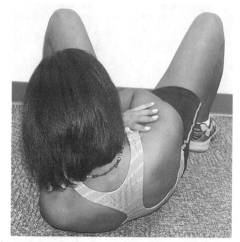

Figure 2-173 Oblique crunch right-shoulder midpoint.

Courtesy of Patrick Hagerman, Ed.D. Quest Personal Training, Inc.

Wall Push-Up

Starting position: Place the hands against a wall with the arms totally straight and at shoulder level. Keep the feet together and the body completely rigid; do not let the hips fall forward during the exercise.

Movement: Bend at the arms, and slowly lower the chest toward the wall. Stop when the head is about an inch from the wall, and push against the wall with both hands to return to the starting position.

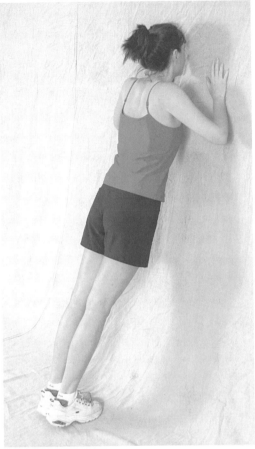

Figure 2-175 Wall push-up midpoint position.
Courtesy of Patrick Hagerman, Ed.D. Quest Personal Training, Inc.

Push-Up

Starting position: Kneel down on the hands and knees, placing the hands directly under the shoulders, arms straight. Straighten the legs and place the feet either together or no more than a few inches apart. The toes and hands will be the only parts of the body touching the floor. Maintain a straight line between the shoulders, hips, and feet.

Movement: Slowly bend at the arms to lower the body down until either the chest comes in contact with the floor or the shoulders are lower than the elbows. Do not go down so far as to lie on the

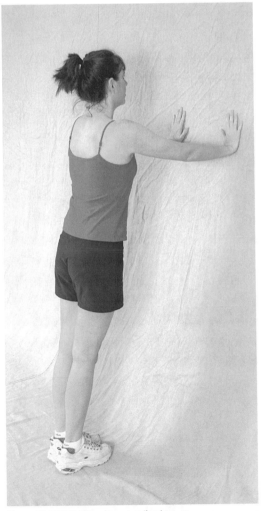

Figure 2-174 Wall push-up start/finish position.
Courtesy of Patrick Hagerman, Ed.D. Quest Personal Training, Inc.

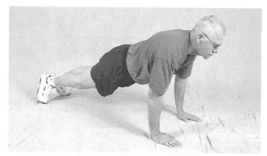

Figure 2-176 Push-up start/finish position.
Courtesy of Patrick Hagerman, Ed.D. Quest Personal Training, Inc.

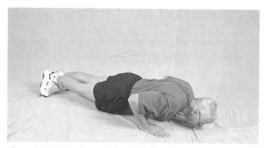

Figure 2-177 Push-up midpoint position.
Courtesy of Patrick Hagerman, Ed.D. Quest Personal Training, Inc.

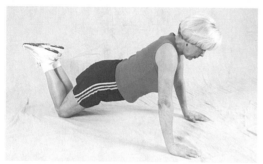

Figure 2-178 Modified push-up start/finish position.
Courtesy of Patrick Hagerman, Ed.D. Quest Personal Training, Inc.

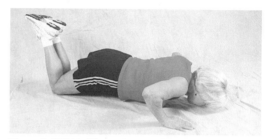

Figure 2-179 Modified push-up midpoint position.
Courtesy of Patrick Hagerman, Ed.D. Quest Personal Training, Inc.

floor. As the elbows bend, point them away from the body. Push against the hands to lift the body back to the starting position; the arms should be straight again.

Variation: A modified push-up places the knees on the floor instead of the toes. Maintain a straight line from the knees to the shoulders during the movement.

Stability Ball Push-Up

Starting position: Place the hands on top of a stability ball in a shoulder-width position, arms straight. Straighten the legs, and create a straight line between the shoulders, hips, and feet.

Movement: Slowly bend at the elbows to lower the body down until the chest is within 1 to 2 inches of touching the ball. As the elbows bend, move them away from the body. Push on the ball until the arms are straight again.

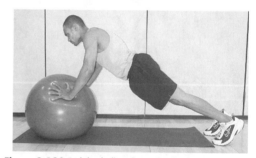

Figure 2-180 Stability ball push-up start/finish position.
Courtesy of Patrick Hagerman, Ed.D. Quest Personal Training, Inc.

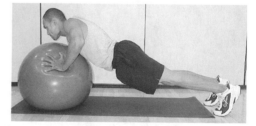

Figure 2-181 Stability ball push-up midpoint.
Courtesy of Patrick Hagerman, Ed.D. Quest Personal Training, Inc.

Medicine Ball Shoulder Press/Push Press

Starting position: Sit on the edge of a bench, or stand with feet shoulder width apart. Hold a medicine ball against the chest, one hand on each side of the ball.

Movement: Press the ball directly overhead until the arms are straight. Slowly lower the ball back to the starting position.

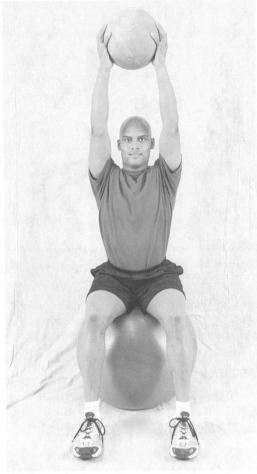

Figure 2-183 Medicine ball shoulder press midpoint position. Courtesy of Patrick Hagerman, Ed.D. Quest Personal Training, Inc.

Medicine Ball Pullover and Throw

Starting position: Sit on top of a stability ball with feet together and tucked close to the ball. Hold a medicine ball overhead in both hands, arms straight. A partner should stand about 10 to15 feet away. Attempt to throw the ball to the partner, aiming for the chest. Start with the partner closer if needed.

Movement: Lower the ball behind the body until the arms are at a 45-degree angle. Pull the ball over the

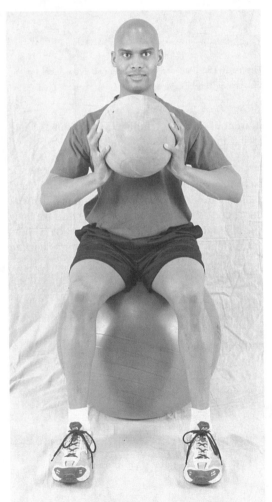

Figure 2-182 Medicine ball shoulder press start/finish position. Courtesy of Patrick Hagerman, Ed.D. Quest Personal Training, Inc.

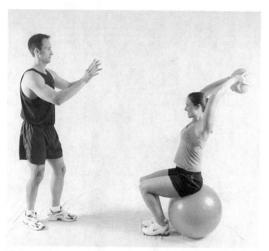

Figure 2-184 Medicine ball pullover and throw start position. Courtesy of Patrick Hagerman, Ed.D. Quest Personal Training, Inc.

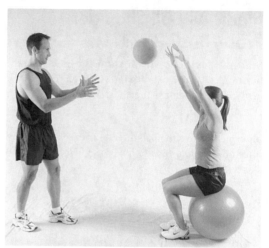

Figure 2-185 Medicine ball pullover and throw finish position. Courtesy of Patrick Hagerman, Ed.D. Quest Personal Training, Inc.

head, and throw it to a partner as hard as possible. When the ball is thrown, keep the torso upright. The partner should catch the ball and hand it back.

Seated Dips

Starting position: Sit on the edge of a chair. Hold on to the front edge of the sides of the seat, and extend the arms to lift the body off the seat. Slide feet out

in front of the body until legs are straight and hips are off the seat.

Movement: Slowly bend at the elbows to lower the body down, until the shoulders are at the same level as the elbows and the upper arms are parallel with the floor. Allow knees and hips to bend so the body moves straight down, but do not lower the body to touch the floor. Push on the hands to rise back to the starting position.

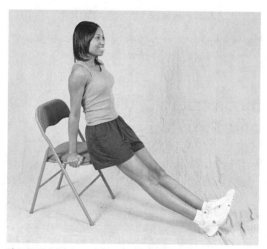

Figure 2-186 Seated dips start/finish position. Courtesy of Patrick Hagerman, Ed.D. Quest Personal Training, Inc.

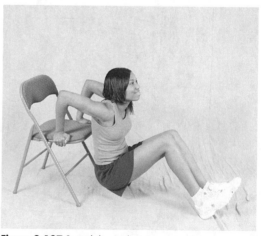

Figure 2-187 Seated dips midpoint. Courtesy of Patrick Hagerman, Ed.D. Quest Personal Training, Inc.

Ankle-Weight Knee Raise

Starting position: Strap an ankle weight to each leg, and stand with the feet a few inches apart. Hold on to something for support and balance if needed.

Movement: Lift one knee as high as possible, and then return it to the floor. Alternate lifting the left knee and right knee until the set is complete.

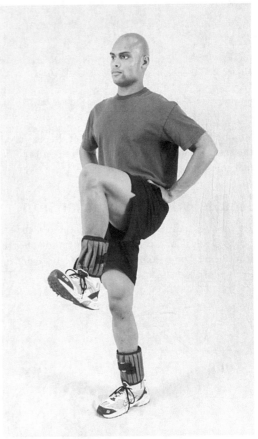

Figure 2-189 Ankle weight knee raise midpoint.
Courtesy of Patrick Hagerman, Ed.D. Quest Personal Training, Inc.

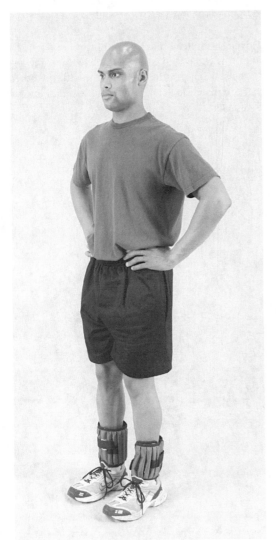

Figure 2-188 Ankle weight knee raise start/finish position.
Courtesy of Patrick Hagerman, Ed.D. Quest Personal Training, Inc.

Ankle-Weight Lateral Leg Raise

Starting position: Strap an ankle weight to each leg, and lie on your side on the floor. Extend the bottom arm, the one that is on the floor, and rest the head on the upper arm. Bend the bottom leg, the one on the floor, so that the knee is in front of the body and the foot is behind the body. The top hand should rest on the hip or waist, and the top leg should be straight and held just off the floor.

Movement: Slowly lift the top leg into the air as far as possible. Lower the leg back toward the floor,

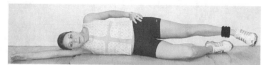

Figure 2-190 Ankle weight lateral leg raise start/finish position.

Courtesy of Patrick Hagerman, Ed.D. Quest Personal Training, Inc.

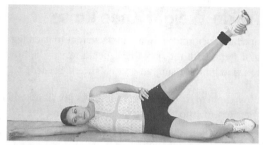

Figure 2-191 Ankle weight lateral leg raise midpoint.

Courtesy of Patrick Hagerman, Ed.D. Quest Personal Training, Inc.

stopping just before making contact. Repeat until the set is complete, then roll over to the other side and complete a set for the other leg.

Ankle-Weight Leg Extension

Starting position: Strap an ankle weight to each leg. Sit on the edge of a chair or bench, feet together in front of the body. Hold on to the sides of the chair for support.

Movement: Extend one leg out in front of the body until it is completely straight. Slowly lower the leg to the starting position, and repeat with the other leg. Alternate the left leg and right leg until the set is complete.

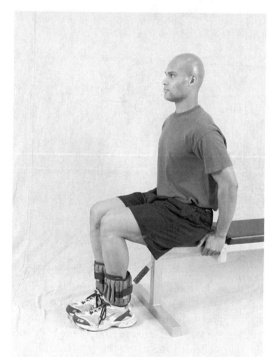

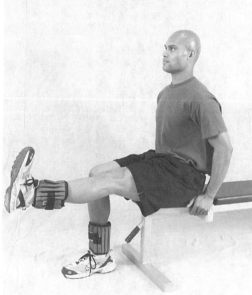

Figure 2-192 Ankle weight leg extension start/finish position.

Courtesy of Patrick Hagerman, Ed.D. Quest Personal Training, Inc.

Figure 2-193 Ankle weight leg extension midpoint.

Courtesy of Patrick Hagerman, Ed.D. Quest Personal Training, Inc.

Ankle-Weight Hip Extension

Starting position: Strap an ankle weight to each leg, and lie in a prone position on the floor. Place the feet together, toes pointed toward the floor.

Movement: Keep the upper body flat against the floor, extending one leg up into the air as high as possible; keep the leg straight at all times. Return the leg to the starting position, and repeat with the other leg, alternating left and right until the set is complete.

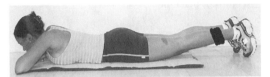

Figure 2-194 Ankle weight hip extension start/finish position.

Courtesy of Patrick Hagerman, Ed.D. Quest Personal Training, Inc.

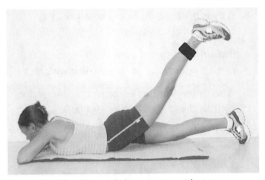

Figure 2-195 Ankle weight hip extension midpoint.

Courtesy of Patrick Hagerman, Ed.D. Quest Personal Training, Inc.

Ankle-Weight Standing Leg Curl

Starting position: Strap an ankle weight to each leg. Stand with the feet a few inches apart, holding on to something for support and balance if needed.

Movement: Shift your body weight to one leg, and bend at the knee of the other leg to pull the foot up and toward the buttocks. Attempt to touch the heel to the buttocks. Return the leg to the starting position, and repeat with the other leg, alternating left and right until the set is complete.

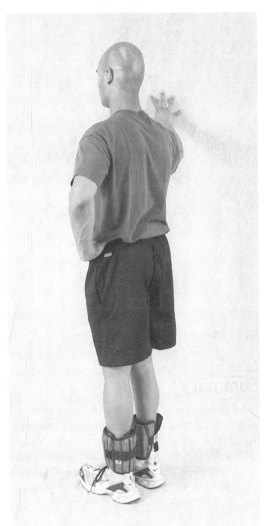

Figure 2-196 Ankle weight leg curl start/finish position.

Courtesy of Patrick Hagerman, Ed.D. Quest Personal Training, Inc.

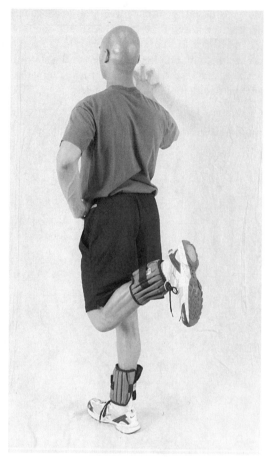

Figure 2-197 Ankle weight leg curl midpoint.
Courtesy of Patrick Hagerman, Ed.D. Quest Personal Training, Inc.

Summary

The student should refer back to this chapter for instructions on how to complete the exercises prescribed for each population. Exercises not specifically prescribed for a population may be used given that there are no contraindications and that the individual has obtained the necessary level of skill needed to safely complete the exercise.

Key Terms

Alternating grip
Ankle weights
Assisting

Barbell
Cable/pulley system
Dumbbell
EZ-curl barbell
High-pulley setup
Low-pulley setup
Medicine balls
Narrow grip
Neutral grip
Normal grip
Plate-loaded machine
Pronated grip
Resistance tubing
Selectorized machine
Spotting
Stability ball
Supinated grip
Tubing–door anchor
Valsalva maneuver
Wide grip

Study Questions

1. Why is it important to examine exercise equipment before using it?

2. Explain the different methods of spotting, and give an example of an exercise that uses each.

3. What is the Valsalva maneuver, and how does it affect the cardiovascular system?

4. Explain the differences in normal, narrow, and wide grips.

References

1. American College of Sports Medicine. ACSM's Guidelines for Exercise Testing and Prescription. 7th ed. Baltimore: Williams & Wilkins. 2005.

2. MacDougall JD, Tuxen D, Dale DG, Moroz JR, Sutton JR. Arterial blood pressure responses to heavy resistance exercise. *J Applied Physiol.* 1985;58:785–790.

3. Wilmore JH, Costill DL. *Physiology of Sport and Exercise.* 3rd ed. Champaign, IL: Human Kinetics. 2004.

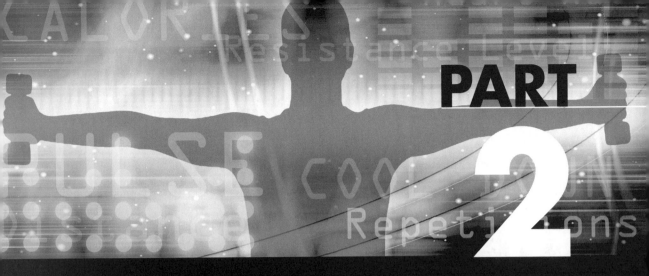

PART 2

RESISTANCE TRAINING STRATEGIES

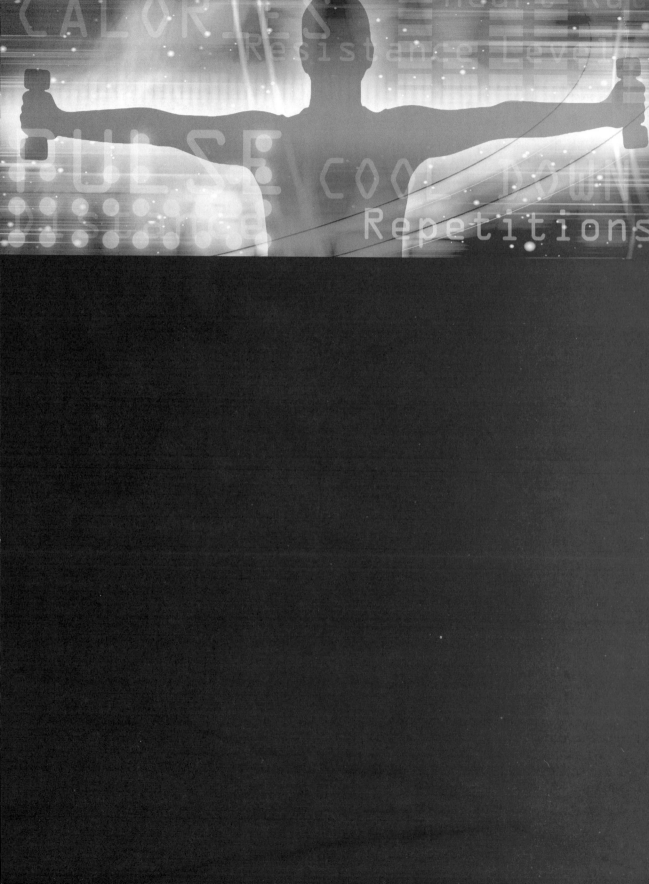

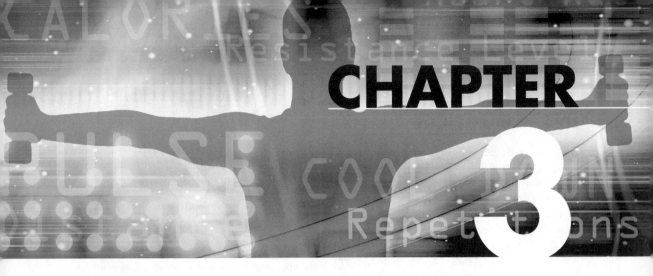

CHAPTER 3

RESISTANCE-TRAINING STRATEGIES FOR OLDER ADULTS

Objectives

Upon completion of this chapter, the reader should be able to:

- Discuss the demographics of the aging population in the United States and the health implications of disability and frailty in this population
- Discuss the role of resistance training to modify age-related functional decline
- Identify key obstacles to resistance training among the older adult population and possible ways to overcome them
- Demonstrate strategies to achieve optimal pre-exercise screening, exercise testing, and exercise prescription in a resistance-training program for older adults.
- Describe the potential role of high-velocity resistance training, or power training, for older adults

INTRODUCTION

Although resistance training benefits adults of all ages, its advantages for older adults are especially noteworthy. Aging is associated with a cascade of morphological and physiological changes that naturally predispose older adults to progressive weakening, functional decline, increased morbidity-associated disability, diminished quality of life, and increased mortality (67). Resistance training is vital therapy that can be used to modify such insidious aging patterns. Not only can resistance training help to stabilize health profiles, it helps preserve and possibly enhance functional capacity, vitality, and quality of life even among those who are very old and those who are already frail (40, 63, 72, 83). Unfortunately, advanced age also presents distinctive obstacles to resistance training. Multiple chronic medical conditions, limited access to appropriate programs, fear of injury, and logistical obstacles are common hindrances to both initiating and sustaining exercise patterns. Moreover, resistance training requires qualified instruction in exercise technique, which also can become a major obstacle due to poor access and failing cognition for many older adults. This chapter discusses the benefits of resistance training for older adults and identifies strategies to overcome age-related barriers to exercise therapy.

PREVALENCE AND ECONOMIC IMPACT OF AGING

The United States Census Bureau estimates that about 35 million Americans are over 65 years old, approximately 12 percent of the total population (76). By 2030, an anticipated 70.3 million adults will be over 65 years old, over 20 percent of the population. Moreover the subgroup aged 85 years and older is expected to grow 3 percent per year over this time (76). Public health implications are profound, especially because this burgeoning population of older adults is intrinsically susceptible to frailty, disease, and dependency. **Frailty** is a condition in which mechanical weakening is compounded by concomitant issues of fatigue, diminished balance and coordination, reduced physical activity, slowed motor processing and performance, social withdrawal, and cognitive decline (82).

Although only a small percentage of older adults develop frailty (84), this group consumes disproportionate health care resources. Medical utilization not only arises from falls and related injuries, but frailty also erodes biological reserves, and detrimental sequences tend to arise even from minor illnesses or procedures. Diminished function, hospital readmissions, and exacerbations of chronic illnesses are all common and costly. Overall, care for frail older adults constitutes 50 percent of all hospital care, 80 percent of home care services, and 90 percent of all nursing home beds in the United States (45).

In 2000, the U.S. government spent $585 billion on health care with approximately 66 percent oriented to older adults (84). Not only are these costs expected to steadily increase for third-party payers—approximately 5.6 percent per year in anticipated cost increases to Medicare, Medicaid, and private insurers—they represent an increasing financial burden to the individuals themselves and to their families. While details vary from individual to individual, Medicare and insurance do not cover a significant portion of total medical costs, because long-term care, prescriptions, and home health aides are usually not covered. A key benefit of resistance training is that it affords the potential to mitigate frailty and to therefore achieve greater cost efficiency in the caregiving for this population.

PHYSIOLOGY OF AGING

Aging is associated with omnipresent changes throughout the body. Key aspects include pervasive loss of fat-free mass (skeletal muscle), as well as increases in body fat, particularly in the abdominal viscera and within muscle itself. **Sarcopenia** is a term used to describe age-related loss of skeletal muscle mass and strength, and it entails progressive atrophy of skeletal tissue with reduced number and size of skeletal myocytes and intrinsic declines in their contractile performance. Changes in muscle mass are considerable, with 0.5 to 1 percent of muscle mass usually lost every year from age 20 to 50, accelerating in the years thereafter (83). For instance, Lexell and colleagues (42) described 25 percent fewer vastus lateralis muscle fibers in 70- to 73-year-old men, compared to men aged 19 to 37 years, with losses climbing to 40 percent among octogenarians (32). Declines in muscle mass and performance predispose older adults to functional limitations. Activities that were once routine often become overwhelming, because small physical tasks require higher proportions of maximal functional capacity. Yet beyond risks of overexertion, the apprehension from such limitation is also a risk, often predisposing a person to progressive fearfulness, depression, and diminished quality of life.

Although sarcopenia predisposes an individual to detrimental functional limitations, accumulating body fat with age adds to clinical risks. Increased body fat predisposes people to metabolic-based morbidities such as insulin resistance, diabetes, dyslipidemia, hypertension, and intrinsic weakening and disability. Furthermore, increased body fat in relation to age is prevalent, because caloric intake tends to be preserved among elderly despite their diminished activity and energy expenditure (44, 77). Multiple studies demonstrate that a higher percentage of body fat, independent of sarcopenia, is a powerful predictor of disability (12, 52, 79), physical limitation (12, 34), and declining mobility and quality of life with higher mortality (71). Furthermore, the ill effects of mounting body fat and sarcopenia typically compound one another to increase overall morbidity and mortality.

Typical age-related cardiovascular changes include transformations of the large central arteries from the pulsatile, dynamic vessels found in most young adults into stiff, pipe-like cylinders in most elderly (38). Whereas the pulsatile character of youthful arteries facilitates an efficient means to propel blood forward, the vascular stiffening of older age means the heart must work harder to push blood downstream: blood no longer propagates itself through the local distension and recoil of pulsatile flow. Consequently, the cardiac workload is paradoxically increased in many older adults, exacerbating exercise intolerance and increased susceptibility to instability. To make matters even worse, many noncardiac diseases—such as COPD, infections, and arthritis—have also been linked to high ambient inflammation (64) and are also common detriments to functional capacity in the elderly.

One common link between sarcopenia, cardiovascular disease, and other morbidities in the elderly is inflammation. Visceral fat is a common source of systemic inflammatory peptides. Many studies highlight correlations between inflammatory/catabolic biomarkers and harmful clinical sequelae that include frailty, morbidity, and functional decline (12, 21, 30, 34, 52, 66, 71, 79, 80, 82). Furthermore, the fat-induced vulnerability to sarcopenia and disease often leads to a vicious cycle, because such diseases undercut exercise tolerance; and it has been found that diminished exercise predisposes a person to greater systemic inflammation (48). Sarcopenia may also add to risk and instability by removing a critical repository of protein in skeletal muscle that normally plays a key role in the capacity to withstand stress and overcoming disease (41).

BENEFITS OF RESISTANCE TRAINING FOR OLDER ADULTS

Although aging predisposes a person to changes in skeletal muscle, body fat, vascular stiffening, infection, comorbidity, and frailty, many aspects of these patterns are modifiable. Exercise training, particularly resistance training, allays muscle weakening and atrophy and can even stimulate muscle growth. Resistance training can reduce body fat, reduce inflammation and catabolism, increase function, diminish frailty, and preserve or restore a more youthful and generally healthier physical profile (15). Consistently, resistance training helps improve affect, social engagement, and even cognition (68, 84), and it mitigates many of the elements underlying frailty. Latham and colleagues (40) reviewed 62 randomized, controlled resistance-training trials (total n = 3674) that compared progressive resistance training to controls in older adults. Moderate to large increases in strength were evident, along with many significant benefits, including moderate increases in gait speed. Table 3-1 outlines the numerous benefits of resistance training for older adults found by Nied and Franklin (53).

Impact on Aerobic Power

A key rationale of resistance training for older adults is that it facilitates increases in overall physical activity (13, 15) and aerobic power. While it is well known that increased activity significantly decreases age-related morbidity and cardiovascular mortality (2, 9, 31, 57, 81), goals to initiate an aerobic exercise routine, no matter how well intended, often seem impractical among individuals who are severely deconditioned or frail (28). Therefore, a key benefit of resistance training is that it

provides a mechanism to safely initiate activity and grow sufficient physical capacity and confidence to gradually achieve broader training goals, including aerobic training. Many studies highlight the benefits of resistance training to increase posture, joint stability, balance, flexibility, and bone strength among older adults (8, 13, 51), benefits essential for improving aerobic power. Consistently, resistance training has been demonstrated to improve capacity for specific tasks required in the course of daily living, such as rising from a chair or lifting legs more vigorously to avoid tripping and falling (43, 67).

Impact on Sarcopenia

Much attention has been focused on the benefits of resistance training to modify sarcopenia, which entails cell atrophy of a variety of skeletal muscle cell types. Both Type I (aerobic) and Type II (anaerobic) fibers decline, and shrinkage of Type II fibers (20, 23) is also notable. A range of theories regard specific mechanisms underlying skeletal muscle aging: high oxidative stress (35), muscle denervation (69), Insulin-like Growth

Table 3-1 Benefits of Resistance Training for Aging Populations

Body Composition	**Cardiovascular**
Increases muscle mass	Improves physiologic parameters (VO_2 peak)
Increases muscle strength	Improves blood pressure
Increases fat-free mass	
Decreases fat mass	
Metabolism	**Osteoporosis**
Improves insulin sensitivity	Increases bone mineral density
Improves glycemic control	Decreases hip and vertebral fractures
Decreases hemoglobin A_{1C} levels	Decreases risk of falling
Improves lipid profile (decreases total cholesterol and LDL-C)	
Neuropsychological Health	**Other**
Improves quality of sleep	Decreases morbidity (all causes)
Improves cognitive function	
Improves Beck depression scores	

Source: Nied RJ, Franklin B. Promoting and prescribing exercise for the elderly. *Am Fam Physician.* 2002;65:419–426.

Factor-1 (IGF-1) resistance (3), increased ambient inflammation (65), and poor nutrition (62, 63) have all been described. In fact, these mechanisms may be interrelated, such that age predisposes people to an increased inflammatory cellular milieu that compounds the effects of high oxidative stress, IGF-1 resistance, and poor nutrition (22, 59). However, IGF-1 resistance seems by most accounts to play a key role within a larger pathophysiological picture by disrupting normal cell-to-cell signaling patterns and triggering sequences of muscle breakdown (3, 25).

In counterbalance, resistance training with nutritional supplementation has been demonstrated to increase IGF-1 effects and thereby attenuate sarcopenia (3, 11, 27). Resistance training increases fiber size, particularly Type II fibers; increases muscle mass and intrinsic strength (29); mitigates oxidative stress (78); increases protective heat-shock proteins (49); and contributes to a pattern of increased overall activity that reduces ambient inflammation (48). All these changes likely induce more healthful gene-to-gene signaling patterns with associated improvements in muscle growth responses.

Multiple studies demonstrate the utility of resistance training to increase muscle mass even among frail older men and women (28, 29, 32, 50, 73, 74, 75). Nelson and colleagues (50) showed an increase in muscle mass by 1.2 kg in strength-trained women aged 50 to 70, versus a decrease of 0.5 kg in the control group after one year of resistance training. Frontera and colleagues (29) showed 11.8 percent increases in muscle cross-sectional area of the mid thigh and muscle strength increases of greater than 100 percent with a 12-week high-intensity resistance-training program in older men with a mean age of 65.4 years.

Impact on Body Fat

Coupled with the benefits for skeletal muscle, resistance training also helps to reduce body fat. Increased muscle mass from resistance training typically leads to higher levels of both physical activity and resting energy expenditure that results in a reduction in fat. Furthermore, fat reduction

tends to occur in a regional distribution such that health benefits are amplified by a disproportionate reduction of visceral fat and the associated risks for insulin resistance and hypertension. Ross and colleagues (62) showed that resistance training and diet reduced visceral fat by about 35 percent. The benefits of resistance training on skeletal muscle consistently enhance insulin sensitivity and decrease inflammation (14), changes that are conducive to weight loss (85).

Impact on Bone Mineral Density

Resistance training for older adults affects bone mineral density and strength in large part due to the healthful effects of increased muscle strength stimulating bone homeostasis. Although aging often predisposes a person to bone demineralization and weakening, a process known as osteopenia, and associated risks of fractures and osteoarthritis, this can be modified with resistance training. Nelson and colleagues (50) conducted a randomized controlled trial of high-intensity resistance training for post-menopausal women aged 50 to 70 to study its benefits on bone. They found that a regimen of 45-minute sessions of high-intensity resistance training 2 days per week, using 80 percent of 1RM and 16 to 17 on the Borg Scale, was adequate stimulus to preserve bone mineral density. In addition, significant improvements were noted in muscle mass, strength, and balance.

Impact on Vasculature

Several investigations raised concerns that resistance training might exacerbate vascular stiffening among older adults (46, 47); however, mechanisms underlying such purported changes were never clarified. Further analysis demonstrated that resistance training does not affect arterial distensibility after 12 weeks of training twice a week. Physiologically this finding is consistent with other resistance-training benefits on body fat and inflammation, which would logically confer predominant vascular benefit.

HETEROGENEITY OF OLDER ADULTS

Exercise strategies for older adults must incorporate a range of strategies that respond to the range of health profiles associated with aging. While many older adults personify issues of frailty, deconditioning, and disability, many older adults are relatively vigorous. Resistance-training goals and regimens need to be adapted to the different aging subtypes. Specific exercises used in a program may not differ; however the volume and progression of resistance will vary considerably.

Frail older adults are characterized by having some type of **mobility disability,** which is related to their capacity to complete purposeful movements at a required speed and maintain balance during these movements. It is often helpful to classify the extent of mobility disability as a means to anticipate frailty and other issues germane to exercise prescription. The **Short Physical Performance Battery (SPPB)** provides a convenient screening tool that can be administered in less than 10 minutes (33). The test is scored as a total of 12 points, 4 points each for timed tests that assess balance, walking speed, and chair-rise time. This test is becoming more widely used in geriatric and physical medicine clinics as an index of disability. Individuals who score between 0 and 6 are considered severely disabled, and scores of 7 to 9 are consistent with moderate disability.

Primary goals of resistance training for frail older adults are oriented to slowing the progression of weakening and disability and even regaining capacity for activities of daily living. Despite these substantial objectives, initial training regimens first emphasize safety and a foundation that fosters behaviors conducive to long-term resistance-training progression. Therefore, resistance training for frail older adults usually starts with very basic movements that are easily learned and performed. Proper warm-up and stretching are essential, as are careful instruction on balance and breathing. Regimens start with very low-intensity resistance, often with body weight alone, slowly progressing

to resistance tubing and bands, ankle weights, and other weights over many weeks and months. Sets are usually short with only one to two sessions a week. As strength increases, exercise is best advanced by first increasing the number of repetitions before increasing the resistance.

Resistance training for older adults who are more vigorous is typically oriented more to strategies that achieve maximum increases in muscle mass, muscle strength, and function. The most common and well-substantiated resistance-training strategy is to progressively overload the muscles to provoke positive adaptations. High-intensity regimens, defined as greater than 80 percent of one-repetition maximum (1RM), have been demonstrated not only to be safe but to be an effective means to achieve beneficial muscle and metabolic changes (1). Many research investigations have demonstrated the benefits of high-intensity resistance training for the elderly. For instance, using high-intensity, slow-speed training, Wieser and colleagues showed 26 to 38 percent improvements in strength, 12 percent improvements in VO_2 peak, gains in fat-free body mass, and reductions in body-fat mass in community-dwelling adults (83). Benefits among men and women were similar.

While the imperative of safety and tempered training regimens for frail older adults has been emphasized, ultimately strong rationale exists to progress toward higher-intensity training goals even among those who are severely disabled at the onset. Fiatarone and colleagues demonstrated the benefits of high-intensity resistance training even for frail nursing home residents, including improved muscle cross-section area (3 to 9 percent), increased strength (>100 percent) and improved functional performance measured as gait speed and stair-climbing ability (28). Similar training and progressive benefits each year during a 2-year program led to conclusions that age and frailty are not barriers to high-intensity resistance training (70). In fact, these studies suggest that relative improvements in skeletal muscle mass and function may be greatest among those who are the most deconditioned and frail at the onset.

Another training consideration for frail and robust elderly relates to velocity of movement, or power. Ongoing research suggests this property may also factor into resistance-training benefits for balance, stability, and function. In the InCHIANTI study, Bean and colleagues compared leg power and maximum strength in adults aged 65 and older, and they demonstrated that power played a more decisive role than maximum strength in determining function (6). Similar studies of elderly populations have demonstrated the impact of muscle velocity on gait acceleration, stair-climbing and descent speeds, get-up-and-go times, and balance assessments (5, 7, 39).

Related studies of myocyte morphology suggest that disproportionate atrophy of Type II skeletal muscle fibers in sarcopenia may underlie lower muscle velocities in older adults. One implication is that certain exercises may be better suited to increasing Type II skeletal muscle fibers (37). Novel studies, like those of Orr and colleagues, are therefore studying benefits of low resistance but higher velocity resistance-training regimens. That study showed improved activity initiation and balance (56). Likewise, Earles and colleagues emphasized benefits of high-velocity training in older adults (26). Their study combined high velocity of movement with moderate or high resistance to attain significant benefits of leg power and endurance.

EXERCISE PRESCRIPTION STRATEGIES FOR OLDER ADULTS

The American College of Sports Medicine (ACSM) guidelines for resistance training suggests training intensity ranging from 12 to 19 on the Borg Scale of Perceived Exertion at a frequency of 2 to 3 days per week and lasting for up to an hour (1, 10). These goals can generally be maintained for older adults with key refinements to preserve suitability of resistance training for those who are frail. The ACSM general recommendation for intensity of resistance training for adults is primarily based on the Borg Scale of exertion. Notably, heart rate is not typically used as a measure of intensity, because the increases in effort with resistance training are disproportionate to heart rate and oxygen consumption. Lower intensities of 12 to 13, which are still somewhat difficult, are well suited to initial training of more vigorous older adults and may even constitute a top training intensity for older adults who are very frail. If resistance training is well tolerated and safe, regimens should ideally advance to 15 to 16 to induce the greatest physiological benefits. As an alternative to the Borg scale, the intensity of resistance training can also be gauged using a percentage of the 1RM as discussed in Chapter 1. However, this method of establishing intensity can be particularly challenging in frail elderly, who are more vulnerable to sprain and injury associated with maximum effort.

ACSM resistance-training guidelines generally recommend two to three training sessions per week, on nonconsecutive days, with a duration that does not exceed 1 hour. Likewise, sessions typically include 8 to 10 exercises to include all the major muscle groups. Nonetheless, frequency of training sessions and the number of repetitions can vary widely, depending on the individual baseline condition and the goals of training. Overall emphasis of training is usually oriented to muscle groups in the upper and lower extremities that help facilitate standing, walking, lifting, and reaching, respectively (see Table 3-2).

Resistance training using exercise machines has advantages for older adults, especially those who are frail, because the range of motion is easier to control, and the margin of safety is increased. However, free weights provide much greater accessibility and cost advantages. Certainly, studies have demonstrated the efficacy of free weights for older adults (50). However, the need to provide the thorough instruction and monitoring required for effective and safe resistance training is often particularly hard when using free weights with frail older adults.

Table 3-2 Resistance-Training Exercises Suitable for the Elderly

Exercise	Equipment Needed*	Muscles Trained	Functional Significance
Triceps press	Chair with armrests, or wheelchair with wheels locked	Chest, triceps and shoulders	Strengthen muscles used to push off from seated positions (chairs, toilet)
Chest press	Resistance band tethered around the back of a chair or person's torso	Chest, triceps and shoulders	Strengthen muscles used to push off from seated positions (chairs, toilet)
Seated row	Resistance band fixed around a pole, door-jamb, or other immovable support	Back and biceps	Strengthens postural muscles
Bicep curl	Resistance band or handheld weights	Biceps	Strengthens muscles used to carry things and self-feed
Side lateral raise	Handheld weights	Shoulders	Strengthens muscles used to reach, carry things, and to self-feed
Seated knee Extension	Chair/wheelchair, ankle weights ranging from 1 to ≥ 10lbs	Quadriceps	Strengthens muscles used to stand, walk, rise from a seated position
Seated hamstring curl	Resistance band or adjustable pulley system	Hamstrings	Strengthens muscles used to stand, walk, rise from a seated position

* Equipment summarized here demonstrates what is typically available in most institutions, however, all of these exercises may be performed on specialized exercise machines.

As has been described for those who are frail, initial exercise intensity, frequency, and goals should be tempered to emphasize safety, especially given frail adults' common predisposition to sprains and injury, and such exercises must occur in an environment that is conducive to participation and adherence to a regimen. Adaptation periods are extended up to 8 weeks, during which minimal resistance can continue without progression to allow concentration on range of motion and breathing. Supervision, monitoring, teaching, and encouragement are paramount, with added benefit when this support comes from people familiar with the special needs of the elderly. If injury or illness should interrupt an exercise routine, resistance training should be resumed with a maximum of 50 percent of the previous intensity, and exercise should only start in a pain-free range of motion.

Factors Influencing Exercise Prescription

There are many factors that impact the safety and efficacy of resistance training for older adults, including the following:

○ Time of day when exercise is completed is especially important with respect to medications that serve to palliate concomitant disease states, such as diabetes. Time of day is also important with respect to the severity of symptoms in conditions such as rheumatoid arthritis, in which discomfort is greatest in the early hours after rising from sleep.

○ Proper clothing and appropriate footwear, such as sturdy shoes or sneakers that help balance during activity, are crucial for safe exercise participation.

○ An appropriate warm-up will help decrease the risk of musculoskeletal injury. The warm-up increases blood flow to the muscles, slightly increases body temperature, and activates joints and muscles to become limber and flexible. Recommended warm-up may include walking on a treadmill or cycling at a brisk pace for 5 minutes, followed by static stretching.

○ The cooldown helps return heart rate to a normal resting state and minimizes exercise-related injuries. Recommended cooldown includes slow walking for at least 5 minutes and static stretching.

○ Static stretching for each muscle group for 20 to 30 seconds may help reduce injuries such as muscle strain and also increases range of motion.

○ Proper breathing during resistance training is important.

Avoiding or minimizing the Valsalva maneuver should be taught to all individuals participating in resistance training.

○ Movements should be rhythmic, performed at a moderate to slow controlled speed, through a full range of motion, and with a normal breathing pattern while lifting as described in Chapter 2.

○ Supervised training on the proper technique and instruction before adding weight will decrease the risk of injury.

○ Initiate resistance training with short sessions, and only advance towards goals as stamina and comfort increase.

○ Use unilateral rather than bilateral movements when possible to increase balance, and decrease the total amount of work being done at any one time.

○ Rest as needed, and avoid rushing through the exercise routine, especially during changes in body position; and avoid rushing through movements between exercises and/or exercise equipment.

○ Utilize the Borg Scale of Perceived Exertion to gauge exercise intensity and guide exercise patterns according to the training goals.

Effects of Cardiovascular, Metabolic, and Pulmonary Diseases on the Exercise Prescription

Clinical assessment, coordinated care with the primary physician, and monitoring are essential for a resistance-training program. A key concern in assessing suitability for resistance training is the presence and/or severity of cardiovascular disease. Since age itself constitutes a risk factor for cardiovascular disease, this disease is extremely common among older adults considering resistance training. Pulmonary and metabolic diseases are also common, as are other age-related diseases including arthritis. Musculoskeletal impairments, sensory limitations, and polypharmacology could also affect the safety of resistance training. However, the presence of cardiovascular disease alone does not prohibit participation in a resistance-training program. Instead, contraindications pertain to signs and symptoms of unstable cardiac conditions, including unstable angina, ECG changes, significant ventricular ectopy, unstable hemodyamics, severe valve dysfunction, high-grade heart blocks, acute congestive heart failure, pulmonary embolism, myocarditis, and pericarditis (1).

To the surprise of many patients, and even many clinicians, resistance training is typically safer for cardiac patients than aerobic training, particularly because the heart rate is usually slower with less cardiac work demands and arrhythmia than with aerobic exercise modalities (18). Similarly, whereas many older adults fear musculoskeletal injury as a consequence of resistance training, risks of a sedentary lifestyle far exceed the risks of carefully supervised and monitored resistance training, even among those with baseline impairments. Similarly, other comorbidities often trigger concerns; however, in most cases the benefits of resistance training are usually predominant. In all cases, supervision and monitoring play key roles in efficacy and safety; therefore older adults should exercise in an environment in which assessment, teaching, feedback, and monitoring are all well integrated.

BARRIERS TO RESISTANCE TRAINING FOR OLDER ADULTS

Despite its touted benefits, the concept of resistance training often overwhelms many older adults. The far-reaching clinical and socioeconomic impacts

of aging often translate into disproportionate fear with diminished self-efficacy and confidence in resistance training. Among the many common age-related concerns, many older adults fear precipitating a cardiac event, such as a myocardial infarction, or they fear musculoskeletal injury or even embarrassment because of incontinence or lack of exercise-related skill. Age-related hearing and visual impairments, cognitive slowing, and economic constraints add to the apprehension. Likewise, many older adults can no longer drive or afford alternate transportation, such as taxis or shuttle services, and many are tethered by caregiver responsibilities to an infirm spouse. Furthermore, many older adults also suffer from poor nutrition and poor sleep quality, which adds to their disinclination to exercise.

Overcoming these barriers requires a stepwise individual approach. Barriers specific to each individual should be identified and the plan tailored accordingly. Individuals with higher exercise self-efficacy expectations tend to maintain positive affects during exercise (16), a quality which has been attributed to confidence in their capacity to succeed and benefit (17). Considering such issues is critical to achieving and sustaining a successful resistance-training program (15, 17, 36). Fears can also be mitigated with education, especially that which helps teach modifiable risks related to resistance training along with insights regarding injury prevention and how to adjust and monitor exercise intensity. Likewise, resistance training can easily be structured as a seated exercise, eliminating most of the fall-related apprehensions.

Muscle soreness is also a common deterrent for resistance training among many older adults. Frequently, muscle soreness is innocuous and transient and can be modified with patience and proper responses. With the initiation of resistance training, there is often a period of physiological adaptation during which muscle soreness occurs. In most individuals this adaptation can take 2 to 3 weeks, but it may take longer in the elderly. Unfortunately, many older adults react to soreness with fear and apprehension and use this as rationale to abandon their fledgling exercise routines. However, if resistance training is modified to include very low-resistance regimens with modest progression, soreness will frequently resolve. Also, regimens that minimize the eccentric phase of muscle contraction typically are conducive to less muscle soreness.

Age-related sensory impairment barriers can be overcome or alleviated through the use of visual aids with large fonts and equipment such as dumbbells that are colored to denote the weight. Posting prominent signage on the rating of perceived exertion (RPE) scale on the wall demarcating the appropriate resistance-training ranges can be helpful as well. Emphasis on consistent room organization and proper lighting will help older adults with visual impairment to locate items needed for their routine. Sensory impairments such as hearing loss can make it difficult to instruct older adults in resistance-training exercise. Speaking loudly and slowly, using visual aids, and demonstrating exercises are all techniques that help participants.

Overcoming economic and transportation challenges can often be particularly difficult. Numerous senior centers in cities throughout the country offer exercise classes daily, but they are of little value to those who lack essential transportation. While many cities offer transportation assistance to get to medical appointments, those benefits rarely apply to exercise classes. Alternatively, it is usually not feasible to expect older adults, particularly those who are frail, to initiate resistance training independently in their own homes. There remains a pressing need to develop resistance-training programs and offer low cost transportation particularly suited for the needs of the growing older population.

has published *Exercise: A Guideline for Adults of All Ages* (54). This publication is offered free to the public and is a useful tool for those who are able to engage in safe home-based resistance training. Still, such home-based exercise presents many problems. Frail older adults, many of whom have never engaged in formal resistance training, will need personal instruction on how to perform the exercises. After initial training it will be necessary and prudent to have periodic reassessment of safety and reinforcement of proper technique by a qualified exercise professional. Lack of emergency care for home-based exercise compounds risk and apprehension.

Community-based exercise takes place in a setting such as a health or fitness center, is usually supervised, and allows several individuals to exercise together or at the same time. Community-based exercise programs specifically oriented to resistance training have been developed that offer several advantages over home-based exercise. In addition to incorporating components of assessment, monitoring, and safety, community-based programs provide opportunities for social reinforcement and encourage participation. Overall, community-based supervised resistance training has consistently achieved more significant increases in lean mass and muscle strength than home-based control groups (24, 51, 60, 61). Furthermore, community-based programs are better suited for older adults with baseline frailty and/or concomitant exercise risks such as neurological, cardiovascular, orthopedic, or pulmonary conditions (1).

HOME-BASED AND COMMUNITY-BASED EXERCISE

Home-based exercise takes place in the individual's residence, is not supervised, and is often conducted alone. The National Institute on Aging promotes home-based exercise for older adults and

BEHAVIORAL ASPECTS OF RESISTANCE TRAINING FOR OLDER ADULTS

Comprehensive behavioral strategies, including social support and positive reinforcement, are essential to helping older adults initiate and maintain physical activity. Most adults know the importance of physical activity, but that alone is insufficient to motivate them to initiate and adhere to an exercise regimen. Hence, it is important to incorporate a comprehensive management strategy to maximize recruitment, increase teaching and safety, increase motivation, and minimize attrition (17). Social support from family, friends, and physicians provides a key component to long-term participation in physical activity (17, 55, 58). The more involved older adults are with their physician, the more likely their physician will facilitate positive exercise behavior, set realistic goals and a course of action, and reinforce a commitment to the exercise routine (17).

Nonetheless, it remains a limitation that many patients rely exclusively on their primary physician to prescribe an exercise training protocol. Dauenhauer and colleagues demonstrated that 47 percent of primary care physicians do not prescribe exercise for older adults, and 85 percent reported having no formal training in exercise prescription (19). Many physicians avoid giving their older patients written instructions due to feeling inadequately prepared to prescribe an exercise regimen based on numerous factors, including complex medical conditions and medication regimens (4, 19).

SAMPLE 24-WEEK PROGRAM

The following is a general outline of a 24-week program, including a pre-exercise physical exam and assessment, an initial exercise plan, and strategies for exercise progression. Exercises follow a standardized format but should be individually modified based on the relative frailty or vigor of each individual.

Week 1

A physical exam by the primary care physician should be performed to determine general medical stability, both cardiovascular and metabolic, and to identify potential exercise-limiting factors such as restrictions to range of motion, orthostatic

hypotension, joint pain, incontinence, and sensory and/or cognitive impairment. Next, a pre-exercise intake by an exercise professional should identify the initial fitness level using strength testing and functional outcome assessment tools such as the Short Physical Performance Battery (SPPB), stair-climbing ability, and exercise self-efficacy questionnaires. Intake also entails clarification of program goals based on baseline status and expectations.

Weeks 2 through 4

Provide instructions on using the Borg Ratings of Perceived Exertion (RPE) scale, and supply guidelines for appropriate resistance training. During this period an RPE of 11 to 13, which is fairly light to somewhat hard, should be used to minimize damage or irritation to joints and connective tissue. Initiate training without any added resistance, focusing on proper form and breathing. Exercise sessions should be kept short, up to 30 minutes maximum, and limited to twice per week. Perform 1 set of 5 to 10 repetitions for each exercise as tolerated in the target RPE range. A sample of possible exercises is listed in Table 3-3.

Weeks 5 through 8

Continue with the above recommendations, but attempt to increase the number of repetitions to 12 or 15. By the end of week 8, attempt to progress to 2 sets, and lengthen exercise sessions up to 1 hour as tolerated.

Weeks 9 through 12

Increase RPE range from 11 to 15 as tolerated. Continue with 2 sets and up to 15 repetitions. At the end of week 12, reassess fitness level and outcomes measured in the first week.

Weeks 13 through 24

Continue to progress resistance according to the RPE scales. Two sets of up to 15 repetitions, 2 days per week is recommended, although for those who are motivated and have no time constraints, 3 sets may be considered, as well as training 3 days per week.

Table 3-3 Exercises That May be Performed and Modified for the Frail or Robust

Exercise Purpose/ Target Muscle Group	Modification for Frail Elderly	Modification for Robust Elderly
Full-body warm-up, strengthen legs	Repeated chair stands (if able to get out of a chair or wheelchair) using arms to help push off	Repeated chair stands with arms folded across the chest
Muscles used to lift/carry	Seated* biceps curls; use very light or no resistance and alternate arms	Standing bicep curls, both arms at the same time
	Seated lateral raise	Standing lateral raise
	Seated triceps push-down using light to medium resistance tubing or band tethered to doorjamb or ballet bar**	Standing triceps pushdown using medium- to heavy-resistance tubing or band tethered to doorjamb or ballet bar**
Postural muscles	Seated rows using light- to medium-resistance tubing or band tethered to doorjamb or ballet bar	Standing rows using medium- to heavy-resistance tubing or band tethered to doorjamb or ballet bar
Abdominals	Seated abdominal contraction coordinated with forced exhalation	Seated or standing abdominal contraction coordinated with forced exhalation
Hip flexors	Seated knee raise with or without added resistance of ankle weights	Standing knee raise with or without added resistance of ankle weights
Muscles used for ambulation	Seated knee extension with or without added resistance of ankle weights	Seated knee extension with ankle weights
	Seated calf raises	Standing calf raises
	Seated hamstring curls using light-resistance tubing or band	Standing hamstring curl using ankle weights or resistance tubing or band
		Standing hip extension with or without resistance
		Standing lateral leg raises with or without resistance

* Seated exercises should be done using a chair without armrests (or placing moveable armrests in the upright position), sitting toward the front of the chair or wheelchair so arms are clear of the armrests.
** Resistance tubing or band can be fixed around any immovable object, such as the legs of a physical therapy plinth.

CASE STUDY

Mrs. W is a 92-year-old woman living in the community. She does not drive and relies on public transportation, such as buses and the subway. She has a history of falls and uses a cane. Her hypertension is well controlled with medication, but her high cholesterol is untreated. She frequently complains of back and leg pain and occasionally sees a chiropractor for treatment. Her primary care provider referred her to an outpatient physical medicine clinic, where she was referred and received medical clearance for a 3-day-per-week exercise program based on the NIH publication *Exercise: A Guide from the National Institute on Aging.* Prior to initiation of the program, Mrs. W underwent a pre-exercise assessment that included the SPPB. Her SPPB score of 5 out of 12 was consistent with moderate to severe mobility impairment.

At the beginning of each exercise session, resting heart rate and blood pressure were measured. During the first exercise session, Mrs. W was shown all the exercise movements but with no added resistance. She used the weight of her own limbs in the exercises, practicing the proper range of motion. She was instructed on how to use the Borg RPE scale. For her first few weeks of training, she would try to exercise in an RPE range of 11 to 13, fairly light to somewhat hard, but the intention was to progress to a level of 13 to 16, somewhat hard to hard. During her first session, in learning the exercise movements, she reported an RPE of 11 to 12. The exercise session was divided into chair-based exercises focused primarily on the upper body and standing exercises focused on the lower body, performed at a ballet bar for balance. One set of 8 repetitions was performed for each exercise. The seated exercises consisted of 1) rising from a chair with arms folded across the chest to strengthen the thighs and buttocks and to provide a whole-body warm-up, 2) lateral raises and shoulder flexion to strengthen the shoulders, 3) bicep curls and triceps extensions to strengthen the arm muscles, and 4) knee extensions to strengthen the quadriceps. The standing exercises consisted of 1) knee flexion to strengthen the hamstrings, 2) hip extension to strengthen the buttocks, 3) lateral leg

raises to strengthen the abductors, 4) hip flexion to strengthen the namstrings and buttocks, and 5) plantar flexion to strengthen the calves. At the end of each session, gentle stretching exercises were performed, targeting each of the muscle groups. Heart rate and blood pressure were measured after stretching.

Mrs. W reported that she was quite tired after the first session, and when she returned for the next session, she reported slight muscle soreness. No resistance was added to her routine for the rest of the week. By the second week of exercise, Mrs. W reported her muscle soreness had resolved, so 1-pound dumbbells were used for her upper-body exercises, and 1.5-pound ankle weights were used for her lower-body exercises. Resistance increased each week, and by week 8, she was using 4 pounds for her upper-body exercises and 5 pounds for her lower-body exercises. Also at 8 weeks, some of the pre-exercise assessments were repeated, including the SPPB, which was improved to a score of 9.

During her tenth week of training, Mrs. W missed several sessions due to a fall in a restaurant and a swollen ankle. X-rays showed no fracture, but her primary care doctor advised her not to do any weight-bearing exercise for several weeks until the swelling and pain subsided. A week after her fall, Mrs. W returned to exercise classes, participating only in the upper-body exercises. When she resumed participation in lower-body exercise several weeks later, she had lost strength, and her ankle weights were decreased to 2 pounds. However, by the end of the third week after rejoining the exercise group, she was back to using 5-pound weights for her lower-body exercises.

Summary

Resistance training has particular advantages for older adults as a means to modify some of the health risks attributable to age-related physiological effects, even in the context of common comorbid diseases. Resistance training is safe for older adults, even for those who are frail, with proven efficacy in preserving and enhancing physical functioning. Properly initiated and reinforced resistance training can become a vital adjunct to medical therapy for a wide range of patients, ranging from older adults who are frail and deconditioned to those who are vigorous and active. Key factors of success relate not only to the particular training but also to the composite needs and limitations of the individuals and their nutrition, logistics, and broader environmental context. Proper supervision, monitoring, and well-informed encouragement and instruction are key components to effective training regimens.

Key Terms

Community-based exercise
Frailty
Home-based exercise
Mobility disability
Osteopenia
Sarcopenia
Short Physical Performance Battery (SPPB)

Study Questions

1. Explain the relationship between velocity of movement and function in older adults.

2. Discuss factors that impact the safety and efficacy of resistance training in older adults.

3. Discuss the safety of resistance training in relation to cardiovascular disease and comorbidities in older adults.

References

1. American College of Sports Medicine. *Guidelines for Exercise Testing and Prescription*. 7th ed. Baltimore, MD: Lippincott, Williams & Wilkins; 2006.

2. American College of Sports Medicine. Position stand: Exercise and physical activity for older adults. *Med Sci Sports Exerc*. 1998;30(6):992-1008.

3. Adamo ML, Farrar RP. Resistance training and IGF involvement in the maintenance of muscle mass during the aging process. *Aging Res Rev*. 2006;5(3):310-331.

4. Andersen RE, Blair SN, Cheskin LJ, Bartlett SJ. Encouraging patients to become more physically active: The physician's role. *Ann of Int Med*. 1997;127:395-400.

5. Bean JF, Kiely DK, Herman S, et al. The relationship between leg power and physical performance in mobility-limited older people. *J Am Geriatr Soc*. 2002;50(3):461-467.

6. Bean JF, Leveille SG, Kiely DK, et al. A comparison of leg power and leg strength within the InCHIANTI study: Which influences mobility more? *J of Gerontol*. 2003;58A:728-733.

7. Bean J, Herman S, Kiely D, et al. Weighted stair climbing in mobility-limited older people: A pilot study. *J of Am Geriat Soc*. 2002;50(4):663-670.

8. Beniamini Y, Rubenstein JJ, Faigenbaum AD, Lichtenstein AH, Crim MC. High-intensity strength training of patients enrolled in an outpatient cardiac rehabilitation program. *J Cardiopulmonary Rehabil*. 1999;19:8-17.

9. Blair SN, Kohl HW III, Paffenbarger RS Jr, Clark DG, Cooper KH, Gibbons LW. Physical fitness and all-cause mortality. A prospective study of healthy men and women. *JAMA*. 1989;262:2395-2401.

10. Borg, G. Borg's Perceived Exertion and Pain Scales. Human Kinetics; 1998.

11. Borst SE, Vincent KR, Lowenthal DT, Braith RW. Effects of resistance training on insulin-like growth factor and its binding proteins in men and women aged 60 to 85. *J Am Geriatr Soc*. 2002;50(5):884-888.

12. Brach JS, Simonsick EM, Kritchevsky S, Yaffe K, Newman AB, for the Health, Aging, and Body Composition Study Research Group. Lifestyle activity and exercise: the association with physical function in the Health, Aging, and Body Composition (Health ABC) Study. *J Am Geriatr Soc*. 2004;52:502-509.

13. Brochu M, Savage P, Lee M, et al. Effects of resistance training on physical function in

older disabled women with coronary heart disease. *J Appl Physiol.* 2002;92:672-678.

14. Brooks N, Layne JE, Gordon PL, Roubenoff R, Nelson ME, Castaneda-Sceppa C. Strength training improves muscle quality and insulin sensitivity in Hispanic older adults with type 2 diabetes. *Int J Med Sci.* 2007;4:19-27.

15. Capodaglio P, Capodaglio EM, Facioli M, Saibene F. Long-term strength training for community-dwelling people over 75: Impact on muscle function, functional ability, and lifestyle. *Eur J Appl Physiol.* 2007;100(5):535-42. Epub 2006 April 25.

16. Conn VS, Burks KJ, Pomeroy SH, Ulbrich SL, Cochran JE. *Women's Health Issues.* 2003;13:158-166.

17. Cress EM, Buchner DM, Prohaska T, et al. Physical activity programs and behavior counseling in older adult populations. *Med Sci in Sports Ex.* 2004;36(11):1997-2003.

18. Daub WD, Knapik GP, Black WR. Strength training early after myocardial infarction. *Cardiopulm Rehabil.* 1996;16(2):100-109.

19. Dauenhauer JA, Podgorski CA, Karuza J. Prescribing exercise for older adults: A needs assessment comparing primary care physicians, nurse practitioners, and physician assistants. *Geronol & Geriat.* 2006;26(3):81-99.

20. Deschenes MR. Effects of aging on muscle fibre type and size. *Sports Med.* 2004;34(12):809-824.

21. Di Iorio A, Abate M, Di Renzo D, et al. Sarcopenia: Age-related skeletal muscle changes from determinants to physical disability. *Int J Immunopathol Pharmacol.* 2006;19(4):703-719.

22. Dirks AJ, Leeuwenburgh C. The role of apoptosis in age-related skeletal muscle atrophy. *Sports Med.* 2005;35(6):473-483.

23. Doherty TJ. Invited review: Aging and sarcopenia. *J Appl Physiol.* 2003;95(4):1717-1727.

24. Dunstan DW, Daly RM, Owen N, et al. Home-based resistance training is not sufficient to maintain improved glycemic control following supervised training in older individuals with type 2 diabetes. *Diabetes Care.* 2005;28(1):3-9.

25. Duscha BD, Schulze PC, Robbins JL, Forman DE. Implications of chronic heart failure on peripheral vasculature and skeletal muscle before and after exercise training. *Heart Fail Rev.* 2008;13(1):21-37.

26. Earles DR, Judge JO, Gunnarsson OT. Velocity training induces power-specific adaptations in highly functioning older adults. *Arch Phys Med Rehabil.* 2001;164(3):259-267.

27. Ferketich AK, Kirby TE, Alway SE. Cardiovascular and muscular adaptations to combined endurance and strength training in elderly women. *Acta Physio Scand.* 1998;164(3):259-267.

28. Fiatarone M, O'Neill E, Ryan N, et al. Exercise training and nutritional supplementation for physical frailty in very elderly people. *New England J of Med.* 1994;330:1769-1775.

29. Frontera, WR, Meredith, CN, O'Reilly, P, Knuttgen, HG, Evans, WJ. Strength conditioning in older men: Skeletal muscle hypertrophy and improved function. *J. Appl. Physiol.* 1998;64:1038-1044.

30. Gordon PL, Vannier E, Hamada K, et al. Resistance training alters cytokine gene expression in skeletal muscle of adults with type 2 diabetes. *Int J Immunopathol Pharmacol.* 2006;19(4):739-749.

31. Gregg EW, Cauley JA, Stone K, Thompson TJ, Bauer DC, Cummings SR. Relationship of changes in physical activity and mortality among older women. *JAMA.* 2003;289: 2379-2386.

32. Grimby G, Saltin B. The aging muscle. *Clin Physio.* 1983;3:209-218.

33. Guralnik JM, Simonsick EM, Ferrucci L, et al. A short physical performance battery assessing

lower extremity function: Association with self-reported disability and prediction of mortality and nursing home admission. *J Gerontol.* 2994;49(2):M85-94.

34. Guralnik JM, Simonsick EM. Physical disability in older Americans. *J Gerontol.* 1993;48 Spec No:3-10.

35. Judge S, Jang YM, Smith A, Hagen T, Leeuwenburgh C. Age-associated increases in oxidative stress and antioxidant enzyme activities in cardiac interfibrillar mitochondria: Implications for the mitochondrial theory of aging. *FASEB J.* 2005;19(3):419-421.

36. King AC, Rejeski WJ, Buchner DM. Physical activity interventions targeting older adults: A critical review and recommendations. *Am J Prev Med.* 1998;15:316-333.

37. Korhonen MT, Cristea A, Alen M, et al. Aging, muscle fiber type, and contractile function in sprint-trained athletes. *J Appl Physiol.* 2006;101(3):906-917.

38. Lakatta EG. Age-associated cardiovascular changes in health: Impact on cardiovascular disease in older persons. *Heart Fail Rev.* 2002;7(1):29-49.

39. Larsson, L. Grimby, G., Karlsson, J. Muscle strength and speed of movement in relation to age and muscle morphology. *J Appl Physiol.* 1979;46:451-456.

40. Latham NK, Bennett DA, Stretton CM, Anderson CS. Systemic review of progressive resistance strength training in older adults. *J Geront.* 2004;59A(1):48-61.

41. Leeuwenburgh C. Role of apoptosis in sarcopenia. *J Gerontol A Biol Sci Med Sci.* 2003;58(11):999-1001.

42. Lexell J, Taylor CC, Sjostrom M. What is the cause of the aging atrophy? Total number, size, and proportion of different fiber types studied in whole vastus lateralis muscle from 15- to 83-year-old men. *J of Neurolog Sci.* 1998;84:275-294.

43. Liu-Ambrose TY, Khan KM, Eng JJ, Gillies GL, Lord SR, McKay HA. The beneficial effects of group-based exercises on fall risk profile and physical activity persist 1 year postintervention in older women with low bone mass: Follow-up after withdrawal of exercise. *J Am Geriatr Soc.* 2005;53(10):1767-1773.

44. Mazzeo RS, Cavanagh P, Evans WJ, et al. Position stand: Exercise and physical activity for older adults. *Med Sci Sports Exerc.* 1998;30(6):992-1008.

45. Mezey M, Fulmer T. Quality care for the frail elderly. *Nursing Outlook.* 1998;46(6):291-292.

46. Miyachi M, Sugawara J, Kawano H, et al. Unfavorable effects of resistance training on central arterial compliance: A randomized intervention study. *Circulation.* 2004;110(18):2858-2863.

47. Miyachi M, Donato AJ, Yamamoto K, et al. Greater age-related reductions in central arterial compliance in resistance-trained men. *Hypertension.* 2003;41(1):130-135.

48. Mora S, Cook N, Buring JE, Ridker PM, Lee IM. Physical activity and reduced risk of cardiovascular events: Potential mediating mechanisms. *Circulation.* 2007;6;116(19):2110-2118.

49. Murlasits Z, Cutlip RG, Geronilla KB, Rao KM, Wonderlin WF, Alway SE. Resistance training increases heat shock protein levels in skeletal muscle of young and old rats. *Exp Gerontol.* 2006;41(4):398-406.

50. Nelson M, Fiatarone M, Morganti C, Trice I, Greenberg R, Evans W. Effects of high-intensity strength training on multiple risk factors for osteoporotic fractures. A randomized controlled trial. *JAMA.* 1994;272(24):1919-1914.

51. Nelson M, Layne J, Bernstein M, et al. The effects of multidimensional home-based exercise on functional performance in elderly people. *J Gerontol A Biol Sci Med Sci.* 2004;59(2):154-160.

52. Newman AB, Kupelian V, Visser M, et al. Sarcopenia: alternative definitions and associations with lower extremity function. *J Am Geriatrics Soc.* 2003;51:1602-1609.

53. Nied RJ, Franklin B. Promoting and prescribing exercise for the elderly. *Am Fam Physician.* 2002;65:419-426.

54. NIH Publication No. 01-4258. Reprinted April 2004. *Exercise: A Guide from the National Institute on Aging.* Available at http://www.nih.gov/nia. Accessed April 15, 2008.

55. Oka R, King A. Sources of social support as predictors of exercise adherence in women and men age 50 to 65 years. *Women's Health.* 1995;1:161-175.

56. Orr R, De Vos NJ, Singh NA, Ross DA, Stavrinos TM, Fiatarone-Singh MA. Power training improves balance in healthy older adults. *J Gerontol A Biol Sci Med Sci.* 2006;61A(1):78-85.

57. Paffenbarger RS Jr, Hyde RT, Wing AL, Lee IM, Jung D, Kampert JB. The association of changes in physical-activity level and other lifestyle characteristics with mortality among men. *N Engl J Med.* 1993;328:538-545.

58. Petrella PJ, Koval JJ, Cunningham DA, Paterson DH. Can primary care doctors prescribe exercise to improve fitness? *Am J Prev Med.* 2003;24(4):316-322.

59. Pistilli EE, Jackson JR, Alway SE. Death receptor-associated pro-apoptotic signaling in aged skeletal muscle. *Apoptosis.* 2006;11(12):2115-2126.

60. Ransdell L, Taylor A, Oakland D, Schmidt J, Moyer-Mileur L, Shultz B. Daughters and mothers exercising together: Effects of home- and community-based programs. *Med. Sci. Sports Exerc.* 2003;35(2):286-296.

61. Ravaud P, Giraudeau B, Logeart I, et al. Management of osteoarthritis (OA) with an unsupervised home based exercise programme and/or patient administered assessment tools. A cluster randomised controlled trial with a 2x2 factorial design. *Ann Rheum Dis.* 2004;63(6):703-708.

62. Ross R, Rissanen J, Pedwell H, Clifford J, Shragge P. Influence of diet and exercise on skeletal muscle and visceral adipose tissue in men. *J Appl Physiol.* 1996;81(6):2445-2455.

63. Roubenoff R. Sarcopenia: A major modifiable cause of frailty in the elderly. *J of Nutri Health and Aging.* 2000;4(3):140-142.

64. Roubenoff R. Catabolism of aging: Is it an inflammatory process? *Curr Opin Clin Nutr Metab Care.* 2003;6:295–299.

65. Schaap LA, Pluijm SM, Deeg DJ, Visser M. Inflammatory markers and loss of muscle mass (sarcopenia) and strength. *Am J Med.* 2006;119(6):526.e9-17.

66. Semba RD, Lauretani F, Ferrucci L. Carotenoids as protection against sarcopenia in older adults. *Arch Biochem Biophys.* 2007;458(2):141-145. Epub 2006 Dec 6.

67. Simons R, Andel R. The effects of resistance training and walking on functional fitness in advanced old age. *J Aging Health.* 2006;18(1):91-105.

68. Singh NA, Clements KM, Fiatarone MA. A randomized controlled trial of progressive resistance training in depressed elders. *J. Gerontol A Biol Sci Med Sci.* 1997;52(1):M27-M35.

69. Siu PM, Alway SE. Mitochondria-associated apoptotic signalling in denervated rat skeletal muscle. *J Physiol.* 2005;15;565(Pt 1):309-323. Epub 2005 Mar 17.

70. Smith K, Winegard K, Hicks AL, McCartney N. Two years of resistance training in older men and women: The effects of three years of detraining on the retention of dynamic strength. *Can J Appl Physiol.* 2003;28(3):462-474.

71. Sternfeld B, Ngo L, Satariano WA, Tager IB. Associations of body composition with physical performance and self-reported functional

limitation in elderly men and women. *Am J of Epidemiol.* 2002;156(2):110-121.

72. Symons TB, Vandervoort AA, Rice CL, Overend TJ, Marsh GD. Effects of maximal isometric and isokinetic resistance training on strength and functional mobility in older adults. *J Geront.* 2005;60A(6):777-781.

73. Tinetti ME, Baker DI, McAvay G, et al. A multifactorial intervention to reduce the risk of falling among elderly people living in the community. *N Engl J Med.* 1994;331:821-827.

74. Tinetti ME, Speechley M, Ginter SF. Risk factors for falls among elderly persons living in the community. *N Engl J Med.* 1988;319:1701-1707.

75. Trappe S, Williamson D, Godard M. Maintenance of whole muscle strength and size following resistance training in older men. *J Gerontol A Biol Sci Med Sci.* 2002;57(4):B138-B143.

76. US Census Bureau: National Population Estimates. Available at http://www.census.gov/popest/national/asrh/NC-EST2005-sa.html. Accessed May 19, 2008.

77. Villareal DT, Banks M, Sinacore DR, Siener C, Klein S. Effects of weight loss and exercise on frailty in obese older adults. *Arch Intern Med.* 2006;166:860-866.

78. Vincent KF, Vincent KH, Braith RW, et al. Resistance exercise training attenuates exercise-induced lipid peroxidation in the elderly. *Eur J Appl Physiol.* 2002;87:416-423.

79. Visser M, Harris TB, Langlois J, et al. Body fat and skeletal muscle mass in relation to physical disability in very old men and women of the Framingham Heart Study. *J Gerontol A Biol Sci Med Sci.* 1998;53(3):M214-M221.

80. Visser M, Pahor M, Taaffe DR et al. Relationship of Interleukin-6 and Tumor Necrosis Factor-alpha with muscle mass and muscle strength in elderly men and women: The Health ABC Study. *J Gerontol A Biol Sci Med Sci.* 2002;57:M326-M332.

81. Vita AJ, Terry RB, Hubert HB, Fries JF. Aging, health risks, and cumulative disability. *N Engl J Med.* 1998;338:1035-1041.

82. Walston J, Hadley EC, Ferrucci L, et al. Research agenda for frailty in older adults: toward a better understanding of physiology and etiology: summary from the American Geriatrics Society/National Institute on Aging Research Conference on Frailty in Older Adults. *J Am Geriatr Soc.* 2006;54(6):991-1001.

83. Wieser M, Haber P. The effects of systematic resistance training in the elderly. *Int J Sports Med.* 2007;28(1): 59-65. Epub 2006 June 8.

84. Young, HM. Challenges and solutions for care of frail older adults. *Online J Issues Nurs.* May 31, 2003.

85. Zoico E, Roubenoff R. The role of cytokines in regulating protein metabolism and muscle function. *Nutr Rev.* 2002;60(2):39-51.

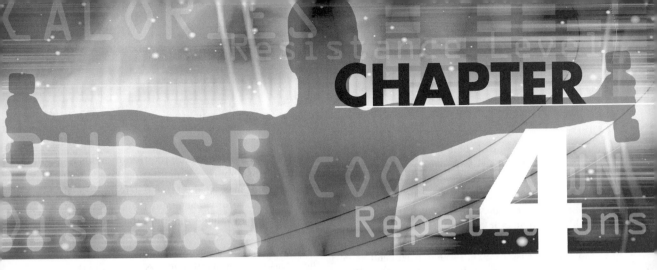

CHAPTER 4

RESISTANCE-TRAINING STRATEGIES FOR INDIVIDUALS WITH OSTEOPOROSIS

Objectives

Upon completion of this chapter, the reader should be able to:

- Recognize the pervasiveness of osteoporosis in society
- Identify risk factors and preventive options for osteoporosis
- Explain the difference between primary and secondary osteoporosis
- Describe the disease process of osteoporosis
- Explain how resistance training impacts osteoporosis
- Develop a safe and effective resistance-training exercise prescription for an individual with osteoporosis

INTRODUCTION

Osteoporosis, or brittle bone disease, is one of the most common diseases impacting the integrity of the skeleton (57). Osteoporosis, which literally means "porous bone," is a disease that erodes bone tissue until it becomes so fragile that it breaks, even without a traumatic accident. Often a precursor to osteoporosis is osteopenia, the term used to describe low bone density (59, 60). While osteopenia is not a disease, but rather a description of a condition that can lead to osteoporosis, both osteopenia and osteoporosis predispose individuals to untimely, unanticipated fractures. Hence, it would appear that early detection and treatment of osteopenia and osteoporosis can help to reduce fracture risk. The focus of this chapter will be to discuss the role of resistance training on encouraging bone maintenance and attenuating the osteoporotic process.

PREVALENCE AND ECONOMIC IMPACT OF OSTEOPOROSIS

In Europe, the prevalence of osteoporosis amounts to 650,000 cases a year, or roughly 1700 fractures daily (22). Annual fracture rates due to weakened bones in the United States has been estimated to involve as many as 1.5 million Americans; an estimated 10 million Americans over 50 years of age have osteoporosis, and another 34 million have osteopenia (57).

The most common fractures occur to the wrist, hip, and spine, with hip fractures proving to be the most devastating. Of the 300,000 hospitalizations yearly due to hip fractures, the mortality rate is 20 percent; another 20 percent lose their independence and must be admitted to a nursing home (57). In 1997, estimates placed the cost of treatment and rehabilitation for osteoporotic fractures as high as $20,000 per incident in some Western countries (21). More recent reports place the cost of lifetime care due to one hip fracture at approximately $80,000. The cost for the care

of bone fractures due to osteoporosis now exceeds $17 billion annually (57).

In the United Kingdom (60), the risk of men sustaining an osteoporotic fracture increased from 7.1 percent of men aged 50 to 8.0 percent of men aged 80; the risk for women more than doubled for the same age and time frame: the fracture risk at age 50 was 9.8 percent, age 80, it was 21.7 percent. Even though men get osteoporosis, statistics show the disease predominantly impacts women, particularly small-framed Caucasian and Asian women. The third National Health and Nutrition Examination Survey (NHANES III, 1988–1994) reported that the lowest rates existed among non-Hispanic Black women, followed by Mexican-American women, at rates of 5 percent and 10 percent, respectively (30). Table 4-1 summarizes the known risk factors for osteoporosis.

Unless effective preventive measures are implemented, estimates predict that half of all Americans aged 50 or older will have osteopenia and/or osteoporosis by the year 2020 (57). The World Health Organization's May 2006 report, issued by the Health Evidence Network on the effectiveness of prevention and screening for osteoporosis, concluded that some evidence showed that nonspecific physical exercise can prevent fractures due to a reduction in falls (22). Furthermore, when combined with nutritional supplementation of calcium and vitamin D and other pharmaceutical approaches, both cost effectiveness and fracture risk reduction was significantly improved in high-risk groups (22).

ETIOLOGY OF OSTEOPOROSIS

Bone is a dynamic living organ that is constantly changing. The bone-shape alterations that occur during puberty and young adulthood are known as **bone modeling**. Puberty is a time of rapid bone growth, with peak **bone mineral density** occurring around 20 years of age (62). Bone mineral density is a measure of the structural integrity and strength of

Table 4-1 Risk Factors for Osteoporosis (9, 38, 39)

Risk Factor	Genetic	Behavioral	Medical	Modifiable
Family history	√			No
Female gender	√			No
Advanced age (> age 65)	√			No
Low-trauma Fx Hx > age 50	√			No
Caucasian or Asian race	√			No
Dietary intake deficiencies		√	√	Yes
Physical inactivity		√		Yes
Smoking		√		Yes
Excessive alcohol use		√		Yes
Low body mass	√	√		Maybe
Low estrogen status	√		√	Maybe
Certain medications†			√	Maybe
Other comorbidities††	√	√	√	Maybe

† Glucocorticosteroids, radiation, chemotherapy, excess thyroxin replacement, antiepileptics, immunosuppressive agents, gonadal hormone suppression agents.

†† Chronic lung disease, diabetes, inflammatory bowel disease, cancer, celiac disease, anorexia nervosa, hyperthyroidism/hyperparathyroidism, liver and kidney disease, sarcoidosis, lactose intolerance, immobility or bed-rest confinement, Cushing disease, multiple sclerosis, rheumatoid arthritis, sarcoidosis, hemochromatosis.

Fx Hx Functional History

an area of bone, and it is maintained by remodeling via the process of **resorption,** the dissolving of bone mineral by osteoclasts, and **deposition,** the rebuilding of bone by osteoblasts (6). Bone has a wide range of functions that include providing structural support for soft tissue, a place of attachment for muscles, whole blood-cell production, calcium maintenance, and a storage site for other minerals (47).

During the second and third decades of life, the remodeling process is usually well balanced across genders, providing that adequate nutrition and physical activity are undertaken. The remodeling process becomes unbalanced when women enter perimenopause, evidenced by a 1 percent loss of bone yearly. When estrogen is no longer produced, either due to the natural cessation of ovarian function with menopause or due to surgical removal of the ovaries, rapid bone loss ensues for up to 5 years (10, 23). Hence, with osteoporosis, the resorption rate exceeds the deposition rate, resulting in less dense bone as illustrated in Figure 4-1.

The adult skeleton comprises two distinct types of bone: 80 percent is **cortical bone,** or compact bone, and 20 percent is **trabecular bone,** or cancellous spongiosa bone. As can be seen in Figure 4-2, the biggest difference between these two bone types is in their density. Cortical bone is 90 percent more dense, with an apparent density of 1.8 g/cm^3, versus trabecular bone, with an apparent density of only 0.2 g/cm^3. As for regional distribution of bone type, over 90 percent of the diaphyseal shaft of long bone is cortical, whereas approximately 70 percent of the central axial skeleton, the spine, is trabecular (5). Therefore, bone loss impacts stature over time as the vertebral column becomes compressed due to loss of critical trabecular bone. The individual not only loses height, but the back may take on a hunched appearance, depicted in Figure 4-1. This usual deformity includes a forward position of the head, rounded spine due to thoracic kyphosis and loss of the normal lumbar lordosis, and rounded shoulders with the scapulae in an abducted position.

However, even within specific bones, the ratio of cortical to trabecular bone varies. For instance, the cortical–trabecular ratio in the trochanteric region of the hip is 50:50, but in the proximal femur of the hip, it is 57:43 (5). Furthermore, although men and women tend to lose similar amounts of cortical bone—about 30 percent—women lose dramatically greater trabecular bone compared to men— 50 percent versus 20 percent (24, 30, 33, 40, 43, 57, 58). Therefore, performing bone density screening on various locations of bone is important. Similarly,

when attempting to impact bone with exercise, the bone sites measured must correspond to the bone sites targeted with exercise. The most common regions affected by osteoporosis include the wrist, spine, and hip; so exercise specifically targeting these regions is particularly critical. Table 4-2 summarizes the World Health Organization's (WHO) classification system for osteoporosis progression in terms of bone mineral density (59, 60).

Osteoporosis is categorized as either primary or secondary, depending on the origin of the disease in the individual (44). **Primary osteoporosis,** which is characterized by a marked acceleration of bone-mass loss, is further categorized into three types: *postmenopausal,* also known as *Type I osteoporosis; senile,* also known as *Type II osteoporosis;* and *idiopathic,* in which the cause of the bone loss is unknown. **Secondary osteoporosis** is a consequential condition resulting from another disease process and/or its treatment, such as corticosteroid treatment for asthma or rheumatoid arthritis (44).

BENEFITS OF RESISTANCE TRAINING FOR INDIVIDUALS WITH OSTEOPOROSIS

Resistance training for individuals with osteoporosis commonly focuses only on the benefits to the skeleton. In adults with osteoporosis, resistance training can assist in maintaining bone mass and can affect bone morphology; that is, it can affect the size and shape of bone, enabling the skeleton to resist the loads that cause fractures. Improving muscular fitness also has the potential to prevent or improve spine deformity and reduce the risk of falls and injuries caused by falls, including fractures. All these benefits contribute to the ultimate goal of keeping individuals with osteoporosis functioning optimally in daily life.

The most obvious way to prevent or reduce osteoporosis risk is through encouraging bone-mass

Osteoporosis

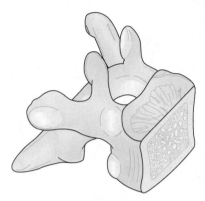

Normal bone

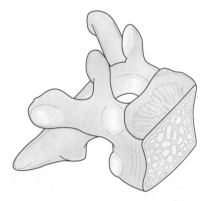

Osteoporotic bone

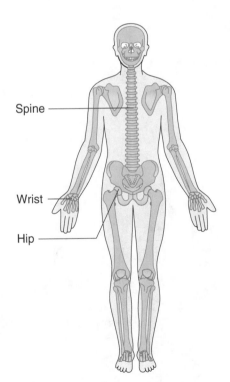

Spine

Wrist

Hip

Common sites
for osteoporosis

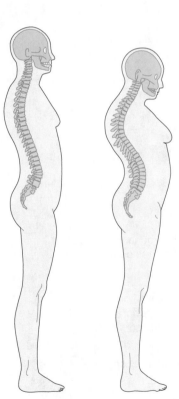

Gradually the bones of the spinal column become thin
and weaken causing a hunch back appearance

Figure 4-1 Osteoporosis "Swiss cheese" appearance, common sites, and effects.

© Delmar/Cengage Learning.

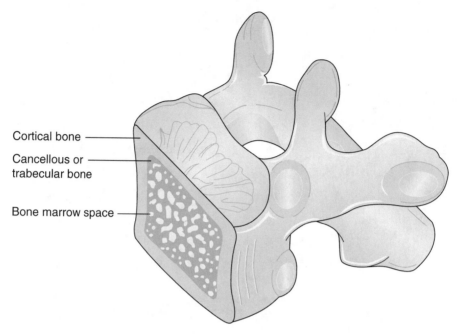

Cortical bone

Cancellous or
trabecular bone

Bone marrow space

Normal bone

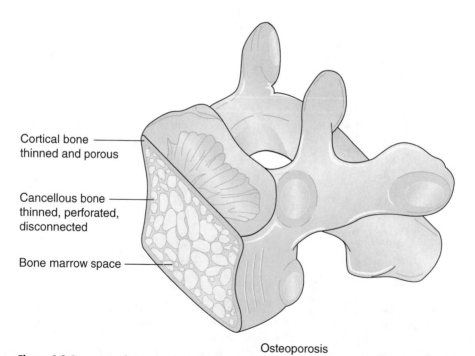

Cortical bone
thinned and porous

Cancellous bone
thinned, perforated,
disconnected

Bone marrow space

Osteoporosis

Figure 4-2 Comparison of cortical and trabecular bone.
© Delmar/Cengage Learning.

Table 4-2 Bone Mineral Density Classification System Based on T Scores† (59, 60)

Category	Description
Normal	BMD within 1 SD of young adult mean (±1 SD)
Osteopenia	BMD 1 to 2.5 SD below young adult mean (–1 to –2.5 SD)
Osteoporosis	BMD 2.5 SD or more below young adult mean (> –2.5 SD)
Severe Osteoporosis	BMD >2.5 SD below young adult mean plus fractures

† The T score is a mathematical representation of distance from the normative healthy population score. Falling below the norm (a negative T score beyond –1.0 SD) suggests that a follow-up medical evaluation is in order.

BMD: Bone mineral density

SD: Standard deviation

accumulation, beginning in puberty and continuing throughout life, via adequate intake of calcium and foods rich in vitamin D, judicious sun exposure, and daily weight-bearing physical activity (57). Once a person has been diagnosed with osteoporosis, the goal is to retard the progression of the disease. Besides pharmaceutical management and aerobic weight-bearing exercise, resistance training can also be incorporated. The premise behind recommending resistance training is the modeling effect it has on bone tissue.

Direct Effects of Training for the Skeleton

Despite the vast amount of research on bone modeling, the exact mechanisms by which exercise training impacts bone morphology remain elusive. However, bone tissue responds to stresses placed on it, especially **strain**; the deformation of bone tissue responds to mechanical loading, thereby resulting in bone hypertrophy. The appropriate amounts, types, and directions of strain result in bone-mass maintenance, bone bone strength through increasing the cross-sectional area, or the size of the bone, and increasing the thickness of cortical bone (28, 49, 50, 56).

Strain causes biochemical signals that influence bone-cell function and keep osteocytes vital (50).

Osteocytes, the cells located beneath the surface of bone in the mineralized matrix, function as strain transducers and communicate with the cells on the surface of bone, where formation and resorption occur (27, 50, 53). In the case of resistance training, muscle contraction deforms the osteocytes that then signal osteoblasts, lining cells, osteoclasts, and other cells to produce or break down bone. Hence, the magnitude of the imposed strain, as well as the frequency and rate of strain, all influence the adaptive response of bone (62).

The stimulation of bone formation due to mechanical strain is not a linear function. The adaptation and desensitization of the mechanoreceptors in bone cells occur swiftly, so that multiple strain repetitions are not required for bone modeling or maintenance (50). In fact, avian research has shown maintenance of bone mass with only 4 repetitions of daily loading and bone building with only 36 repetitions of daily loading (50, 53). However, the number of repetitions is not the only loading parameter that must be met for building bone. Strain magnitude and rates must be higher than the typical or habitual force exertion to signal bone production (27, 50).

The human body experiences thousands of strains on a daily basis, predominantly consisting of smaller strains under 10 $\mu\varepsilon$, or microstrains, and a few larger strains exceeding 1000 $\mu\varepsilon$ (62). Only dynamic stimuli are **osteogenic,** or bone building, so strains held at a constant static level, where the strain rate equals zero, do not encourage bone modeling (62). Physical inactivity results in bone loss. Patients who are bedridden, and those who have immobilized extremities, lose bone at high rates (50). One study documented that patients put on total bed rest lost bone at a rate of nearly 1 percent per week. Further, the rate of bone recovery was only 1 percent a month, far slower than the rapid rate of initial loss (27). On the opposite end of the spectrum, the microstrain damage threshold hovers about 3000 $\mu\varepsilon$. Repeated microdamage to the bone from vigorous prolonged exercise, such as marathon training, can result in athletically induced stress fractures. Definitive bone fractures occur at about 25,000 $\mu\varepsilon$ (11).

Increased bone resorption occurs when mechanical strain rates fall below 700 $\mu\varepsilon$ (11, 37, 50). Most exercise in middle-aged to older adults' daily activities, including resistance training, tend to fall between 700 and 1500 $\mu\varepsilon$ (11). These strains are sufficient to maintain bone mass but not high enough to build new bone. Only impact exercise provides a high enough strain rate and magnitude (1500 to 3000 $\mu\varepsilon$) to build new bone; and the impact activity ideally should load the bone from multiple, atypical directions (11). Results from numerous randomized clinical trials have shown that weight-bearing activity, resistance training, and impact activities—such as one- and two-footed jumping and long-term racquet sport participation—preserves or increases bone density in the activity-specific limbs (4, 19, 29, 35, 50, 61). The benefits of a well-designed resistance-training program are self-evident and include stronger bones, improved muscular strength, improved balance and stability, improved self-efficacy, a reduction in the risk of falls, and a likely reduction in bone fractures.

Of particular importance is that the bone-building effects of exercise are transient. Once bones have become accustomed to resistance training, any significant interruption in that training routine will disrupt the bone-maintenance process. In short, the bone tissue will consider itself to be in a state of disuse and remodeling, and removal of the bone

tissue gained will ensue due to perceived lack of need (11, 36). Thus, resistance training must become a regular lifestyle component to retain any gains accrued in bone mineral density.

Review of Research Supporting Resistance Training for Osteoporosis

Several excellent, comprehensive reviews on osteoporosis provide viewpoints from the disciplines of epidemiology, medicine, rehabilitative therapy, and sports medicine (5, 8, 22, 34, 50, 60). The consensus is that regular, progressive resistive exercise two to four times per week increases bone density at the hip and spine by 0.5 percent to 3 percent in both young and postmenopausal women (4, 7, 19, 26, 29, 50, 61). Therefore, even small gains in bone mass from resistive exercise—as little as 0.5 to 1 percent per year—can be clinically relevant (50).

Table 4-3 provides a synopsis of the few studies (18, 25, 26, 41, 48, 54) that utilized classical resistance-training (weight lifting) paradigms without confounding exercise co-therapies. Subject populations included not only those with diagnosed osteoporosis but also those with osteopenia. Training studies investigating the impact of lifting on bone mineral density in healthy populations, those not defined as at risk for osteoporosis, were not included in this table. The reader is referred to the actual referenced articles for additional study details.

Although overwhelming evidence supports strengthening the bones and maintaining bone density through exercise for osteoporosis prevention and management, the majority of the research has been confounded by the inability to adequately separate out the impact of multiple therapies. Furthermore, men are not adequately represented, even though they are susceptible to osteoporosis, albeit fewer men have the disease. An additional problem lies in the difficulty of retaining subjects; the few that did have a relatively pure resistance-training component also had higher attrition rates than those utilizing other therapies, especially in older female populations.

Table 4-3 Impact of Classical Weight-Lifting Protocols on Strength and Bone Mineral Density (18, 25, 26, 41, 48, 54)

Author (Date)	n	Mean Age, Gender	Program Length	Modes and Intensity	Strength and BMD Outcomes
Hartard (1996)	16	64, F	6 mo 2x/wk	11 muscle groups, 70%1RM 8–12 reps, 1–2 sets	40–75% improvement in strength; neck of femur ↓ in controls but maintained in treatment group
Kerr (1996)	23	55, F	1 yr 3x/wk	Unilateral, 10 exercises 3 sets x 8RM	Strength gains positively correlated w/BMD, $p < .01$; high-load low reps improved BMD
Kerr (2001)	42 Str. 42 Fit.	60, F 59, F	2 yr 3x/wk	S: 9 exercises, 3 sets x 8RM progressive overload F: 9 exercises; minimal load, No progressive overload, added bicycling	No significant difference in BMD between groups @ forearm, lumbar spine, whole body sites; ~ 1% increase in hip BMD for Str. whereas F & C hip BMD ↓ and spine BMD ↓ (all groups)
Nelson (1994)	T 20	57, F	1 yr 2x/wk	High-intensity weight lifting; Five exercises, 80% 1RM 3 sets x 8 reps	↑ strength, neck and spine BMD
Ryan (1998)	T 21	62, F	16 wks 3x/wk	90% 3RM; 11 machines 12–15 reps Upper body: 1 set Lower body: 2 sets	BMD did not change in any location; 36–63% ↑ upper-body strength; 32–98% ↑ lower-body strength
Stengel (2005)	Str. 28 Pwr. 25	58, F 58, F	1 yr 2x/wk	All: 12-week intervals 90% 1RM 4-5 wks 50% 1RM; 11 machines; plus low to high-impact aerobics, gymnastics; home program Strength group: SLOW lifting (4 sec CON, 4 sec ECC) Power Group: FAST lifting ("explosive" CON, 4 sec ECC)	Power: maintained BMD at hip and spine Strength: ↓ BMD hip, spine Neither group had pain; Strength gains similar between groups

BMD: Bone mineral density
1RM: One-repetition maximum
ECC: Eccentric
CON: Concentric
Str: Strength

Pwr: Power
T: Training Group
F: Female
Fit: Fitness Group

The terms *strength training, weight-bearing, weighted exercise, resistive training, resistance training, weight training,* and *weight lifting* are used interchangeably in the literature such that it is difficult to determine the actual impact "traditional" weight lifting, with external free weights or machines, has had on bone in the osteoporotic individual. The literature is further complicated by intermingling subjects with osteopenia, osteoporosis, and those with either no or a low risk of low bone density. While reducing bone fractures is the ultimate goal for management of osteoporosis, no study has yet proven that resistance training actually reduces fracture risk. Neither has a study been published that has shown that participating in a supervised resistance-training program, incorporating the latest resistance-training techniques, actually caused a fracture.

DESIGNING A RESISTANCE-TRAINING PROGRAM FOR INDIVIDUALS WITH OSTEOPOROSIS

A regular program of resistance training is critical for improving and maintaining overall muscular strength and bone health of older adults. Equally important is the benefit of resistance training on the physical functioning and mobility in this population. The negative cycle of **sarcopenia**, loss of muscle mass, includes loss of bone mass, increased risk for falls, and subsequent disability; but it is not necessarily an inevitable aspect of aging. In fact, numerous studies indicate that aging-related decreases in muscular strength and bone health outcomes can be reversed, prevented, or delayed with resistance training (12, 32).

For older adults with osteopenia or osteoporosis, an appropriately designed resistance-training program can positively impact the negative sequelae that often accompany these health conditions. Clinical trials employing high-intensity resistance training have demonstrated a significant beneficial impact on

strength, balance, and fracture risk in osteoporotic older adults (31). In addition, resistance training may reduce the risk of falls and the severity of fall-related injuries in those with osteoporosis (55), and it improves quality of life in osteoporotic older women with prevalent vertebral fractures (42). Given the evidence and expert recommendations for resistance training as a crucial aspect of the primary and secondary prevention of osteoporosis, the rationale for a regular program of strengthening in osteoporotic older adults is to improve strength and functioning and reduce the risk of falls and vertebral fractures.

Although numerous exercise options are available to healthy older adults, those with osteoporosis need to take into account not only their specific goals to maintain bone mass but also their health status. Although regular exercise affords a host of health benefits, there are also associated health risks, such as exacerbating existing medical problems, increasing muscle and joint injuries, and in rare instances, inducing heart attack (1). Furthermore, a program that may be beneficial for a person with osteopenia may be too aggressive for the osteoporotic individual. In fact, some exercises that are indicated for osteopenia are contraindicated for osteoporosis (38). Thus, exercise programs for these two conditions, though having similar goals, are not readily interchangeable. Exercise programs for osteoporosis need to be designed to capitalize on bone-maintenance benefits while avoiding or minimizing the potential risks of untoward health complications or fractures (32).

Understanding bone loading, unloading, and overloading principles, along with understanding the accompanying risks, will enable the exercise professional to design safe resistance-training protocols for individuals with osteopenia or osteoporosis (34). The general resistance-training guidelines for older adults outlined in Chapter 3 must be modified to manage the specific medical issues that accompany the varying severities of osteoporosis. Of particular concern is the perplexing problem of strengthening fracture-risk areas that have no direct muscular attachments, such as the mid to lower thoracic spine and the neck of the femur. Besides simply protecting the area, another possible solution to this dilemma is focusing on improving body alignment with the secondary hope of gaining bone mass in the process (34).

As with any exercise program, individuals should first check with their physician for advice concerning the progression of their specific type of osteoporosis. Understanding the limits of their disease and how various therapies may impact their disease process, as well as their overall health and well-being, is critical. Resistance-training programs designed to prevent osteoporosis in individuals diagnosed with osteopenia will likely be more aggressive and will have more training options. As discussed earlier with osteoporosis, a more cautionary approach to resistance training and physical activity in general is necessary due to the increased likelihood of incurring fractures with higher impact, twisting, and bending activities. The severity of the disease will dictate the degree of aggressiveness of the exercise program.

Preventing or Improving Spine Deformity

Degenerative changes of the spine and osteoporotic vertebral fractures that occur with aging cause loss of height and spine deformity. Resistance training should focus on strengthening the abdominal, neck, erector spinae, scapular, and gluteal muscles to minimize spine deformity and help the individual resume a more erect posture. Along with resistance training, exercise that stretches the anterior structures of the body, such as the pectoral and hip flexor muscles, will improve thoracic and lumbar extension flexibility. Spinal extension exercises may also improve postural alignment (15, 20, 50). An exercise study involving older women, with a mean age 81 years and a history of vertebral fractures, demonstrated that group exercise classes held three times per week for 6 months could improve trunk extension strength (13). Furthermore, two observational studies by Sinaki and colleagues suggested that spinal-extension exercise was associated with a lower incidence of vertebral fractures in postmenopausal women (51, 52). However, exercise professionals must be alert to warning signs that indicate the resistance-training program may be too aggressive, such

as if the individual is unable to maintain proper alignment, or they are losing height (50).

Strength-Testing Considerations

The following guidelines are suggested when considering exercise testing for individuals with osteoporosis (1, 2, 17):

○ Obtain physician clearance prior to testing.

○ Ensure a safe environment to reduce the risk of falls.
  ○ Provide clean, dry, nonslip floors, adequate lighting, and so.
  ○ Offer walking assistance or assistive devices when appropriate.
  ○ Recognize that those with severe kyphosis are predisposed to balance instability due to a forward shift in their center of gravity.

○ All testing should be done in an upright posture.

○ Ten-repetition maximum testing for strength assessment is recommended.

○ Maximal isometric muscle strength assessment—such as with handgrip dynamometry and handheld, manual muscle testers—is recommended if not contraindicated due to hypertension.

○ Falls risk assessment should include evaluations of gait speed, tandem gait, and balance.

○ If the patient is suspected of also being at risk for heart disease, a cardiopulmonary exercise test should be done.
  ○ Cycle ergometry is the preferred mode for aerobic capacity testing.
  ○ If treadmill testing is used, handrails should be installed and other precautions instituted to prevent tripping or falling.

○ Premature test termination may occur due to pain or reduced ventilatory capacity.
○ Supplemental oxygen should be available.

○ Contraindicated tests:
  ○ Spinal flexion
  ○ Sit-and-reach
  ○ One-repetition maximum strength assessment

○ Standard emergency medical procedures should be in place.

Program Components and Exercise Selection

Resistance-training programs may be more beneficial for bone modeling than classic weight-bearing activity such as walking, due to the ability to

impact the upper-body extremities as well as the lower body. All exercises should be done with slow, controlled movements to avoid muscle strain and fractures. Flexibility exercises should be performed almost daily, and all activity should be preceded by a 5- to 10-minute light dynamic warm-up on an upright cycle ergometer with no load, followed by a 10- to 20-minute cooldown stretching program (1, 2, 17). Table 4-4 and Table 4-5 outline specific guidelines for designing a resistance-training program for individuals with osteoporosis.

Progression of the program should follow the American College of Sports Medicine guidelines for clinical populations and for older adults (1, 3) with special considerations for osteoporotic older adults. For instance, any strengthening exercises that require lumbar flexion, such as seated rows and abdominal crunches, should be avoided. While significant strength gains can be observed in as little as

Table 4-4 Resistance Training Guidelines (1, 2, 17)	
Modes:	Free weights, machines, calisthenics, elastic color-coded resistance bands
Frequency:	2 to 3 days a week, allowing 48 to 72 hours rest between training days, ideally on days alternating with aerobic conditioning days
Duration:	8 to 15 repetitions completed in a continuous, rhythmic fashion (~3 sec concentric, per repetition; ~3 sec eccentric, per repetition)
	8 to 10 exercises targeting the entire body; 1 to 3 sets with 1.5-minute rests between sets and 2-minute rests between exercise stations, or when breathing returns to normal (about 12 breaths/minute)
Intensity:	RPE of 13 to 15 (somewhat high to high)
	Resistance bands: check the color-coded chart for level of difficulty 30 to 50 or 70% of 10RM, depending upon disease severity
Progression:	Increase load ~2 to 10% every 2 to 3 weeks or when RPE rating drops below 13 for 2 to 3 consecutive training sessions
Tips:	Maintain normal breathing pattern and avoid Valsalva maneuver (breath holding)
	Train with a partner
	For pain or improper body alignment, stop and reassess exercise station and rate of overload progression.

RM = Repetition Maximum

Table 4-5 Activity Participation Guide for Patients with Osteoporosis (2, 34, 50)

Activities to Avoid:

- High-impact aerobics (e.g., running, aerobic dance)
- Racquet sports, golf, bowling
- Single-leg jumps
- Rowing
- Rebounding (e.g., mini-trampoline)
- Spine *flexion* exercises
- Bending from the torso or dynamic abdominal exercises (e.g., toe touches, sit-ups, squats with free weights)
- Aerobic equipment requiring the involvement of both the arms and legs (e.g., cross-country ski machine)
- Trunk twisting or rotation-type stretches or exercises
- Any activity with a high risk of falling (e.g., rollerblading, mountain biking, wall climbing)
- Any hyperextension of the back due to risk of incurring fractures in the vertebrae

Activities to Perform with Caution:

- Use of aerobic equipment utilizing both the arms and legs may be performed, providing that use of the arms is not mandatory (e.g., Airdyne-type cycle ergometers, elliptical trainers)
- Treadmill walking: use slower speeds and secure handrails

Suggested Activities:

- Swimming, walking, walking with weighted vest, cycling indoors on a stationary bike
- Cautious resistance training with free weights, including appropriate alignment for bicep curl and triceps extension, resistance bands, and machines
- Balance training
- Quadriceps strengthening
- Seated spine *extension* exercises
- Calisthenic toning/stretches and exercises that do not involve trunk rotation or bending over
- Stair-climbing machine, provided no hip or ankle problems exist

8 to 12 weeks, bone remodeling resulting in only modest increases in bone mineral density (1 to 2 percent) may take 6 to 18 months to see. Individuals with a goal of improving bone mineral density should be made aware of a modest at best resistance-training effect on bone mineral density, and the numerous other health benefits mentioned previously can be stressed for motivational purposes.

Assessments of physical performance measures at baseline and at 12-week intervals are recommended to determine the effectiveness of the program on mobility and strength. As an example, the Fullerton Functional Performance Test Battery developed by Rikli and Jones (45, 46) includes individual components that measure mobility and upper- and lower-body strength for men and women over the age of 60. The individual test components of the Fullerton battery that measure mobility and strength are:

- The 30-second chair-stand test (leg strength)
- The 30-second arm-curl test (upper body strength)
- The 8-foot up-and-go test (dynamic balance and mobility)

Additionally, the Fullerton battery has age- and gender-matched national normative data for each test component, which allows meaningful interpretation of test results.

A twice-per-week program focused on high-force loading is the desired resistance-training frequency and intensity in osteoporotic older adults; however, due to likely significant deconditioning of the individual, an initial 2- to 4-week period of acclimatization may be necessary to focus on proper exercise form and technique rather than intensity. Following acclimatization, a program progressing from 1 to 2 sets of 8 repetitions at a progressive load that maintains a rating of perceived exertion (RPE) of "somewhat hard" to "hard"—an RPE of 13 to 15 on a 6 to 20 scale—should be the goal. All major muscle groups should be targeted with an additional emphasis on lower-body and back extensor (erector spinae) strengthening.

SAMPLE 24-WEEK PROGRAM

The following program was designed with the older (60+) osteopenic/osteoporotic individual as the focus. The program should generally follow a schedule of 2 days per week with 48 to 72 hours of rest between training sessions. Table 4-6 outlines the exercises used in this program.

Weeks 1 through 2

Assessment and Orientation

○ The individual must obtain physician clearance and provide a health history that includes any falls, medications, current medical conditions, and symptoms with particular emphasis on osteoporosis information.

○ Resting heart rate, blood pressure, weight, and height measurements are taken. In addition, ask the individual to recall their height at age 25; a loss of more than four centimeters in height from full adult height may indicate prevalent vertebral fractures (14).

○ Functional performance assessments are made, including measures of balance, mobility, and strength. Examples of balance and mobility measures include noting the time it takes to walk 10 meters at normal walking pace or the 8-foot up-and-go test, the time it takes to rise from a chair, walk around a cone 8 feet away, and return to a seated position in the chair. Strength may be measured using a chair-stand test, which measures the number of stands in 30-seconds or the time it takes to complete five chair stands as quickly as possible (16).

○ One set of 8 to 10 repetitions for 5 to 6 exercises is encouraged, including unloaded half squats or sit-back squats, chest presses, lat pulldowns, shoulder presses, lower-back extensions, and seated or supine isometric abdominals. Intensity should be light to somewhat hard with an RPE of 11 to 13. The focus of this set is exercise form and technique rather than intensity. When orienting to machines or dumbbells, start with the lightest resistance possible and increase load in the smallest possible increments until the desired RPE of 11 to 13 is achieved.

Weeks 3 through 6

Training Intensity Focus

○ One set of 8 repetitions for 6 to 8 exercises is initiated, including leg presses, unloaded half squats or sit-back squats, chest presses,

Table 4-6 Facility and Home-Based Strengthening Exercises for Older Adults with Osteoporosis

Muscle Group(s)	Facility-Based	Home-Based
Hip/Thigh	Leg-press machine, knee extension, leg curl	Half squats, sit-back squats, chair stands, stair climbing
Calf	Seated calf-raise machine	Standing calf raise
Chest	Chest-press machine or chest fly; supine dumbbell presses	Seated chest press with resistance tubing and/or bands
Upper back	Lat pulldown machine	Lat pulldown or standing rows (posture focused) with resistance tubing/bands
Shoulders	Seated overhead-press machine; seated/standing overhead dumbbell presses	Seated/standing overhead presses with resistance tubing/bands or dumbbells
Arms, biceps	Bicep-curl machine*; Standing/seated* dumbbell curls	Standing/seated curls with resistance tubing/bands or dumbbells
Arms, triceps	Triceps-extension machine or triceps cable pushdown	Standing arm extension with resistance tubing/bands
Abdominal	Seated isometric abdominals; supine abdominal isometrics on floor	Seated isometric abdominals; supine abdominal isometrics on floor
Lower back	Back bridges; erector lifts on floor	Back bridges; erector lifts on floor

*Avoid seated bicep curls, including bicep curl machine in those who have hyperkyphosis.

Source: Mansfield E. Designing exercising programs to lower fracture risk in mature women. *Strength and Conditioning Journal.* 2006;28:24-29.

lat pulldowns, shoulder presses, lower-back exercises, and seated or supine isometric abdominals. Intensity should be somewhat hard to hard, with an RPE of 13 to 15.

Weeks 7 through 12

Incorporate All Major Muscle Groups

○ One set of 8 repetitions for 8 to 10 exercises is undertaken, including leg presses, unloaded

half squats or sit-back squats, toe raises, chest presses, lat pulldowns, shoulder presses, triceps extensions, biceps curls, lower-back extensions, and seated or supine isometric abdominals. Intensity should be somewhat hard to hard, with an RPE of 13 to 15.

○ Reassess weight, height, and physical performance at week 12, and interpret test results with emphasis on gains and opportunities for program changes in deficit areas.

Weeks 13 through 18

Progression

○ Two sets of 8 repetitions for 8 to 10 exercises begin, including leg presses, unloaded half squats or sit-back squats, toe raises, chest presses, lat pulldowns, shoulder presses, triceps extensions, biceps curls, lower-back extensions, and seated or supine isometric abdominals. Intensity should be somewhat hard to hard with an RPE of 13 to 15.

○ Begin to educate the individual on appropriate progression and possible alterations to the program for a home routine if the current program is facility based.

Weeks 19 through 24

Continued Focus on High-Load Training

○ Continue training program with alterations as needed.

○ Continue education on appropriate progression based on maintaining an RPE of 13 to 15, which will generally follow a 2 to 10 percent increase in resistance bi-weekly and a home-based routine if facility-based training is no longer an option.

○ Reassess weight, height, and physical performance at week 24; interpret test results with an emphasis on gains, and recommend program changes in deficit areas.

○ Perform final program review.

CASE STUDY

The following case study is modified from a referral-based, outpatient exercise and health-promotion program for older adult veterans located at the Durham Veteran's Affairs Medical Center (36). Mrs. S is 83 years old with multiple medical conditions, including osteoporosis of the hip and spine, coronary heart disease, hypertension, and bilateral osteoarthritis of the knees. She is 60 inches tall and weighs 100 pounds (BMI = 18). She has a history of non-injurious falls with two falls in the last 12 months. She is widowed, lives independently, and has full driving privileges. Her goals are to remain living independently and to have the strength to get through the day without feeling tired and weak. A recent stress test revealed an aerobic capacity of 6 Metabolic Equivalents of Task (METS), indicating extreme deconditioning. Baseline physical performance testing indicated that Mrs. S was at or below the fifteenth percentile compared to women her age in lower- and upper- body strength and mobility according to the Fullerton Test Battery.

A resistance-training program was implemented with an initial focus on form and technique. Following a brief stretching and warm-up period prior to each session, the twice-per-week sessions for weeks 1 and 2 consisted of a single set of 8 to 10 repetitions of half-squats with hands on a secure object for balance and support, a chair beneath, and close spotting; seated machine chest presses (10 lbs.); machine lat pulldowns (10 lbs.); seated machine shoulder presses with no added weight; bridges for the lower back; and seated isometric abdominals. The amount of initial resistance on the machines was set with the pin removed to be as light as possible, with minimal increases (10 lbs. each) to elicit an RPE of no greater than somewhat hard (RPE<14) during the first week of the 2-week acclimatization period. The client was instructed to walk at a comfortable pace for 5- to 10-minute intervals and to progress as tolerated on the off-training days, 5 days per week. Progression of intensity and volume was a focus starting at week 3, with reassessment of physical performance at weeks 12 and 24. Additional lower-body (seated leg presses, chair stands), lower-back and abdominal (back erector lifts and supine abdominal isometrics), and upper-body exercises (triceps extensions and biceps curls) were gradually added over the 24-week period with a continued focus on high-force loading equivalent to a perceived exertion of somewhat hard to hard with an RPE of 13 to 15.

Mrs. S had clinically meaningful gains in all physical performance measures, in the twenty-fifth percentile or better, and reported ease in carrying out daily activities. These gains were observed despite a 2-week absence due to illness. She reported no falls during the 24-week period and had no change in bone mineral density according to her last DXA scan results: all her previous scans showed a progressive loss of density.

This case reveals several important points: 1) older adults with osteoporosis often have multiple concurrent health conditions; 2) goals for training often are not fitness related, therefore the exercise professional will often need to provide education on how the resistance-training program can positively affect daily life; 3) perceived exertion is a simple way to train at the appropriate intensity; 4) a focus on high-force loading and progression is necessary to impact osteoporotic-related health outcomes such as bone mineral density, fractures, and falls; and 5) older adults with a complex medical history and multiple health conditions can substantially benefit from a safe and appropriate high-intensity resistance-training program.

Summary

Resistance training is a critical therapeutic modality for the prevention and treatment of osteoporosis. Even though it is often difficult to differentiate specific benefits gained from resistance training due to confounding co-therapies, the fact remains that bone benefits from resistance training that incorporates a prudent progressive overload. Exercise professionals should apply resistance-training modalities to ensure the development of safe and effective programs for both osteopenic and osteoporotic patient populations.

Key Terms

Bone mineral density
Bone modeling
Cortical bone
Deposition
Osteocytes

Osteogenic
Osteopenia
Osteoporosis
Primary osteoporosis
Resorption
Sarcopenia
Secondary osteoporosis
Strain
Trabecular bone

Study Questions

1. What are the various subcategories of osteoporosis, and which populations are likely to be affected?

2. How does resistance training improve bone structure and function?

3. What is the difference between *osteopenia* and *osteoporosis*? Compare and contrast resistance training for these two conditions.

4. What are the safety issues one must consider when developing a resistance-training program for patients with osteoporosis?

References

1. Senior Editor Mitchell H. Whaley. ACSM Guidelines for Exercise Testing and Prescription. 7th ed. New York: Lippincott, Williams & Wilkins; 2006.

2. Mazzeo RS, Cavanagh P, Evans WJ et al. ACSM's Resources for Clinical Exercise Physiology: Musculoskeletal, Neuromuscular, Neoplastic, Immunologic, and Hematologic Conditions. New York: Lippincott, Williams & Wilkins; 2002.

3. Mazzeo RS, Cavanagh P, Evans WJ et al. American College of Sports Medicine. Exercise and physical activity for older adults. *Med Sci Sports Exerc.* 1998;30:992-1008.

4. Bassey J, Ramsdale S. Increase in femoral bone density in young women following high-impact exercise. *Osteoporos Int.* 1994;4:72-75.

5. Borer KT. Physical activity in the prevention and amelioration of osteoporosis in women. *Sports Medicine.* 2005;35(9):779-830.

6. Buckwalter JA, Glimcher MJ, Cooper RR, et al. Bone biology II: Formation, form, modeling, remodeling, and regulation of cell function. *Instr Course Lect.* 1996;45:387-399 Review.

7. Dalsky PG, Stocke KS, Ehsani AA, et al. Weight-bearing exercise training and lumbar bone mineral content in postmenopausal women. *Ann Intern Med.* 1988;108:824-828.

8. Downey PA, Siegal MI. Bone biology and the clinical implications for osteoporosis. *Physical Therapy.* 2006;86(1):77-91.

9. Duchman RL, Berg KE. The implications of genetics and physical activity on the incidence of osteoporosis in pre- and postmenopausal women: A review. *Strength and Conditioning Journal.* 2006;28(2):26-32.

10. Ensrud KE, Palermo I, Black DM, et al. Hip and calcaneal bone loss increase with advancing age: Longitudinal results from the study of osteoporotic fractures. *J Bone Miner Res.* 1995;10:1778-1787.

11. Frost HM. Why do marathon runners have less bone than weight lifters? A vital biomechanical view and explanation. *Bone.* 1997; 20:183-189.

12. Gillespie LD, Gillespie WJ, Robertson MC, Lamb SE, Cumming RG, Rowe BH. Interventions for preventing falls in elderly people. *Cochrane Database of Systematic Reviews.* 2003, Issue 4. Art No.: CD000340. DOI: 10.1002/14651858.CD000340.

13. Gold DT, Shipp KM, Pieper CF, et al. Group treatment improves trunk strength and psychological status in older women with vertebral fractures: results of a randomized clinical trial. *J Amer Geriatr Soc.* 2004;52:1471-1478.

14. Green A, Colon-Emeric C, Bastian L, Drake M, Lyles K. Does this woman have osteoporosis? *JAMA.* 2004;292:2890-2900.

15. Greendale GA, McDivit A, Carpenter A, Seeger L, Huang MH. Yoga for women with hyperkyphosis: Results of a pilot study. *Am J Public Health.* 2002;92:1611-1614.

16. Guralnik JM, Simonsick EM, Ferrucci L, et al. A short physical performance battery assessing lower-extremity function: Association with self-reported disability and prediction of mortality and nursing home admission. *J Gerontol.* 1994;49:M85-M94.

17. Haff, GG. Roundtable discussion: resistance training the older adult. *Strength and Conditioning Journal.* 2005;27(6):48-68.

18. Hartard M, Haber P, Ilieva D, Preisinger E, Seidl G, Huber J. Systematic strength training as a model of therapeutic intervention: A controlled trial in postmenopausal women with osteopenia. *Am J Phys Med Rehabil.* 1996;75:21-28.

19. Heinonen A, Kannus P, Sievanen H, et al. Randomised controlled trial of effect of high-impact exercise on selected risk factors for osteoporotic fractures. *Lancet.* 1996;348:1343-1347.

20. Itoi E, Sinaki M. Effect of back-strengthening exercise on posture in healthy women 49 to 65 years of age. *Mayo Clin Proc.* 1994;69: 1954-1959.

21. Johnell O. The socioeconomic burden of fractures: Today and the 21st century. *Am J Med.* 1997;103(2A):20S-26S.

22. Johnell O, Hertzman P. What evidence is there for the prevention and screening of osteoporosis? Copenhagen, WHO Regional Office for Europe. Health Evidence Network Report, 2006. Available at: http://www.euro.who.int/document/e88668.pdf. Accessed May 18, 2006.

23. Jones G, Nguyen T, Sambrook P, et al. Progressive loss of bone in the femoral neck in elderly people: Longitudinal findings from the Dubbo osteoporosis epidemiology study. *BMJ.* 1994;309:691-695.

24. Kenny AM, Prestwood KM. Osteoporosis: Pathogenesis, diagnosis, and treatment in older adults. *RheumDis Clin North Am.* 2001; 26:569-591.

25. Kerr D, Ackland T, Maslen B, Morton A, Prince R. Resistance training over 2 years increases bone mass in calcium-replete postmenopausal women. *J Bone Miner Res.* 2001;16:175-181.

26. Kerr D, Morton A, Dick I, et al. Exercise effects on bone mass in postmenopausal women are site-specific and load-dependent. *J Bone Min Res.* 1996;11:218-225.

27. Krolner B, Toft B. Vertebral bone loss: An un-heeded side effect of therapeutic bed rest. *Clin Sci.* 1983;64:537-540.

28. Lanyon LE. Using functional loading to influence bone mass and architecture: Objectives, mechanisms, and relationship with estrogen of the mechanically adaptive process in bone. *Bone.* 1996;18:37S-43S.

29. Layne JE, Nelson ME. The effects of progressive resistance training on bone density: A review. *Med Sci Sports Exerc.* 1999;31:25-30.

30. Looker AC, Orwoll ES, Johnston CC, et al. Prevalence of low femoral bone density in older US adults from NHANES III. *J Bone Miner Res.* 1997;12:1761-1768.

31. Mansfield E. Designing exercising programs to lower fracture risk in mature women. *Strength and Conditioning Journal.* 2006;28:24-29.

32. Marks, BL. Physiologic responses to exercise in older women. *Topics in Geriatric Rehabilitation.* 2002;18(1):9-20.

33. McClung MR. Prevention and management of osteoporosis. *Best Pract Res Clin Endocrinol Metab.* 2003;17:53-71.

34. Meeks SM. The role of the physical therapist in the recognition, assessment, and exercise intervention in persons with, or at risk for, osteoporosis. *Topics in Geriatric Rehabilitation.* 2005;21(1):42-56.

35. Mitchell MJ, Baz MA, Fulton MN, et al. Resistance training prevents vertebral osteoporosis in lung transplant recipients. *Transplantation.* 2003;76:557-562.

36. Morey M, Crowley GM, Robbins MS, Cowper PA, Sullivan RJ. The Gerofit Program: a VA innovation. *South Med J.* 1994;87:S83-S87.

37. Mosekilde L. Osteoporosis and exercise. *Bone.* 1995;17:193-195.

38. National Institutes of Health Osteoporosis and Related Bone Diseases. The National Resource Center. Osteoporosis red flags. Available at: http://www.osteo.org/redflags.html. Accessed July 28, 2006.

39. National Osteoporosis Foundation. *Boning up on Osteoporosis. A Guide to Prevention and Treatment.* Washington, DC; 1997.

40. National Institutes of Health Consensus Development Panel on Osteoporosis Prevention, Diagnosis, and Therapy. Osteoporosis, prevention, diagnosis, and therapy. *JAMA.* 2001;285:785-795.

41. Nelson ME, Fiatarone MA, Morganti CM, Trice I, Greenberg RA, Evans WJ. Effects of high-intensity strength training on multiple risk factors for osteoporotic fractures. A randomized controlled trail. *JAMA.* 1994;272:1909-1914.

42. Papaioannou A, Adachi J, Winegard K, et al. Efficacy of home-based exercise for improving quality of life among elderly women with symptomatic osteoporosis-related vertebral fractures. *Osteoporos Int.* 2003;14:677-682.

43. Parsons LC. Osteoporosis: Incidence, prevention, and treatment of the silent killer. *Nurs Clin North Am.* 2005;40:119-133.

44. Riggs BL, Melton LJ. Evidence for two distinct syndromes of involutional osteoporosis. *Am J Med.* 1983;75:899-901.

45. Rikli RE, Jones CJ. Development and validation of a functional fitness test for community-residing older adults. *J Aging Phys Activ.* 1999;7:121-161.

46. Rikli RE, Jones CJ. Functional fitness normative scores for community-residing older adults, ages 60-94. *J Aging Phys Activ*. 1999;7:162-181.

47. Rodan GA. Introduction to bone biology. *Bone*. 1992;13:S3-S6.

48. Ryan AS, Treuth MS, Hunger GR, Elahi D. Resistive training maintains bone mineral density in postmenopausal women. *Calcif Tissue Int*. 1998;62:295-299.

49. Seeman E. Editorial: An exercise in geometry. *J Bone Miner Res*. 2002;17:373-380.

50. Shipp KM. Osteoporosis and aging females. Clinical commentary. *J of Women's Health Physical Therapy*. 2005;19(3):42-52.

51. Sinaki M, Mikkelsen BA. Postmenopausal spinal osteoporosis: Flexion versus extension exercises. *Arch Phys Med Rehabil*. 1984;65:593-596.

52. Sinaki M, Wahner HW, Wollan P, et al. Stronger back muscles reduce the incidence of vertebral fractures: A prospective 10-year follow-up of postmenopausal women. *Bone*. 2002;30: 836-841.

53. Skerry TM, Suva LJ. Investigation of the regulation of bone mass by mechanical loading: From quantitative cytochemistry to gene array. *Cell Biochem Funct*. 2003;21:223-229.

54. Stengel SV, Kemmler W, Pintag R, et al. Power training is more effective than strength training for maintaining bone mineral density in postmenopausal women. *J Appl Physiol*. 2005;99(1):181-188.

55. Suominen H. Muscle training for bone health. *Aging Clin Exp Res*. 2006;18:85-93.

56. Turner CH, Robling AG. Designing exercise regimens to increase bone strength. *Exerc Sport Sci Rev*. 2003;31:45-50.

57. US Department of Health and Human Services. *Bone Health and Osteoporosis: A Report of the Surgeon General*. USHHS, Office of the Surgeon General, 2004.

58. Van der Voort DJ, Geusens PP, Dinant GJ. Risk factors for osteoporosis related to their outcomes: Fractures. *Osteoporos Int*. 2001;12:630-638.

59. WHO. Assessment of fracture risk and its application to screening for postmenopausal osteoporosis. Report of a WHO study group. World Health Organ Tech Rep Ser. 1994; 843: 1-129 Review.

60. Woolf AD, Pfleger B. Burden of major musculoskeletal conditions. *Bulletin of the World Health Organization*. 2003;81(9):646-656.

61. Wolff I, Van Croonenborg JJ, Kemper HCG, et al. The effect of exercise training programs on bone mass: A meta-analysis of published controlled trials in pre- and postmenopausal women. *Osteoporos Int*. 1999;9:1-12.

62. Zernicke RF, Wohl GR, LaMothe JM. The skeletal-articular system. In *ACSM Advanced Exercise Physiology*. C. Tipton (Ed.). New York: Lippincott, Williams & Wilkins; 2006.

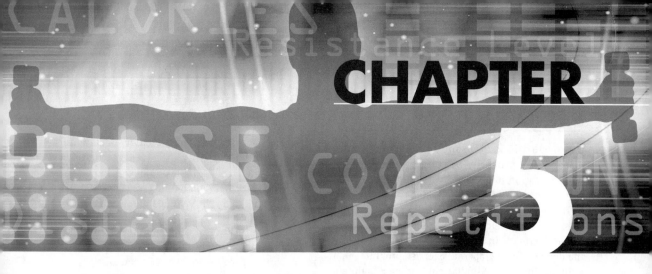

CHAPTER 5

RESISTANCE TRAINING STRATEGIES FOR INDIVIDUALS WITH OSTEOARTHRITIS

Objectives

Upon completion of this chapter, the reader should be able to:

- Identify the widespread prevalence of lower-extremity osteoarthritis and its associated economic impact
- Describe the etiology and progression of osteoarthritis
- Discuss the beneficial role of physical activity and exercise in regulating symptoms and progression of osteoarthritis
- Describe the relationship between decline in muscle strength and progression of osteoarthritis
- Design a resistance-training program for individuals with osteoarthritis

INTRODUCTION

Osteoarthritis is a chronic, degenerative joint disease that primarily affects lower-extremity, weight-bearing joints such as the hips, knees, and spine. Among older adults, osteoarthritis is one of the most prevalent and disabling chronic conditions. As the percentage of adults over 65 years of age increases in future decades, an increase in the demand for therapeutic exercise programs that minimize functional limitations and help maintain joint and muscle health can be anticipated. Resistance-training programs offer a proven strategy to increase muscle strength and improve function.

The exact etiology of osteoarthritis is unknown. The progressive breakdown of joint cartilage and decreased synovial fluid results in pain during weight-bearing activities, such as walking and standing. Limitations in movement due to pain can lead to disuse and atrophy of regional muscles. Ligaments may also become more lax. Resistance training to gradually and progressively develop skeletal muscle strength can help control impact to the joints and provide significant functional benefits. Resistance-training programs have also been demonstrated to reduce symptoms of osteoarthritis.

PREVALENCE AND ECONOMIC IMPACT OF OSTEOARTHRITIS

Arthritis is an inflammatory condition of the joints characterized by pain, swelling, heat, redness, and limitation of movement. Nearly 40 million Americans, 15 percent of the United States population, have some form of arthritis (45). By the year 2020, 18.2 percent of the United States population—59.4 million people—are expected to have arthritis (45); and by the year 2030, this projection increases to 25 percent, or 67 million (36). Arthritis accounts for approximately 750,000 hospitalizations and 36 million physician visits

each year (36). These numbers can be expected to increase given the prevalence of arthritis in older adults and the aging population. Activity limitations due to arthritis currently affect approximately 7 million Americans (45). This number is expected to increase to 11.6 million by the year 2020 (45, 71) and to 25 million by the year 2030 (36).

Osteoarthritis is the most common form of arthritis, impacting approximately 21 million Americans (23), the majority of whom are over 45 years of age (1). Prevalence of osteoarthritis increases with age (2, 4, 14, 15), often affecting individuals during the peak working ages of 45 to 65 years. Osteoarthritis is equally prevalent in all ethnic and demographic groups (18, 38). An estimated 480,000 new cases of osteoarthritis are diagnosed in the United States population each year (70), and this number is expected to increase as the population ages. Among adults aged 30 or older, 6 percent reported symptomatic knee osteoarthritis, and 3 percent reported symptomatic hip osteoarthritis; severe or moderate osteoarthritis of the hip has been found to affect an estimated 3.1 percent of all individuals between the ages of 65 and 74 (48).

Osteoarthritis accounts for more dependency in walking, stair climbing, and other lower-extremity tasks than any other disease (30). In addition, osteoarthritis is the leading cause of work-related disability and the leading cause of disability in persons over 65 years of age in the United States (39). Osteoarthritis of the knees and hips is implicated in decreased physical functioning and mobility, greater risk for falls and joint dislocations, and is associated with greater social costs and disability than degenerative changes of other joints (31). Approximately 60 to 80 percent of patients with osteoarthritis experience limitations in activities due to their musculoskeletal symptoms (69).

The total annual cost of osteoarthritis in the United States is estimated at $15.5 billion (23). On an individual basis, the 6-month costs related to osteoarthritis are estimated at $2,856 excluding the cost of comorbid conditions (46). In a study in which quality of life aspects were investigated, hip patients with osteoarthritis reported quality of life as being at least as adversely affected as that reported by hemodialysis patents with anemia (44). Thus, when considering all the associated costs related to arthritis, psychological cost should be included in addition to social and economic costs.

ETIOLOGY OF OSTEOARTHRITIS

Osteoarthritis primarily affects the lower-extremity, weight-bearing joints of the hips, knees, and spine; less commonly it affects the hands, feet, elbows, and shoulders. Excessive biomechanical loading due to injury, accident, or overuse—and abnormal biomechanical properties of joint tissues such as articular cartilage, subchondral bone, or a combination of these factors—play a role in the pathogenesis of osteoarthritis; but the exact etiology of osteoarthritis is unknown. In contrast to the puffy joint swelling typically seen in rheumatoid arthritis, joint swelling in osteoarthritis is firm due to overgrowth of bone and cartilage. Osteoarthritis is characterized by the breakdown of **joint cartilage,** which acts to cushion the ends of bones. The increased release of matrix-degrading enzymes in articular cartilage may lead to morphologic changes such as pitting, fibrillation, and thinning of tissue, resulting in diminished ability to dissipate mechanical load. Once cartilage breaks down, the cushioning effect is minimal or absent, allowing bones to come in contact with each other, causing pain and loss of movement. Disability results most often when the disease affects the spine, knees, and hips. The progression of osteoarthritis varies among individuals, and although pathologic joint damage is irreversible, symptoms may be experienced intermittently. Age seems to be a dominant and unavoidable risk factor for osteoarthritis, but it is not the sole precondition. Obesity, joint injuries due to sports or work-related activities, nerve injury, lack of physical activity, and genetics are all contributing factors that may lead to increased risk of developing osteoarthritis (4).

BENEFITS OF RESISTANCE TRAINING FOR OSTEOARTHRITIS

Empirical evidence supports the role of exercise in reducing pain and disability for individuals with arthritis by improving muscle strength, stability, range of motion in joints, and improving aerobic fitness (41, 72). Since the mid 1980s, a growing number of scientific studies have been published examining the efficacy and benefits of various therapeutic exercise interventions for the management and treatment of arthritis. These studies have unanimously agreed that therapeutic exercise, including resistance training, is beneficial in the treatment and management of patients with osteoarthritis (12, 27, 41, 51-53, 61, 65).

Resistance-training programs for the treatment of arthritis have evolved over the past three decades, from conventional programs consisting of isometric resistance training and range of motion exercises to progressive programs advocating moderate- to high-intensity resistance training and aerobic conditioning. Throughout this evolution, resistance training has remained the core foundation of therapeutic exercise programs. Randomized controlled trials have shown that lower-extremity resistance training for individuals with osteoarthritis leads to significant reductions in reports of pain at rest (32, 55), pain at night (59), and pain experienced during functional activities such as walking, stair climbing, and bending (32, 52, 64).

Literature Review of Research Supporting Resistance Training for Osteoarthritis

Gains in muscle strength and in performance of activities of daily living as a result of resistance training and increased physical activity are well established. A randomized controlled trial compared 16 weeks of isometric muscle strengthening versus dynamic resistance training versus control conditions on knee functioning in patients with knee osteoarthritis (64). In the isometric group, time to descend and ascend a flight of stairs, and time to get down and up from the floor significantly increased by 16 to 23 percent. In the dynamic-resistance training group, time to descend and ascend stairs decreased by 13 to 17 percent. In a study by Huang and associates (37), individuals with osteoarthritis of the knee were randomly assigned to a control group or one of three resistance-training groups: isokinetic, isotonic, or isometric muscle strengthening. Exercises were performed three times per week for 8 weeks. Initial resistance was set at 60 percent of average peak torque and incrementally increased over 24 training sessions. Mean peak torque for knee flexion and extension in concentric and eccentric action improved significantly at the end of 8 weeks in the isokinetic and isotonic resistance-training groups, and all three training groups exhibited increased strength at the end of the training period compared to no change in the control group. Similar results were evident for improvement in gait speed, with all three resistance-training groups exhibiting significant improvements in gait speed at the end of the training period. Furthermore, results were maintained by each resistance-training group at one year.

Other studies have also demonstrated significant improvements in gait speed, gait parameters, and stair-climbing time following participation in lower-extremity resistance training (16, 28, 32). These results are consistent with the findings of several evidence-based reviews of randomized controlled trials and clinical controlled trials, which have determined that strong evidence exists to support resistance training in the treatment and management of osteoarthritis (40, 52, 58, 62).

Foley and colleagues (25) compared isometric quadriceps strength, gait speed, and distance walked in 6 minutes among three groups of adults with knee or hip osteoarthritis who were randomly assigned to one of three resistance-training programs: hydrotherapy resistance exercise, gym-based resistance exercise, or a control condition receiving no exercise. The resistance-exercise groups participated in three, 30-minute sessions

for 6 weeks. At the end of 6 weeks, mean isometric quadriceps strength was significantly improved in the resistance-exercise groups when compared with the control group, with results favoring the gym-based resistance-training group. Walking speed and distance walked were also significantly improved in both resistance-exercise groups. Other research has demonstrated that walking programs can improve gait speed (19, 49), stair-climbing time (56), and heart rate (49). Thus, resistance-training programs that incorporate functional activities may provide added benefit.

For individuals with osteoarthritis, the setting in which exercise occurs does not appear to influence outcomes; significant benefits can be realized through group or one-on-one programs (27, 41). Green and colleagues (29) reported that a clinic-based hydrotherapy program for individuals with osteoarthritis of the hip was as effective as a home-based training program. More recently, Evcik (21) found that compared to a walking intervention, a home-based resistance-training program for the quadriceps femoris muscle resulted in significantly less pain and greater function and mobility. Hakkinen and colleagues observed that patients with early rheumatoid arthritis who participated in a 2-year, home-based resistance-training program reported reduced pain and exhibited increased peak muscle strength, and these improvements were maintained 3 years after completion of the training program (33, 34, 35). Table 5-1 presents a summary of resistance-training studies for individuals with osteoarthritis.

BEHAVIORAL ISSUES AND GOAL SETTING

Individuals with osteoarthritis commonly adopt a sedentary lifestyle as a result of increased pain, reduced mobility, and loss of independence in performing activities of daily living. These factors affect physical function and can lead to distressing emotions, such as anxiety and depression. A study conducted by van Baar and colleagues found

Table 5-1 Studies Incorporating Resistance Training for Individuals with Osteoarthritis

Authors	Population Data	Exercise Program	Frequency/ Duration	Outcome Measures
Topp, et al. 2002 (64)	OA = Knee Mean age = 63 N = 102 Experimental (2) and control (1) groups	Dynamic and isometric resistance using elastic bands	3 x per week for 4 months	Pain, time to ascend/descend stairs, time to get down and up from the floor, WOMAC
Gur, et al. 2002 (32)	OA = Knee Mean age = 56 N = 23 Experimental (2) and control (1) groups	Concentric extension and flexion	3 x per week for 8 weeks	Pain, time to rise from a chair, time to ascend/descend stairs, time to walk 15 meters
O'Reilly, et al. 1999 (50)	OA = Knee Mean age = 62 N = 191 Experimental (1) and control (1) groups	Isometric or isotonic quadriceps femoris contraction in full extension	1 x per day for 6 months	Isometric quadriceps femoris strength, WOMAC, self-report health status
van Baar, et al. 1998 (65)	OA = Hip and Knee Mean age = 68 N = 191 Experimental (1) and control (1) groups	Progressive resistance exercises to increase strength and muscle length	1 to 2 x per week for 12 weeks	Pain, range of motion, hip and knee strength
Deyle, et al. 2005 (17)	OA = Knee Mean age = 64 N = 134 Clinically supervised (1) and home-exercise (1) groups	Manual therapy, range of motion, strengthening and stretching, stationary bicycle	2 to 8 supervised sessions, followed by home exercise prescription	Time to complete 6-minute walk, WOMAC

(continued)

Table 5-1 Studies Incorporating Resistance Training for Individuals with Osteoarthritis (continued)

Authors	Population Data	Exercise Program	Frequency/ Duration	Outcome Measures
Huang, et al. 2003 (37)	OA = Knee, bilateral Mean age = 62 N = 132 Experimental (3) and control (1) groups	Isotonic muscle strength, isokinetic muscle strength, isometric muscle strength	3 x per week for 8 weeks	Pain, isokinetic peak torque during flexion and extension, time to walk 50 meters, self-reported disability
Rogind, et al. 1998 (59)	OA = Knee Mean age = 71 N = 25 Experimental (1) and control (1) groups	Progressive resistance exercises, stretching, balance	6 x per week for 12 weeks (2 x per week in group setting; 4 x per week at home)	Isokinetic and isometric strength, pain, function, and gait speed
Foley, et al. 2006 (25)	OA = Hip and Knee Mean age = 71 Experimental (2) and control (1) groups	Hydrotherapy: walking, hip and knee flexion and extension, hip abduction/adduction, knee cycling Gym-based program: seated bench press, hip abduction/adduction, knee extension, and double-leg press	3 x per week for 6 weeks	Quadriceps strength, 6-minute walk, WOMAC, Adelaide Activities Profile, SF-12 Health Survey, and Arthritis Self-Efficacy Questionnaire
Evcik and Sonel 2002 (21)	OA = Knee Mean age = 56 N = 81 Experimental (2) and control (1) groups	Home program: isometric and isotonic exercises Walking program	Home exercise group: 2 x per week for 12 weeks; Walking group: 10 min, 3 x per week, gradually increased to 30 min.	Nottingham Health Profile, WOMAC, pain

Table 5-1 Studies Incorporating Resistance Training for Individuals with Osteoarthritis (continued)

Authors	Population Data	Exercise Program	Frequency/ Duration	Outcome Measures
Ettinger, et al. 1997 (21)	OA = Knee Mean age = 69 N = 103 Experimental (2) and control (1) groups	Aerobic training group: warm-up, 40 min. walking at 50–80% of HR reserve, cool down Resistance-training group: upper- and lower-body exercises using dumbbells and cuff weights	3 x per week for 18 months (3-month facility-based program followed by 15-month home program	Gait speed, cadence, stride length, and stance time

that after controlling for articular factors, muscular and psychological characteristics in patients with osteoarthritis were associated with self-reported disability (66). Individuals with osteoarthritis may not realize the health benefits that can be experienced as a result of exercise. They may also have unrealistic expectations and may need assistance in setting appropriate exercise goals. The chronic nature of osteoarthritis, and the progressive loss of independence that some individuals experience, can lead to perceived barriers to exercise. **Perceived barriers** are perceptions an individual has that psychologically prevent them from exercising. These barriers should be identified, and individuals should be encouraged to develop a personal strategy for managing barriers that prevent them from engaging in resistance training. If an individual has unrealistic perceptions of the barriers to participating in a resistance-training program, he or she may never begin such a program or may perceive any setback in exercise behavior or outcomes as an insurmountable barrier to realizing goals. An important component of any training program is educating the client at the outset on the benefits of exercise specific to the individual's health status and presentation of osteoarthritis. Exercise professionals who become

alert to statements such as "My joints feel too stiff to exercise" can help individuals overcome such a perceived barrier by addressing the benefits of training through factual statements, such as "Exercise can relieve stiffness and soreness." This can also be achieved by reshaping individual perceptions; for example, "A little soreness means your muscles are getting stronger."

Development of realistic and attainable training goals and identification of personal preferences regarding resistance training are also important factors in program design for the individual with osteoarthritis. Goals should be significant, measurable, attainable, related to the individual, and must include a time frame. Two examples of well-stated training goals for the individual with osteoarthritis are:

○ After 8 weeks of resistance training, I will be able to lift myself out of a bathtub without assistance.

○ After 10 weeks of resistance training, I will be able to climb a flight of 20 stairs in under 15 seconds with no pain.

DESIGNING RESISTANCE-TRAINING PROGRAMS FOR INDIVIDUALS WITH OSTEOARTHRITIS

As detailed earlier, randomized controlled trials have demonstrated that different types of exercise programs have the potential to reduce joint pain and improve muscle strength and function in individuals with osteoarthritis. However, two recent consensus statements are in agreement that the optimal exercise regimen for the management of osteoarthritis has yet to be determined (52, 58). A focused consensus statement (52, 58) on the evidence regarding the role of exercise in managing hip or knee osteoarthritis put forth the following recommendations based on rigorous categories of empirical evidence:

○ Both resistance training and aerobic exercise have a similar effect on reducing pain and improving function and health status in patients with knee and hip osteoarthritis.

○ To be effective, exercise programs should include advice and education to promote positive lifestyle changes that include increases in overall physical activity.

○ Group exercise and home-based exercise programs are equally effective.

○ Strategies to improve and maintain adherence to exercise regimens should be incorporated into the exercise program; these must include frequent monitoring and review and inclusion of a family member or spouse.

Interestingly, literature has failed to support a number of commonly held beliefs and recommendations made to individuals with osteoarthritis about exercise programs. Limited or no evidence is present in the literature to support the idea that weight reduction among individuals with osteoarthritis reduces pain and increases functioning, or that the severity of disease progression based upon radiographic evidence predicts the effectiveness of an exercise intervention among individuals with osteoarthritis.

Exercise Testing Considerations

A preprogram evaluation of any individual with osteoarthritis should be completed to ensure the safety of the individual as well as to collect data needed to formulate the exercise prescription. Since individuals with osteoarthritis tend to be older adults, the American College of Sports Medicine (ACSM) recommendation of a physician-supervised stress test for anyone over the age of 50 years who wants to begin a vigorous training program (3) should be followed. However, a number of factors—including progression of disease, deconditioning, muscle weakness, and joint pain (5, 6, 47)—may prohibit individuals with osteoarthritis from achieving minimal levels of exertion while completing a stress test. Because of these factors, Evans (20) recommends that if an older adult wishes to begin resistance training, a maximum exercise test may be substituted with a series of health-related questions prior to beginning a resistance-training program (20). Table 5-2 provides some sample screening questions that are appropriate for this population.

If an older adult responds "yes" to any of these questions, he or she should not begin a resistance-training program until a medical history, comprehensive physical, and medical clearance are received from a physician.

Individuals with osteoarthritis will exhibit varying degrees of disease progression, deconditioning, muscle weakness, and joint pain, and they should be individually assessed in terms of their capacity to engage in resistance training. After obtaining medical clearance, capacity for engaging in resistance training should be determined before prescribing resistance training. Capacity to engage in resistance

Table 5-2 Screening Questions for Resistance Training (20)

If the individual responds "yes" to any of the following questions, medical clearance from a physician is needed before beginning a resistance-training program.

1. Do you get chest pains while at rest and/or during exertion?
2. Have you ever had a heart attack?
3. Do you have high blood pressure?
4. Are you short of breath after extremely mild exertion and sometimes even at rest or at night in bed?
5. Do you have any ulcerated wounds or cuts on your feet that do not seem to heal?
6. Have you lost 10 or more pounds in the past 6 months without trying?
7. Do you get pain in your buttocks or the back of your legs, thighs, or calves when you walk?
8. While at rest, do you frequently experience fast, irregular heartbeats or, at the other extreme, very slow beats?
9. Are you currently being treated for any heart or circulatory condition, such as vascular disease, stroke, angina, hypertension, congestive heart failure, poor circulation in the legs, heart valve disease, blood clots, or pulmonary disease?
10. Have you fallen more than twice in the past year (no matter what the reason)?
11. Do you have diabetes?

Source: Evans WJ. Exercise training guidelines for the elderly. *Med Sci Sports Exerc.* 1999;31:12-17

training is commonly assessed using a 1RM strength assessment (8). Testing can be completed for any resistance-training exercise that involves isotonic resistance training, including weight machines, free weights, or progressive resistance devices such as elastic bands. Once the preprogram evaluation has been completed, an exercise prescription can be developed for the individual.

Exercise Training Considerations

The objective of a resistance-training program for individuals with osteoarthritis is to reduce pain in the affected joints and improve muscle strength and functional ability. Physical activity has also been shown to reduce medical costs (68). Despite these benefits, many arthritic patients remain physically inactive. Data from the Centers for Disease Control and Prevention's Behavioral Risk Factor Surveillance Survey (BRFSS)

indicates that nearly 62 percent of U.S. adults with arthritis are either physically inactive or engage in insufficient levels of physical activity (26).

The most important factor to consider when designing resistance-training programs for individuals with osteoarthritis is that of individual variation in the manifestation of joint pain, restricted range of motion, muscle weakness, and endurance. The pathology of osteoarthritis results in deterioration of the articular cartilage, which stimulates increased bone growth and results in pain with and following use. This pain results in disuse of the joint and atrophy of the contractile tissue surrounding the joint. Thus, care should be taken when prescribing resistance training for individuals with osteoarthritis to avoid further injuring the affected joints through compressive or shearing forces introduced during training.

A resistance-training program must be flexible in accommodating individual needs based on the joints involved and the health and exercise status of each individual. Although moderate-intensity physical activities—such as walking, swimming, and bicycling—are gentle to the joints and can be performed on a regular basis by individuals with osteoarthritis, the frequency, duration, and intensity will vary among individuals. Identifying present and past fitness activity levels may assist in identifying modes of training the individual may or may not be likely to comply with in the future. For example, an adult who has led an active lifestyle and participated in exercise training may be more compliant with resistance training.

Program Components and Exercise Selection

In individuals with osteoarthritis, muscles adapt to resistance training in a manner similar to healthy younger adults (42). Resistance training for individuals with osteoarthritis may include concentric, muscle-shortening actions; eccentric, muscle-lengthening actions; and isometric actions that produce no change in muscle length. Of these three, eccentric actions produce the greatest maximal torques, and concentric actions produce the lowest maximal torques. As presented in Chapters 1 and 2, these actions can be further divided into closed- and open-chain exercises. Closed-chain exercises involve movements in which the distal segment is relatively fixed, such as squats or push-ups; open-chain exercises involve movements in which the distal segment is relatively free to move, such as seated knee extensions or lateral dumbbell raises. In regard to the individual with osteoarthritis, **joint compression** forces tend to be higher during weight-bearing, closed-chain exercises, and **shear forces** tend to be higher with open-chain exercises. Joint compression occurs when two joints are pressed into one another, causing the anatomical space between them to decrease. Shear forces are found during the movement of joints, especially when bones move across each other in a sliding motion.

A combination of open- and closed-chain exercises within a pain-free range of motion for individuals with osteoarthritis is recommended. Using the knee joint as an example, the open-chain seated knee extension tends to increase shear forces over the last 30 degrees of extension, and the closed-chain squat movement tends to increase patellar–femoral joint compression forces as the knee approaches 90 degrees of flexion. Selecting an exercise range of motion that avoids excessive shear or compression forces is essential. Therefore, resisted seated knee extensions should not be performed through the last 30 degrees of the extension range by individuals with osteoarthritis, particularly if they are experiencing knee pain or discomfort. Similarly, squats should not be performed deeper than 90 degrees of knee flexion.

Another approach to minimizing compression and shear forces in the joint during resistance training is to introduce isometric exercises. Isometric exercises require the individual to maintain a fixed joint angle while increasing the tension in the involved muscle over 5 to 8 seconds. Isometric exercises require the muscle to generate maximal tension while not changing in length during the training. Thus, the capacity to engage in isometric resistance training includes generating maximal muscle tension at a specific joint angle that is unaffected by pain and not restricted by limited range of motion during the muscle contraction. By flexing the extensors and flexors of a joint in a non–weight-bearing position, muscle activation can be maximized, and joint compression and shearing forces can be kept to a minimum. The limitation of isometric resistance training is that strength gains are found only at the joint angle at which the training takes place. This concept is commonly termed **joint-angle specificity** (24). Isometric exercises may be introduced at the joint angle that results in pain from joint compression or shearing forces during isotonic resistance training.

By combining open- and closed-chain isotonic exercises with isometric exercises, an effective resistance-training program can be developed to achieve individual training goals. The activities stated as goals should be consistent with the muscle actions articulated in the resistance-training prescription. For example, if the training goal involves going down stairs, the prescription should involve eccentric exercises of the quadriceps and hamstrings focusing on the range of motion involved with this activity.

As discussed in Chapter 1, load and volume components of a resistance-training program are critical components that promote the neuromuscular adaptations associated with resistance training for osteoarthritis. **Load** refers to the amount of weight assigned to an exercise set, and it is probably the most important variable in resistance-training program design (7). Rhea and colleagues (57) conducted a meta-analysis and concluded that among untrained and trained individuals, an 8 to 12 repetition maximum elicited the greatest gains in strength, and multiple sets of an exercise resulted in superior gains in strength compared to a single set of the exercise. Multiple sets of 8RM to 12RM of a resistance-training exercise may be difficult for an untrained individual with osteoarthritis to attain initially, although numerous investigators have designed resistance-training programs that progress individuals to this volume of training after 4 to 8 weeks.

Specific exercises can be classified as either single- or multiple-joint exercises. Single-joint exercises isolate a specific muscle group and are generally safer for individuals with osteoarthritis, because they require less coordination. However, single-joint exercises produce slower gains in strength, because fewer muscles are involved in the exercise, and less resistance can be prescribed (42). Multiple-joint exercises place more demands on the nervous system to coordinate the movement and are considered more effective at increasing overall body strength, because they enable greater weights to be lifted (3). A majority of functional tasks do not involve the movement of a single joint. If the training goal includes a functional task, such as stair climbing or carrying a laundry basket, single-joint exercises do not conform well to the training principle of specificity. Depending on initial ability, the individual with osteoarthritis may be unable to perform a multiple-joint exercise and may need to train using single-joint exercises until sufficient strength and neuromuscular adaptations

allow them to engage in the multiple-joint exercise. Thus, a resistance-training program for individuals with osteoarthritis should include exercises specific to the fitness goals of the individual. If these goals include functional tasks, then the prescription should progress the individual to engage in multiple-joint exercises that train the muscles involved in the particular functional task.

The sequence of the resistance exercises performed during a single training session should maximize the training stimulus while minimizing fatigue. For individuals with osteoarthritis, it is recommended that a session of resistance training begin with multiple-joint movements involving large muscle groups first, followed by single-joint exercises or exercises that involve small muscle groups with 3 to 5 minutes rest between sets. The effectiveness of this sequencing has been validated by Sforzo and Touey, who report that 25 percent greater loads could be lifted when training order progressed from large muscle mass to small muscle mass exercises (60). Performing large muscle, multiple-joint exercises early in the session has been found to significantly elevate anabolic hormones and may facilitate greater gains in strength among small muscle groups (43, 67).

Frequency of training will also affect the rate at which training goals are attained. The duration of time between sessions must be sufficient to allow for muscular adaptation and recuperation while minimizing the potential for injury due to overtraining (10). A number of previous investigators have reported the benefits of resistance-training frequencies, ranging from one to seven times per week, in eliciting gains in strength and functioning among individuals with osteoarthritis (9, 17, 50, 63). However, these empirical studies do not provide a clear consensus on the optimal frequency of resistance training for individuals with osteoarthritis; thus, resistance-training frequency guidelines for the general population may also be appropriate for individuals with osteoarthritis. Feigenbaum and Pollock (22) conducted a review of the literature and recommended that resistance training be performed 2 days per week. This frequency of training results in 80 to 90 percent of the gains in strength of more frequent training programs (11, 13, 54), is less time consuming, and may reduce the chance of injury and increase adherence to the program (10). Two days per week appears to be the appropriate frequency for resistance training for trained individuals, but untrained individuals respond more favorably to a training frequency of 3 days per week (54). Based on these studies, 3 days per week of resistance training is recommended for individuals with osteoarthritis who are beginning a resistance-training program. Once training goals are achieved, frequency can be decreased to 2 days per week for a maintenance program.

Table 5-3 summarizes the exercise program components, and Table 5-4 provides a sample of resistance-training exercises for patients with hip and knee osteoarthritis.

Osteoarthritis of the upper extremities is a relatively infrequent disorder compared to osteoarthritis of the lower extremities. To date, no exercises for the upper extremities have been developed and empirically tested, and thus it is premature to make unfounded exercise recommendations for individuals with upper-extremity osteoarthritis.

SAMPLE 24-WEEK PROGRAM

The sample 24-week resistance-training program outlined here provides a template for developing a resistance-training program for individuals with osteoarthritis in hip, knee, and ankle joints.

Table 5-3 Exercise Program Components for Individuals with Osteoarthritis

Factor	Initial Prescription	Target Prescription
Muscle action	Consistent with fitness goals Minimize shear and compression forces Minimize motion which causes pain Open/closed chain Isotonic/isometric	Consistent with fitness goals Minimize shear and compression forces Minimize motion which causes pain Open/closed chain Isotonic/isometric
Loading and volume	- 8–12 repetitions, 1 set - 60–70% 1RM - 6–7 (Borg 10-point scale)	8–12 repetitions 1 set for maintenance 2–3 sets for improvement 70–80% 1RM 7–8 (Borg 10-point scale)
Exercise selection and order	Consistent with fitness goals Large muscle groups and multiple-joint exercises first Small muscle groups and single-joint exercises last	Consistent with fitness goals Large muscle groups and multiple-joint exercises first -Small muscle groups and single-joint exercises last
Rest periods	- 5 minutes between sets	- 2 minutes between sets
Frequency	- 3 times per week	- 2 times per week for maintenance - 3 times per week for improvement

Table 5-4 Resistance-Training Exercises for Knee and Hip Osteoarthritis

Exercise	Techniques Specific to Knee and Hip OA	Potential Fitness Goal
Chair squat	Avoid flexing knee over 100° Avoid flexing hip over 100° Avoid bending over while rising from a chair Avoid dropping into chair May need to initially use arms to rise and control descent into chair	Rising and descending from a chair Ascending and descending stairs Knee movement with reduced pain
One-leg squats on stairs	Avoid flexing involved knee over 45° May need to initially use arms for support	Ascending and descending stairs
Standing hamstring curls	Use arms for support Only flex the lower leg; do not flex at the waist or hip Flex knee to 90°	Ambulating Standing for extended periods
Hip flexion Hip extension	Avoid hip flexion beyond 90°	Ambulation Hip movement with reduced pain
Hip abduction Hip adduction	Maintain balance with hand supports	Lateral ambulation
Ankle dorsi flexion	Exercise through the entire range of motion	Postural stability and balance
Ankle plantar flexion	Exercise through the entire range of motion	Postural stability and balance
Seated sit-ups	Focus on contracting abdomen muscles; do not raise feet or legs higher than 6 inches	Core stability Hip flexors

Weeks 1 through 2

Preprogram evaluation should be followed by a training frequency of three times per week with at least one rest day between training days. Use a resistance that produces an intensity rating of 6 to 7 (somewhat hard) out of 10 on the Borg scale. Complete one set of 8 to 12 repetitions of the following exercises: chair squats, one-leg squats on stairs, standing hamstring curls, hip flexion/ extension, hip abduction/adduction, ankle dorsi/ plantar flexion, and seated sit-ups. Rest 5 minutes between sets.

Weeks 3 through 8

Continue a frequency of three times per week with at least one rest day between training days, using a resistance that produces a rating of 8 (hard) on the Borg scale. Attempt to increase resistance during weeks 3 and 6. Increase volume to 1 set of 12 repetitions.

Weeks 9 through 24

Continue a frequency of three times per week with at least one rest day between training days. Increase intensity to a resistance that produces a rating of 8 to 9 (hard to very hard) on the Borg scale. Increase resistance during week 9 and every 3 weeks thereafter. Volume is increased to 2 sets of 8 to 12 repetitions.

CASE STUDY

Mrs. T is a 62-year-old female with osteoarthritis of the right knee. She is 159 cm tall, weighs 82.7 kg, and has a BMI of 33. She does not participate in any form of regular exercise and has been scheduled for total knee replacement in 5 weeks. Her orthopedic surgeon has recommended that she participate in a prehabilitation resistance-training program to improve her strength, flexibility, and functioning prior to surgery, thus improving her outcomes during recovery and rehabilitation.

Mrs. T participated in three exercise sessions per week for 4 weeks, for a total of 12 sessions. Each session consisted of 10 minutes of warm-up exercises, such as walking and static stretching; 30 minutes of resistance-training exercises, including nine lower-body exercises, a minimum of 1 set of 10 repetitions with resistance bands; 10 minutes of step training, with a minimum of 1 set of 8 repetitions that included forward, backward, and lateral movements, with the step height increased progressively; and 5 minutes of light static stretching for cooling down. One session per week was supervised by an exercise professional and performed at an exercise facility. This supervised session allowed reinforcement of proper form and progression of sets and repetitions as needed. Resistance was progressively increased through a selection of heavier resistance bands. The remaining two sessions of each week were performed at home. Mrs. T was asked to keep an exercise log to monitor her compliance and progress.

Over 12 sessions, Mrs. T demonstrated a 14 percent decrease in the amount of time required to complete a 6-minute walk, and an improvement of 33 percent was observed in the 30-second sit-to-stand exercise. She also reported that she felt less pain and substantially less stiffness in her knee as a result of participating in the program. Overall physical function also improved, and she expressed that she felt stronger

and had more energy and less pain. These positive health changes were obtained without making any alterations to her diet or pharmacological regimen.

Summary

Osteoarthritis is a chronic condition associated with aging. As the aging population continues to increase, osteoarthritis and associated comorbidities will increase in prevalence. Various types of resistance-training programs have been demonstrated to significantly reduce the symptoms of osteoarthritis, increase strength, and maximize independence in performance of activities of daily living.

This chapter has presented factors that are critical to consider when developing a resistance-training program for individuals with osteoarthritis. One of the most important elements of any training program is assessment of the individual and development of a tailored exercise program adapted to the individual's health status and training goals.

Key Terms

Arthritis
Joint-angle specificity
Joint cartilage
Joint compression
Load
Osteoarthritis
Perceived barriers
Shear forces

Study Questions

1. What is the prevalence of lower-extremity osteoarthritis and its associated economic impact?

2. What is the etiology and progression of osteoarthritis?

3. What effect does physical activity and exercise have in regulating the symptoms and progression of osteoarthritis?

4. What is the relationship between decline in muscle strength and progression of osteoarthritis?

5. What are the key components of a resistance-training program for individuals with osteoarthritis?

References

1. Ades, PA, Savage, PD, Cress ME, Brochu M, Lee NM, Poehlman ET. Resistance training on physical performance in disabled older female cardiac patients. *Med Sci Sports Exerc.* 2003;35(8):1265-1270.

2. American College of Rheumatology. *Clinical Care in the Rheumatic Diseases.* Atlanta, GA: Wagener T; 1996.

3. American College of Sports Medicine. *Guidelines for Exercise Testing and Prescription.* 6th ed. Baltimore, MD: Williams and Wilkins; 2000.

4. Arthritis Foundation. *Osteoarthritis fact sheet, 2005.* Available at: http://www.arthritis.org/conditions/fact_sheets/oa_fact_sheet.asp.

5. Astrand PO. Aerobic work capacity in men and women with special reference to age. *Acta Physiol Scand.* 1960;49:1-12.

6. Astrand PO. Physical performance as a function of age. *JAMA.* 1968;205(11):729-733.

7. Baechle, TR, Earle RW, Wathen D. Resistance training. In *Essentials of Strength Training and Conditioning.* Baechle TR, Earle RW (Eds.) 2nd ed. Champaign, IL: Human Kinetics; 2000.

8. Baechle TR. *Essentials of Strength and Conditioning.* 1st ed. Champaign, IL: Human Kinetics; 1994.

9. Baker KR, Nelson ME, Felson DT, Layne JE, Sarno R, Roubenoff R. The efficacy of home-based progressive strength training in older adults with knee osteoarthritis: A randomized controlled trial. *J Rheumatol.* 2001;28: 1655-1665.

10. Bird SP, Tarpenning KM, Marino FE. Designing resistance training programmes to enhance muscular fitness: A review of the acute programme variables. *Sports Med.* 2005;35(10):841-851.

11. Braith RW, Graves JE, Pollock ML, Leggett SL, Carpenter DM, Colvin AB. Comparison of 2 vs 3 days/week of variable resistance training during 10- and 18-week programs. *Int J Sports Med.* 1989;10(6):450-454.

12. Brosseau L, Pelland L, Casimiro L. Efficacy of fitness exercise for osteoarthritis, part II: A meta-ananlysis. *Phys Ther Rev.* 2004;10:125-131.

13. Caroll TJ, Abernathy PJ, Logan PA, Barber M, McEniery MT. Resistance training frequency: Strength and myosin heavy chain responses to two and three bouts per week. *Eur J Appl Physiol.* 1998;78(3):270-275.

14. Centers for Disease Control and Prevention. Arthritis prevalence and activity limitations— United States, 1990. In *Morb. Mortal. Wkly Rep.* 1994, June 24;43(24):433-438.

15. Centers for Disease Control and Prevention. Prevalence of disabilities and associated health conditions among adults—United States, 1999. In *Morb. Mortal. Wkly Rep.* 1999;48:120-125.

16. Deyle GD, Allison SC, Matekel RL, et al. Physical therapy treatment effectiveness for osteoarthritis of the knee: A randomized comparison of supervised clinical exercise and manual therapy procedures versus a home exercise program. *Phys Ther.* 2005;85(12):1301-1317.

17. Deyle GD, Henderson NE, Matekel RL, Ryder MG, Garber MB, Allison SC. Effectiveness of manual physical therapy and exercise in osteoarthritis of the knee: A randomized, controlled trial. *Ann Intern Med.* 2000;132:173-181.

18. Dominick KL, Baker TA. Racial and ethnic differences in osteoarthritis: Prevalence, outcomes, and medical care. *Ethn Dis.* 2004;14(4):558-566.

19. Ettinger WH, Burns R, Messier SP, et al. A randomized trial comparing aerobic exercise and resistance exercise with a health education program in older adults with knee

osteoarthritis: The Fitness Arthritis and Seniors Trial (FAST). *JAMA*. 1997;277(1):25-31.

20. Evans WJ. Exercise training guidelines for the elderly. *Med Sci Sports Exerc*. 1999;31:12-17.

21. Evcik D, Sonel B. Effectiveness of a home-based exercise therapy and walking program on osteoarthritis of the knee. *Rheumatol Int*. 2002;22(3):103-106.

22. Feigenbaum MS, Pollock ML. Prescription of resistance training for health and disease. *Med Sci Sports Exerc*. 1999;31(1):38-45.

23. Felson D, Zhang Y. An update on the epidemiology of knee and hip osteoarthritis with a view to prevention. *Arthritis Rheum*. 1998;41(8):1343-1355.

24. Fleck SJ, Kraemer WJ. *Designing resistance training programs*. Champaign, IL: Human Kinetics; 2004.

25. Foley A, Halbert J, Hewitt T, Crotty M. Does hydrotherapy improve strength and physical function in patients with osteoarthritis? A randomized controlled trial comparing a gym-based and a hydrotherapy-based strengthening programme. *Ann Rheum Dis*. 2003;62(12):1162-1167.

26. Fontaine KR, Heo M, Bathon J. Are US adults with arthritis meeting public health recommendations for physical activity? *Arthritis Rheum*. 2004;50(2):624-628.

27. Fransen M, McConnell S, Bell M. Exercise for osteoarthritis of the hip or knee. *Cochrane Database Syst Rev* 2003;(3):CD4286 Review.

28. Fransen M, Crosbie J, Edmonds J. Physical therapy is effective for patients with osteoarthritis of the knee: A randomized controlled clinical trial. *J Rheumatol*. 2001;28(1):156-164.

29. Green J, McKenna F, Redfern EJ, Chamberlein MA. Home exercises are as effective as outpatient hydrotherapy for osteoarthritis of the hip. *Br J Rheumatol*. 1993;32:812-815.

30. Guccione AA, Felson DT, Anderson JJ, Anthony JM, Zhang Y, Wilson PW. The effects of specific medical conditions on functional limitations of elders in the Framingham Study. *Am J Public Health*. 1994;84:351-358.

31. Gunther KP, Sturmer T, Sauerland S, et al. Prevalence of generalized osteoarthritis in patients with advanced hip and knee osteoarthritis: The Ulm Osteoarthritis Study. *Ann Rheum Dis*. 1998;57:717-723.

32. Gur H, Cakin N, Akova B, Okay E, Kucukoglu S. Concentric versus combined concentric-eccentric isokinetic training: Effects on functional capacity and symptoms in patients with osteoarthrosis of the knee. *Arch Phys Med Rehabil*. 2002;83(3):308-316.

33. Hakkinen A. Effectiveness and safety of strength training in rheumatoid arthritis. *Curr Opin Rheumatol*. 2004;16(2):132-137.

34. Hakkinen A, Sokka T, Hannonen P. A home-based two-year strength training period in early rheumatoid arthritis led to good long-term compliance: A 5-year follow-up. *Arthritis Rheum*. 2004;15;51(1):56-62.

35. Hakkinen A, Sokka T, Kautiainen H, Kotaniemi A, Hannonen P. Sustained maintenance of exercise-induced muscle strength gains and normal bone mineral density in patients with early rheumatoid arthritis: A 5-year follow up. *Ann Rheum Dis*. 2004;63(8):910-916.

36. Hootman JM, Helmick CG. Projections of US prevalence of arthritis and associated activity limitations. *Arthritis Rheum*. 2006;54(1):226-229.

37. Huang MH, Lin YS, Yang RC, Lee CL. A comparison of various therapeutic exercises on the functional status of patients with knee osteoarthritis. *Semin Arthritis Rheum*. 2003;32(6):398-406.

38. Ibrahim SA, Siminoff LA, Burant CJ, Kwoh CK. Variation in perceptions of treatment and self-care practices in elderly with osteoarthritis: a comparison between African-American

and white patients. *Arthritis Care Res.* 2001;45:340-345.

39. Jones ML, Sanford J. People with mobility impairments in the United States today and in 2010. *Assist Technol.* 1996;8:43-53.

40. Jordan KM, Arden NK, Doherty M, et al. EU-LAR Recommendations 2003: An evidence-based approach to the management of knee osteoarthritis: Report of a task force of the Standing Committee for International Clinical Studies Including Therapeutic Trials (ESCISIT). *Ann Rheum Dis.* 2003;62(12):1145-1155.

41. Kettunen JA, Kujala UM. Exercise therapy for people with rheumatoid arthritis and osteoarthritis. *J Med Sci Sports.* 2004;14:138-142.

42. Kraemer WJ, Adams K, Cafarelli E, et al. American College of Sports Medicine position stand: Progression models in resistance training for healthy adults. *Med Sci Sports Exerc.* 2002;34(2):364-380.

43. Kraemer WJ, Ratamess NA. Endocrine responses and adaptations to strength and power training. In *Strength and Power in Sport.* 2nd ed. Komi PV (Ed.) Oxford, England: Blackwell Science Ltd; 2003.

44. Laupacis A, Bourne R, Rorabeck C, et al. The effect of elective total hip replacement on health-related quality of life. *J Bone Joint Surg Am.* 1993;75A(11):1619-1626.

45. Lawrence RC, Helmick CJ, Arnett FC, et al. Estimates of the prevalence of arthritis and selected musculoskeletal disorders in the United States. *Arthritis Rheum.* 1998;41(5):778-799.

46. Maetzel A, Li LC, Pencharz J, Tomlinson F, Bombardier C. The economic burden associated with osteoarthritis, rheumatoid arthritis, and hypertension: A comparative study. *Ann Rheum Dis.* 2004;63(4):395-401.

47. Martinez-Caro D, Alegria E, Lorente D, Azpilicueta J, Calabuig J, Ancin R. Diagnostic value of stress testing in the elderly. *Eur Heart J.* 1984;11(5)suppl:E63-E67.

48. Minor MA. Exercise in the management of osteoarthritis of the knee and hip. *Arthritis Care Res.* 1994;7(4):198-204.

49. Minor MA, Hewett JE, Webel RR, Anderson SK, Kay DR. Efficacy of physical conditioning exercise in patients with rheumatoid arthritis and osteoarthritis. *Arthritis Rheum.* 1989;32(11):1396-1405.

50. O'Reilly SC, Muir KR, Doherty M. Effectiveness of home exercise on pain and disability from osteoarthritis of the knee: A randomised controlled trial. *Ann Rheum Dis.* 1999;58(1):15-19.

51. Ottawa Panel. Ottawa panel evidence-based clinical practice guidelines for therapeutic exercises and manual therapy in the management of rheumatoid arthritis. *Phys Ther.* 2004;84(10):934-972.

52. Ottawa Panel. Ottawa panel evidence-based clinical practice guidelines for therapeutic exercises and manual therapy in the management of osteoarthritis. *Phys Ther.* 2005;85(9):907-917.

53. Pelland L, Brosseau L, Casimiro L. Efficacy of strengthening exercise for osteoarthritis, part I: a meta-analysis. *Phys Ther Rev.* 2004;9:77-108.

54. Peterson MD, Rhea MR, Alvar BA. Applications of the dose-response for muscular strength development: A review of meta-analytic efficacy and reliability for designing training prescription. *J Strength Cond Res.* 2005;19(4):950-958.

55. Pettrella RJ. Is exercise effective treatment for osteoarthritis of the knee? *Br J Sports Med.* 2000;34(5):326-331.

56. Rejeski WJ, Ettinger WH, Martin K, Morgan T. Treating disability in knee osteoarthritis with exercise therapy: A central role for self-efficacy and pain. *Arthritis Care & Res.* 1998;11(2):94-101.

57. Rhea MR, Alvar BA, Burkett LN, et al. A meta-analysis to determine the dose response for strength development. *Med Sci Sports Exerc.* 2003;35:456-464.

58. Roddy E, Zhang W, Doherty M., et al. Evidence-based recommendations for the role

of exercise in the management of osteoarthritis of the hip or knee–the MOVE consensus. *Rheumatology.* 2005;44(1):67-73.

59. Rogind H, Bibow-Nielsen B, Jensen B, Moller HC, Frimodt-Moller H, Bliddal H. The effects of a physical training program on patients with osteoarthritis of the knees. *Arch Phys Med Rehabil.* 1998;79(11):1421-1427.

60. Sforzo GA, Touey PR. Manipulating exercise order affects muscular performance during resistance exercise training. *J Strength Cond Res.* 1996;10:20-24.

61. Stenstrom CH, Minor MA. Evidence for the benefit of aerobic and strengthening exercise in rheumatoid arthritis. *Arthritis Rheum.* 2003;49(3):428-434.

62. Taylor NF, Dodd KJ, Damiano DL. Progressive resistance exercise in physical therapy: a summary of systematic reviews. *Phys Ther.* 2005;85(11):1208-1223.

63. Thomas KS, Muir KR, Doherty M, Jones AC, O'Reilly SC, Bassey EJ. Home-based exercise programme for knee pain and knee osteoarthritis: Randomized controlled trial. *BMJ.* 2002;325(7367):752.

64. Topp R, Woolley S, Hornyak J, Khuder S, Kahaleh B. The effect of dynamic versus isometric resistance training on pain and functioning among adults with osteoarthritis of the knee. *Arch Phys Med Rehabil.* 2002;83(9):1187-1195.

65. van Baar ME, Assendelft WJJ, Dekker J, Oostendorp RA, Bijlsma JW. Effectiveness of exercise therapy in patients with osteoarthritis of the hip or knee: A systematic review of randomized clinical trials. *Arthritis Rheum.* 1999;42:1361-1369.

66. van Baar ME, Dekker J, Oostendorp RA, et al. The effectiveness of exercise therapy in patients with osteoarthritis of the hip or knee: A randomized clinical trial. *J Rheumatol.* 1998;25(12):2432-2439.

67. Volek JS, Kraemer WJ, Bush JA, et al. Testosterone and cortisol in relationship to dietary nutrients and resistance exercise. *J Appl Physiol.* 1997;82:49-54.

68. Wang G, Helmick CG, Macera C, Zhang P, Pratt M. Inactivity-associated medical costs among US adults with arthritis. *Arthritis Rheum.* 2001;45:439-445.

69. Stein CM, Griffin MR, Brandt KD. Osteoarthritis. In *Clinical Care in the Rheumatic Diseases.* Wegner ST, Gall EP (Eds) Atlanta, GA: American College of Rheumatology; 1996.

70. Wilson MG, Michet CJ, Istrum DM, Melton LJ. Idiopathic symptomatic osteoarthritis of the hip and knees: A population-based incidence study. Mayo Clin Proc. 1990 Sep;65(9): 1214-1221.

71. Yelin E, Callahan LF. The economic cost and social and psychological impact of musculoskeletal conditions. National Arthritis Data Work Groups. Arthritis Rheum. 1995;38(10): 1351-1362.

72. Zinna EM, Yarasheski YE. Exercise treatment to counteract protein wasting of chronic diseases. *Curr Opin Clin Nutr Metab Care.* 2003;6:87-93.

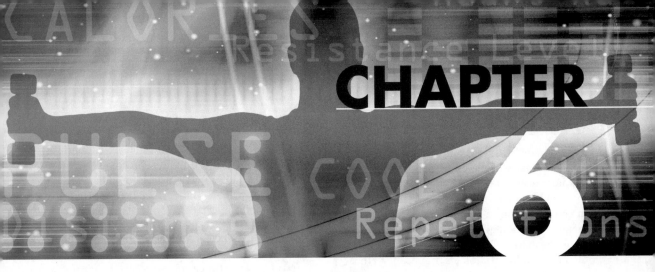

CHAPTER 6

RESISTANCE-TRAINING STRATEGIES FOR INDIVIDUALS WITH LOW BACK PAIN

Objectives

Upon completion of this chapter, the reader should be able to:

- Identify the prevalence of low back pain in the United States and the associated economic cost of this condition
- State the etiology of low back pain, including the numerous pathologic conditions that may cause it
- Explain the current research and limitations of research evaluating the impact of resistance training on low back pain
- Discuss the role of resistance training in the treatment of low back pain
- Identify the different methods of resistance training and understand special considerations to enhance participant safety during exercise testing and training
- Describe program variables used in the design and periodization of a resistance-training program for individuals with low back pain
- Design a safe, effective, and appropriate resistance-training program for individuals with low back pain

INTRODUCTION

An estimated 500 anatomic sites in the back can cause pain, dysfunction, and disability. This chapter focuses primarily on nonspecific acute **low back pain,** a complex and misunderstood interaction of physical, social, and psychological factors (53). Although exercise is used extensively in the treatment of low back pain during physical therapy, significant debate surrounds the efficacy, effectiveness, and timeliness of treating low back pain with exercise (24, 25, 53). Many of the different approaches to the treatment of low back pain, and the results achieved, are due in part to the use of exercise as a modality in the treatment of acute, subacute, or chronic low back pain. This chapter will present the latest research in the use of resistance training and exercise techniques that may impact the overwhelming problem of low back pain. The chapter will not address the acute exercise therapy that may be effective in treating the initial low back injury, but rather it will focus on resistance-training exercise that can be safely and effectively used with those individuals who have chronic low back pain. As with any medical condition, individuals diagnosed with low back pain should see their physician prior to starting a resistance-training program to be sure that the demands of the exercise program will not cause any additional complications. Of all the conditions described in this text, resistance training can probably cause more harm than good if performed incorrectly by individuals who suffer from chronic low back pain.

PREVALENCE AND ECONOMIC IMPACT OF LOW BACK PAIN

Low back pain affects over 80 percent of the people in the world at some point in their lives (18, 50, 63). At any given time, over 35 percent of the population suffers from some form of low back pain dysfunction (50), and the average adult can expect between one to three episodes of low back pain

every year (53). The rate of increase in low back pain is 14 times greater than the population growth (19). As many as 15 percent of individuals with low back pain will have their dysfunction progress to a permanent disability, and 60 percent of individuals with low back pain will suffer from a recurrence of their pain within 1 year (50).

The prognosis for people with acute low back pain is usually good. **Acute low back pain** is defined as activity intolerance of less than 3 months duration due to pain in the low back (63). Almost 90 percent of people with acute low back pain will recover to their previous level of activities of daily living within 1 month (8, 63). Because of this fact, the implementation of an exercise and resistance-training program after the initial acute low back pain subsides has been shown to not only reduce the incidence of low back pain but also to reduce the intensity of the pain (39, 43, 55).

Low back pain is the most expensive disorder to treat and is the most common cause of disability for Americans under the age of 45 (8). Frymoyer and Gordon (18) and Luo and colleagues (40) reported that between $60 billion to $90 billion is spent each year treating low back pain, and over $27 billion is spent related to permanent disability.

ETIOLOGY OF LOW BACK PAIN

When the number of joints, ligaments, muscles, tendons, fascia, vasculature, cartilage, articular surfaces, and vertebral bodies are taken into consideration, the potential etiology of low back pain is difficult to comprehend. One of the most significant factors in the prevalence of low back pain is improper movement or body mechanics. For a great number of people who experience low back pain, the initial injury is due to an improper movement and, most often, a series of repetitive improper movements or mechanics rather than a single traumatic event (8, 38, 44, 50, 63). For most people with low back pain, a combination of two or more defective structures results in the sensation of pain (44, 50, 53). Zusman (73) reports that until the defective structure has been corrected, normal function is impossible and may even be dangerous.

A recent review, as well as other studies of low back pain (1, 37, 51, 52, 63), found two primary functional deficits related to low back pain: weakness of the trunk musculature and compromised **proprioceptive acuity,** or limited awareness of body position. Norris (49, 50) describes the consequences of muscle imbalance between the abdominals and back extensors, and the body's attempt to compensate for these muscle imbalances, as a major cause of disability. A third complication of low back pain is muscle adaptation to injury and immobilization (44, 49, 50, 53, 57). Finally, once an individual recovers from a low back injury, the back is more susceptible to reinjury while performing even the simplest activities of daily living (26, 38, 42, 55, 60).

Symptoms of low back pain include localized or generalized pain of variable duration, frequency, and intensity. The pain may also radiate along the course of the particular nerve that is irritated by some particular pathologic condition (44, 50). Associated symptoms that include weakness, numbness, or other sensory changes in the lower extremities may be due to a specific pathology (50).

There are several risk factors that may exacerbate low back pain. Poor muscular endurance of the back extensor muscles, decreased flexibility of the back and lower extremities, decreased low back and abdominal muscle strength, obesity, sedentary occupations, improper body mechanics during occupational and recreational activities, and prolonged sitting are all common risk factors that may cause low back pain (2, 7, 25, 31, 44, 50). These risk factors occur over time and are part of the reason for the high incidence of low back pain in people over 30 years of age (33, 38, 41, 43).

If low back pain is caused by structural deformities—such as a herniated intervertebral disc or a **spondylolysis** or **spondylolisthesis,** a shifting of the vertebral bodies—the exercise program must be

carefully monitored, and it may not be appropriate to exercise at all until the structural deformity is corrected, either by physical therapy or surgery. By far the most common treatment for low back pain is rest, although recent studies have suggested that prolonged rest may actually increase the severity of low back pain (67). Medications, including injections, are also used in conjunction with carefully designed exercise programs to help relieve the symptoms. For most people, the last resort when all other conservative treatments fail is surgery (44, 69). Waddell (69) found that surgery was only effective in a very small group of patients with low back pain. However, surgical techniques are improving constantly, utilizing less invasive techniques that alter fewer structures, and the results of these newer techniques are very promising (44, 53, 56).

If an individual does require surgical intervention for the relief of low back pain, he or she will need to undergo an extensive rehabilitation program prior to beginning resistance training. Those individuals may also need to utilize a back brace for a prolonged period of time after surgery. When this is the case, the back brace may actually cause the individual to lose more of the abdominal and back extensor strength and muscular endurance (46, 57, 59), because the brace acts to limit movement to the surgically corrected area to allow for proper healing. This limited motion results in the trunk musculature becoming weaker as the brace replaces the muscle in controlling the spine during activities of daily living (46, 59). In fact, Reddell (57) has shown that baggage handlers had a greater risk of injury if they stopped using a back brace belt after wearing one for some time. One of the systems that the back brace or lifting belt impacts both positively and negatively is the proprioception system, which is responsible for an awareness of body position. From a positive perspective, the brace or belt signals the trunk musculature to fire because of the pressure on the muscles from the belt (23). However, several studies have found (46, 57, 58, 59) that prolonged use of a brace or belt may actually compromise the acuity of the proprioceptors and may put the individual at greater risk for low back injuries.

BENEFITS OF RESISTANCE TRAINING FOR INDIVIDUALS WITH LOW BACK PAIN

A comprehensive conditioning program that includes resistance training, dynamic flexibility training, muscular endurance training, and cardiovascular conditioning can significantly reduce many of the risk factors associated with low back pain (1, 3, 7, 9, 12, 13, 15, 16, 31, 37). Lee (37) found that patients with less back extensor muscle strength compared to abdominal strength were at significantly greater risk for low back injuries. Alaranta (2) compared the muscular endurance of the back extensors in individuals with and without low back dysfunction and found a significant increase in low back pain in the group with lower muscular endurance of the back extensors. Nourbakhsh and colleagues (51) investigated the association between 17 different mechanical factors and the incidence of low back pain and found that decreased muscular endurance of the back extensors was the greatest predictor of low back pain. Also found were high correlations between back extensor muscle length and muscle strength imbalance between the abdominal muscles and back extensors and between hip flexors and hip adductors (51, 63). Balance and proprioceptive deficits are also linked to low back pain and dysfunction (50, 53, 56, 63). Poor proprioception has been suggested to result in a disruption or delay in the patterns of trunk muscle activation (26, 48, 56, 63). Individuals with low back pain showed delayed muscle response times in the dynamic stabilizing muscles of the spine when compared to control subjects (56). Each of these consequences of low back pain can be addressed and improved through a specific, progressive resistance-training program.

Education regarding proper body mechanics during activities of daily living should be incorporated into the initial physical therapy treatment and reinforced during exercise and resistance training after the low back injury (15, 38, 44, 53, 63). Although resistance training has been proven to be effective in increasing strength, endurance, proprioception, and functional mobility, these improvements for the individual with low back pain only occur if the resistance-training exercises are done with proper form, proper progression, and in supervised exercise sessions and training (6, 9, 14, 31, 44, 50).

Literature Review of Research Supporting Resistance Training for Low Back Pain

A review of the literature pertaining to exercise training for low back pain can be divided into four different classifications: (1) therapeutic exercise training as part of a physical therapy rehabilitation program, (2) dynamic resistance training, (3) lumbar spine stability training, and (4) isometric resistance-training programs. For this review, physical therapy and rehabilitation exercise programs are beyond the scope of this chapter and therefore will not be discussed. Table 6-1 lists the studies that have examined the role of resistance training for improvements in muscular strength and muscular endurance of the trunk musculature for those individuals with low back pain. Table 6-2 lists the studies that have examined lumbar stability training programs.

Several reviews have addressed the role of exercise in individuals with low back pain. Malkia and colleagues (41, 42) reviewed many of the earlier investigations that looked at the role of exercise in the treatment and prevention of low back pain and found a positive effect on physical impairments and functional limitations. Winett and Carpinelli (72) have also shown that as few as two training sessions of 15 to 20 minutes each utilizing a sensible, low-intensity resistance-training program can reduce the complications of low back pain. Kraemer, Ratamess, and French (31) further discuss the role of incorporating resistance training into the overall, comprehensive fitness program and the potential benefits on health and performance for a wide variety of factors, including the reduction of low back pain. Durall and Manske (15) have provided an excellent review of techniques to avoid injury to the

Table 6-1 Studies of Dynamic Resistance Training for Low Back Pain

Author	n	Training/Exercise	Training Variable	Results
Carpenter(10)	20	Progressive Resistance	1 set, 8 to 15 reps 1 day/wk	Increased strength Decreased pain
Liu-Ambrose(39)	98	Resistance Agility Static stretching	Circuit training Cone drills Static stretching	Increased strength, decreased pain Increased strength, decreased pain No change
Pollock(54)	25	Resistance Isometric	1 set 6 to 15 reps 1 set at 7 angles	Increased lumbar extensor strength Increased lumbar extensor strength
Tucci(66)	50	Resistance Resistance Resistance Resistance Resistance	1 day/wk 12 wks 2 days/wk 12 wks 3 days/wk 12 wks 1 day every 2 wks 1 day every 4 wks	Increased strength Increased strength Increased strength No reduction in strength No reduction in strength
Verna(68)	36	Roman chair	3 days/wk 8 wks	Increased Back Extension Endurance Increased Back Extension Isometric Strength
Wilson(71)	19	Neuro-reeducation + resistance training MET + resistance	2 days/wk 8 wks 2 days/wk 8 wks	No Change Increased Function Decreased Disability

back during resistance-training exercise, discussing modifications of common resistance-training exercises, such as the squat and leg press, to keep the lumbar region of the spine in the correct position, thereby reducing the likelihood of low back pain. These authors also suggest some other low-intensity exercises done without resistance to reduce the risk of injury to the back. An article by Stephenson and Swank (64) provides an excellent overview of the components of a trunk or core-training program

that can be undertaken to enhance stability and flexibility of the trunk muscles and improve strength of the core musculature to provide a stable base of support. It also discusses the use of an unstable environment during resistance-training exercises, a relatively new concept in resistance training. Hayden and colleagues (24, 25) performed a meta-analysis of over 60 randomized controlled trials and found that resistance training was effective at decreasing pain and improving function in adults with chronic

Table 6-2 List of Studies of Lumbar Stability and Resistance Training for Low Back Pain

Author	n	Exercise	Training Variable	Results
Carter(11)	20	3 stability ball	2x/wk for 10 wks Increased reps from 10 to 20 over 10 wks.	Increased back endurance
Graves(22)	77	Various resistance	1x/wk 8 to 12 reps 12 wks of training	Increased isometric strength
Kavcic(28)	10	8 stabilization	Spine kinematics EMG External force	Rank order of spine stability established
Kavcic(29)	7	7 stabilization	Spine kinematics EMG External force	Roles of 14 muscles during common stability exercise shown to change with movements during exercise

low back pain. However, for people with acute low back pain, resistance training was as effective as no treatment or other conservative treatments. Hayden and colleagues (25) concluded that when resistance training is individually designed and performed in a supervised environment, a significant reduction in low back pain, as well as a significant increase in exercise compliance, resulted.

Three investigations examined the effects of dynamic resistance training on isometric strength of the trunk musculature and the impact on individuals with low back pain (14, 21, 22). DeMichele and colleagues (14) found that performing dynamic resistance-training exercises for the trunk rotators as little as twice per week resulted in significant increases in isometric strength after 12 weeks of dynamic resistance training. Graves and colleagues (21, 22) performed two very interesting investigations. First, the effect of dynamic resistance training, with a frequency of either once every 2 weeks, once a week, twice a week, or three times per week was examined (21). When isometric strength of the

back extensors, a measure of spinal stability, was evaluated, a training frequency as low as once per week produced significant improvements. In the second investigation (22), the effect of dynamic resistance training once per week on pelvic stabilization was examined. Dynamic resistance training in conjunction with pelvic stabilization exercises produced the most significant increase in the strength of the lumbar extensor musculature.

Because of the vast differences in the etiology and severity of low back pain, clinical trials looking at exercise as a treatment modality have some significant limitations. The subject pool changes rapidly due to reinjury or noncompliance due to decreased pain. Initial evaluation of subjects can be difficult due to the stage of their low back pain (acute, subacute, or chronic), and as such, pre- and post-test comparisons can be questioned. Finally, the length of the exercise program is typically up to 12 weeks, and this may not be enough time to make the positive changes in muscle strength, endurance, and function that years of low back pain have altered in the first place.

DESIGNING RESISTANCE-TRAINING PROGRAMS FOR INDIVIDUALS WITH LOW BACK PAIN

The American College of Sports Medicine (ACSM) and the National Strength and Conditioning Association (NSCA) have developed guidelines for the implementation of safe and effective resistance training programs (3, 6, 16). An individual with low back pain should obtain physician clearance to begin a resistance-training program. One of the key issues in designing an appropriate and safe resistance-training program is to identify what structures are responsible for causing the low back pain. The exercise professional should be informed by the individual, as well as the individual's physician, as to the exact structure or structures that are causing the low back pain so that an appropriate resistance-training program can be established. In general, movements that cause pain should be avoided until they can be done through a pain-free range of motion (8, 11, 15, 19), but movements in the pain-free range of motion are encouraged. As the individual increases strength in the pain-free range, and works on improving the range of motion in the painful range, resistance training can be used to assist in the development of better body control and improved body mechanics.

One of the special considerations for exercise in this population is that the low back pain may have caused a significant level of deconditioning, resulting in an inability to participate in a regular exercise program (44, 50, 53). To that end, prevention of overtraining the severely deconditioned person is important. Unfortunately, **overtraining** is a common occurrence with this population. **Undertraining** is better than overtraining, because with undertraining, the individual can always do more exercise during the next training session. But once someone is overtrained, they may very well need to stop training completely until they are able to fully recover. The other aspect of overtraining that is detrimental to the individual with low back pain is the fact that as the muscles

fatigue, exercise technique is compromised. With any resistance-training exercise, the use of proper form during the movement is critical, but it may be even more so with the individual who has a history of low back pain.

Another special consideration for the individual with low back pain are the types of exercises that may be contraindicated based on the etiology of their particular low back pain. For example, pain may be exacerbated by performing trunk flexion activities and exercises. For these individuals, most of their exercise program should be done with a neutral spine position, progressing to movements and exercises for trunk extension (49, 50, 67). As the individual improves in strength and stability and is able to perform flexion movements in a pain-free range, exercises in the pain-free range may be added to the program.

A final consideration is that the vast majority of individuals who experience low back pain are going to be on some form of pain medication to reduce their pain to manageable levels so that they can perform activities of daily living in more comfort. Many times, these same individuals have other concomitant diseases—such as hypertension, diabetes, cardiovascular, or respiratory conditions—that also require different medications for effective treatment. Although exercising when taking a pain medication is not contraindicated, some form of pharmaceutical interaction between the pain medications and other medications an individual is taking is not uncommon. This potential interaction is one of the main reasons for seeing a physician to get medical clearance prior to starting a resistance-training program.

Exercise Testing Considerations

Traditional testing to establish a baseline level of strength and muscular endurance utilizes a one-repetition maximum protocol. Although this technique for determining the appropriate loading for each exercise works very well for healthy individuals, it is contraindicated for the person with low back pain because of the deconditioned state, the limited range of pain-free motion, and the novelty of performing resistance-training exercises. Two other forms of exercise testing prior to beginning a resistance-training program are recommended for the individual with low back pain: the Rule of 20 and the OMNI RPE scale.

The first method of determining the appropriate resistance, the **Rule of 20**, involves finding a weight that can be lifted safely and with proper form for 20 repetitions (70). With this technique, it is more important to lift a lighter weight correctly than to lift a heavier weight fewer times. Once the individual finds the weight that can be lifted correctly for 20 repetitions, he or she will stay at that intensity, using the same weight and the same number of repetitions, for three to five sessions. This is particularly true for individuals unfamiliar with resistance training. After this initial period of lifting a lighter weight 20 times, the resistance can be increased and the number of repetitions decreased. The individual should maintain this new resistance until 20 repetitions can be performed correctly at the new weight before increasing the intensity. In addition to this gradual and progressive loading of the muscular system, the Rule of 20 will also improve muscular endurance, which is critical for a return to pain-free functioning.

The other method of setting the intensity of the resistance exercise is with the **OMNI RPE scale** (61, 62). The OMNI RPE scale is similar to the Borg RPE scale, except that it is a 10-point scale. Zero is classified as "not tired at all" or "extremely easy," and 10 is classified as "very, very tired" or "extremely hard." The OMNI RPE scale also includes pictures of a person either running, cycling, or stair climbing so that the individual has not only a number to rate their feelings of perceived exertion by but a small "snapshot" of what that level of exertion might feel like (61, 62). Faigenbaum and colleagues (17) have successfully used a similar rating of perceived exertion scale during resistance testing and training with children. The OMNI RPE scale method of selecting the training intensity is appropriate for individuals with low back pain in that they control how much resistance is perceived to be too much, and they can select a training intensity that will not cause them pain or discomfort.

Lifting-Belt Usage for Individuals with Low Back Pain

One last consideration is the use of a **lifting belt** while performing resistance-training exercises. A recent review by Renfro and Ebben (58) provides a summary of the use of lifting belts in both the occupational setting as well as during various types of resistance training. Two of the earliest investigations by Harman and colleagues (23) and Lander and colleagues (34, 35) suggest that the use of a lifting belt during resistance training would increase the intra-abdominal pressure, which is believed to reduce the disc compressive force and improve lifting safety while reducing injuries to the low back area. A lifting belt should be worn during resistance exercises that load the trunk and place stress on the low back—such as squats, deadlifts, and overhead presses—or when lifting maximal or near maximal loads. But the belt should be removed when performing resistance-training exercises that do not load the trunk or stress the lumbar spine (6, 16, 23, 34, 35). Harman and colleagues (23) suggest that if a person uses a lifting belt while performing all resistance-training exercises, the muscles of the trunk may become unaccustomed to performing their normal functional action of supporting the torso during exercise and activities of daily living.

The most recent controversy about the use of some form of lumbar support comes from occupational medicine investigations. Although several studies have suggested that the use of a lifting belt is recommended during work in the occupational setting (20, 27, 32, 45, 65), other studies have shown minimal benefit (36, 47), and several investigators have shown that the use of a lifting belt in the workplace might actually be harmful and could increase the risk of low back injury, pain, and dysfunction (46, 57, 59). Results from these investigations suggest that the use of lifting belts might increase the risk of injury when not wearing the belt after a lifting belt had been worn (45, 57). Reyna and colleagues (59) found that the use of a lumbar belt did not enhance the isometric strength of the back extensor muscles, nor did it increase dynamic lifting capacity.

To summarize, use of a lifting belt is suggested when performing load-bearing resistance exercises or during maximal or near-maximal resistance training. However, the lifting belt should be removed when performing other resistance-training exercises. Regarding the use of a lifting belt during other activities of daily living, individuals with low back pain are advised to discuss this with health care professionals, including their physician, surgeon, and physical therapist and to follow their recommendations.

Program Components and Exercise Selection

The design of a progressive resistance-training program for individuals with low back pain should consist of a full-body, periodized training program that not only enhances muscular strength development but muscular endurance development as well. The other somewhat unique aspect of the resistance-training program designed for individuals with low back pain is the use of nontraditional exercise tools, such as stability balls, balance boards, and other proprioceptive training devices that provide the individual with the most appropriate and functional resistance-training program (4, 5).

A resistance-training program should be divided into three phases, each phase 8 weeks in length. The training program should manipulate training variables such as the number of exercises, number of repetitions, number of sets, rest intervals between sets, and frequency of training to allow for adequate recovery time between training days. Because most individuals with low back pain will have some degree of deconditioning, the progression of the resistance training protocol must be very slow. Importance should be placed on performing exercises safely and without pain or further injury. If individuals remain free of pain and injury, they are more likely to continue the resistance-training program.

The first 8 weeks of the resistance-training program for the individual with low back pain must be designed to accomplish two goals: First, the proper exercise techniques must be learned. Second, the foundation must be laid for muscular strength and muscular endurance to build upon. If an individual with low back pain has just finished formal physical therapy, he or she might be able to progress somewhat faster with the training program. But for the individual who has not exercised in many years due to back pain and dysfunction, the first 8-week cycle is critical to establish good technique, proper training mentality, and to allow progressive adaptation of the neural and musculoskeletal system to the additional demands of the resistance-training protocol.

Following the recommendations of the ACSM and NSCA, a program consisting of 1 to 3 sets of 8 to 15 repetitions, with 1 to 2 minutes rest between sets, is recommended for individuals with low back pain. Exercise selection should begin with those exercises that do not produce pain and only include the range of motion that is pain free.

SAMPLE 24-WEEK PROGRAM

Weeks 1 through 8

Begin with a frequency of 2 days per week with at least 2 days rest between sessions. Perform 1 set of 20 repetitions for the following exercises, with 1 to 2 minutes rest between sets:

Back	Wide-Grip Lat Pulldown
Seated Row	
Chest	Dumbbell Bench Press
	Dumbbell Fly
Arms	Seated Bicep Curl on Stability Ball
	Standing Triceps Pushdown
Legs	Seated Leg Extension
	Seated Leg Flexion
Trunk	Bent-Knee Sit-Ups
	Stability Ball Rolling

Weeks 9 through 16

Increase frequency to 3 days per week with 1 day of rest between sessions. Complete 1 set of 10 to 15 repetitions per exercise, with 1 to 2 minutes of rest between sets on the first and third session of the week, and 2 sets of 8 to 10 repetitions per exercise, with 1 to 2 minutes of rest between sets, on the second session of the week. Include the following exercises each session:

Back	Narrow-Grip Lat Pulldown Prone Dumbbell Fly on Stability Ball Superman on Stability Ball
Chest	Barbell Bench Press Incline Dumbbell Fly Standing Cable Crossover
Arms	Standing Biceps Curl with E-Z Curl Bar Stability Ball Push-Ups Medicine Ball Push Press
Legs	Leg Press Standing Lunge with Dumbbells Seated Calf Raises
Trunk	Horizontal Side Support Bent-Knee Sit-Up over Stability Ball Low Back Extension Machine

Weeks 17 through 24

Continue with three sessions per week, increasing to 2 to 3 sets of 8 to 10 repetitions per exercise, with 1 minute of rest between sets on all days. Include the following exercises:

Back	Roman Chair Deadlift Vee-Handle Lat Pulldown
Chest	Stability Ball Cable Crossover Bench Press (Dumbbells 2 days, Barbell 1 day) Stability Ball Supine Fly
Arms	Medicine Ball Shoulder Press Standing Dumbbell Curls on Wobble Board Stability Ball Dumbbell Shoulder Press
Legs	Squats (Dumbbell to start, progressing to Back Squats with Barbell) Stability Ball Bridge and Hamstring Roll Standing Calf Raise with Dumbbells
Trunk	Trunk Flexion Machine Oblique Sit-Ups with Twist Stability Ball Medicine Ball Pullover and Throw

CASE STUDY

Mr. K was a 42-year-old law enforcement officer with a 15-year history of chronic low back pain. He fell while in the military in his early 20s and strained the multifidus and erector spinae muscles from L2 through L5 on the right side of his spinal column. His pain is not constant, and he has exacerbated his low back pain an average of three to four times per year. He treats the acute pain with ibuprofin, bed rest, and the use of a back belt while riding in his police patrol car. Mr. K used to lift weights as a high school and college athlete but has not done any resistance training for the past 12 years for fear of reinjuring of his low back.

Mr. K spends approximately 4 to 5 hours a day sitting, either in his patrol car or at a desk. The rest of his workday is spent walking a beat, and walking seems to make his back feel better. He has a difficult time sleeping most nights, primarily due to his job stresses. And when he strains his back, bed rest and ibuprofin are the only things that relieve his pain. He has tried heat and cold locally over his lumbar region, but neither seems to offer much relief.

Approximately 6 months before Mr. K was to take his test for a promotion to the next rank on the police force, he came to the local fitness facility to start a resistance-training program so he could pass the physical exam for his promotion. Mr. K had been to physical therapy when he first injured his back 15 years earlier but had not been since then. The evaluation of Mr. K's range of motion showed a slight limitation in all planes of approximately 5 to 10 degrees, limited only by tightness, not pain, in his lumbar region. His strength was graded as good, but the muscular endurance of his lumbar extensors was very poor.

Mr. K was given a resistance-training program to help him regain his muscular strength and muscular endurance to prepare for the physical tests required for his promotion. The recommendation was for an 8-week program consisting of visits three times per week. The program was similar to the 24-week program described previously, with the first 8 weeks consisting primarily of low-intensity, high-repetition resistance training. One set of each exercise was performed, and Mr. K only performed his resistance training 2 days per week.

Because he wanted to do more exercise, he was given an adjustable weight vest that he wore while performing a 30-minute fitness walk every night. The use of a weight vest during walking has been shown to increase caloric expenditure, cardiovascular endurance, local muscular endurance, and to reduce back pain due to a more upright walking posture (30, 53). This form of aerobic conditioning may provide a multitude of benefits for individuals with low back pain.

After the first 8 weeks, Mr. K increased the number of days per week he lifted weights, as well as increasing the load in his weight vest to almost 15 percent of his body weight. He also started using his stability ball at home while watching television or working on his computer, performing simple movements and balancing exercises on the stability ball.

During the final 8 weeks of the resistance-training program, Mr. K reinjured his back climbing a fence to apprehend a suspect. However, because of the previous 16 weeks of resistance training, his low back pain was significantly reduced compared to previous exacerbations, and he was able to return to the fitness facility in approximately 10 days. When he first returned, he added water walking in the hot tub to his training routine each day after he lifted weights, and he reduced the load in his weight vest back to 10 percent of his body weight for 3 weeks, until he was pain free in all planes of movement.

Mr. K not only passed his physical exam, he scored the third-highest score in the group. He received his promotion and continues his resistance training at least 2 days per week, as well as his walking each evening he is not on duty with his weight vest. Mr. K saw what resistance training and conditioning did, not only for his back, but for his overall feeling of well-being. As a result, he made the commitment to make regular exercise part of his daily activities.

Summary

Although the incidence of low back pain continues to impact approximately 80 percent of the population, many investigations have shown that resistance training is indeed an effective modality in the treatment, rehabilitation, and prevention of low back pain. With proper instruction and supervision, as well as proper progression of the intensity and volume of resistance-training exercises, individuals with low back pain can safely and effectively incorporate resistance-training exercises into their overall fitness program. Once they do, most people who have a history of low back pain will find that they not only have less pain, but they are able to recover from an exacerbation of their low back pain significantly faster.

Key Terms

Acute low back pain
Lifting belt
Low back pain
OMNI RPE
Overtraining
Proprioceptive acuity
Rule of 20
Spondylolysis
Spondylolisthesis
Undertraining

Study Questions

1. Explain the effect that lifting belts or back braces have on abdominal strength and low back pain.

2. Discuss why low back pain is so prevalent in our society and how resistance training can lower the incidence and severity of low back pain.

3. Describe the risk factors for low back pain and how exercise, and specifically resistance-training exercise, can play a role in the reduction of those risk factors

4. List the components of a comprehensive resistance-training program for individuals with low back pain, and explain how to safely progress the volume and intensity of the resistance-training program for these individuals.

References

1. Abenhaim L, Rossignol M, Valat JP, et al. The role of activity in therapeutic management of back pain. Report of the International Paris Task Force on Back Pain. *Spine.* 2000;15:(suppl 25, pt 4):1S-33S.

2. Alaranta H, Luoto S, Heliovaara M, Hurri H. Static back endurance and the risk of low back pain. *Clin Biomech* 1995;10:323-326.

3. American College of Sports Medicine. *ACSM's Guidelines for Exercise Testing and Prescription.* 6th ed. Philadelphia: Lippincott, Williams and Wilkins; 2000.

4. Arokoski JP, Balta T, Airaksinen O, Kankaanpaa M. Back and abdominal muscle function during stabilization exercises. *Arch Phys Med Rehabil.* 2001;82:1089-1098.

5. Axler CT, McGill SM. Low back loads over a variety of abdominal exercises: Searching for the safest abdominal challenge. *Med Sci Sports Exerc.* 1997;29:804-811.

6. Baechle TR, Earle RW. Resistance training exercise techniques. In: Earle RW, Baechle TR, eds. *NSCA's essentials of personal training.* 2004;298-299.

7. Behm DG, Anderson KG. The role of instability with resistance training. *J Strength Cond Res.* 2006;20:716-722.

8. Bigos SJ, Bowyer OM, Braen GS. *Acute Low Back Pain Problems in Adults. Clinical Practice Guidelines Quick Reference Guide.* US Department of Health; 1994. AHCPR Publication No. 95-0643.

9. Bigos SJ, Davis GE. Scientific application of sports medicine principles for acute low back pain. *J Orthop Sports Phys Ther.* 1996;24: 192-207.

10. Carpenter DM, Nelson BW. Low back strengthening for the prevention and treatment of low back pain. *Med Sci Sports Exerc.* 1999;31: 18-24.

11. Carter JM, Beam WC, McMaha SG, Barr ML, Brown LE. The effects of stability ball training on spinal stability in sedentary individuals. *J Strength Cond Res.* 2006;20:429-435.

12. Danneels LA, Cools AM, Vanderstraeten GG, et al. The effects of three different training modalities on the cross-sectional area of the paravertebral muscles. *Scand J Med Sci Sports.* 2001;11:335-341.

13. Danneels LA, Vanderstraeten GG, Cambier DC, et al. Effects of three different training modalities on the cross-sectional area of the lumbar multifidus muscle in patients with chronic low back pain. *Br J Sports Med.* 2001;35:186-191.

14. DeMichele PL, Pollock ML, Graves JE, et al. Isometric torso rotation strength: Effect of training frequency on its development. *Arch Phys Med Rehabil.* 1997;78:64-69.

15. Durall CJ, Manske RC. Avoiding lumbar spine injury during resistance training. *Strength Cond J.* 2005;27:64-72.

16. Earle RW, Baechle TR. Resistance Training and Spotting Techniques. In: Baechle TR, Earle RW, eds. *Essentials of Strength Training and Conditioning.* Champaign, IL: Human Kinetics; 2000:346-347.

17. Faigenbaum AF, Milliken L, Cloutier G, Westcott W. Perceived exertion during resistance training in children. *Perceptual Motor Skills.* 2004;98:627-637.

18. Frymoyer JW, Cats-Baril WL. An overview of the incidences and costs of low back pain. *Orthopaedic Clinics of North America.* 1991;22:263-270.

19. Frymoyer JW, Gordon, SL. Symposium on new perspectives on low back pain. American Academy of Orthopaedic Surgeons; 1989; Park Ridge, IL.

20. Giorcelli RJ, Hughes RE, Wassell JT, Hsiao J. The effect of wearing a back belt on spine kinematics during asymmetric lifting of large and small boxes. *Spine.* 2001;26:1794-1798.

21. Graves JE, Pollock ML, Foster DN, et al. Effect of training frequency and specificity on isometric lumbar extension strength. *Spine.* 1990;15:504-509.

22. Graves JE, Webb DC, Pollock ML, et al. Pelvic stabilization during resistance training: Its effect on the development of lumbar extension strength. *Arch Phys Med Rehabil.* 1994;75:210-215.

23. Harman EA, Rosenstein RM, Frykman PN, Nigro GA. Effects of a belt on intra-abdominal pressure during weight lifting. *Med Sci Sports Exerc.* 1989;21:186-190.

24. Hayden JA, van Tulder MW, Malmivaara AV, Koes BW. Meta-analysis: Exercise therapy for nonspecific low back pain. *Ann Intern Med.* 2005;142:765-775.

25. Hayden JA, van Tulder MW, Tomlinson G. Systematic review: strategies for using exercise therapy to improve outcomes in chronic low back pain. *Ann Intern Med.* 2005;142:776-785.

26. Hodges P, Richardson C. Altered trunk muscle recruitment in people with low back pain with upper limb movement at different speeds. *Arch Phys Med Rehabil.* 1999;80:1005-1012.

27. Jonai H, Villanueva MB, Sotoyama M, Hisanaga N, Saito S. The effect of a back belt on torso motion: Survey in an express package delivery company. *Ind Health.* 1997;35:235-242.

28. Kavcic N, Grenier S, McGill SM. Determining the stabilizing role of individual torso muscles during rehabilitation exercises. *Spine.* 2004;29:1254-1265.

29. Kavcic N, Grenier S, McGill SM. Quantifying tissue loads and spine stability while performing commonly prescribed low back stabilization exercises. *Spine.* 2004;29:2319-2329.

30. Knapik JJ, Reynolds KL, Harman, EA. Soldier load carriage: historical, physiological, biomechanical and medical aspects. *Mil Med.* 2004;169:45-56.

31. Kraemer WJ, Ratamess NA, French DN. Resistance training for health and performance. *Curr Sports Med Rep.* 2002;1:165-171.

32. Kraus JF, Schaffer KB, Rice T, Maroosis J, Harper J. A field trial of back belts to reduce the incidence of acute low back injuries in New York City home attendants. *Int J Occup Environ Health.* 2002;8:97-104.

33. Kuukkanen T, Malkia E. Muscular performance after a 3-month progressive physical exercise program and 9-month follow-up in subjects with low back pain. A controlled study. *Scand J Med Sci Sports.* 1996;6:112-121.

34. Lander JE, Simonton RL, Giacobbe JF. The effectiveness of weight belts during the squat exercise. *Med Sci Sports Exerc.* 1990;22:117-126.

35. Lander JE, Hundley JR, Simonton RL. The effectiveness of weight belts during multiple repetitions of the squat exercise. *Med Sci Sports Exerc.* 1990;24:603-609.

36. Lavender SA, Shakeel K, Andersson GB, Thomas JS. Effects of a lifting belt on spine movements and muscle recruitments after unexpected sudden loading. *Spine.* 2000;25:1569-1578.

37. Lee J. Trunk muscle imbalance as a risk factor of the incidence of low back pain: a 5-year

prospective study. *Neuromusculoskeletal Syst.* 1999;7:97-101.

38. Linton S, van Tulder MW. Preventive interventions for back and neck pain problems: What is the evidence? *Spine.* 2001;26:778-787.

39. Liu-Ambrose TY, Khan KM, Eng JJ, Lord SR, Lentle B, McKay HA. Both resistance and agility training reduce back pain and improve health-related quality of life in older women with low bone mass. *Osteoporos Int.* 2005; 16:1321-1329.

40. Luo X, Pietrobon R, Sun S, Liu G, Hey F. Estimates and patterns of direct health care expenditures among individuals with back pain in the United States. *Spine.* 2004;29:79-86.

41. Malkia E, Kannus B. Low back pain: to exercise or not to exercise? *Scand J Med Sci Sports.* 1996;6:61-62.

42. Malkia E, Ljunggren AE. Exercise programs for subjects with low back disorders. *Scand J Med Sci Sports.* 1996;6:73-81.

43. Manniche C. Clinical benefit of intensive dynamic exercises for low back pain. *Scand J Med Sci Sports.* 1996;6:82-87.

44. McGill S. Low back disorders: Evidence-based prevention and rehabilitation. Champaign IL: Human Kinetics; 2002.

45. McIntyre DR, Bolte KM, Pope MH. Study provides new evidence of back belt's effectiveness. *Occup Health Saf.* 1996;65:39-41.

46. Minor SD. Use of back belts in occupational settings. *Phys Ther.* 1996;76:403-408.

47. Mitchell LV, Lawler FH, Bowen D, Mote W, Asundi P, Purswell J. Effectiveness and cost-effectiveness of employer-issued back belts in areas of high risk for back injury. *J Occup Med.* 1994;36:90-94.

48. Newcomer K, Jacboson T, Gabriel D, Larson D, Brey R, An K. Muscle activation patterns in subjects with and without low back pain. *Arch Phys Med Rehabil.* 2002;86:816-821.

49. Norris CM. Spinal stabilization: limiting factors to end-range motion in the lumbar spine. *Physiotherapy.* 1995;81:4-12.

50. Norris CM. *Back stability.* Champaign, IL: Human Kinetics, 2000.

51. Nourbakhsh M, Arab A. Relationship between mechanical factors and incidence of low back pain. *J Orthop Sports Phys Ther.* 2002;32: 447-460.

52. Payne N, Gledhill N, Katzmarzyk P, Jamnik V. Health-related fitness, physical activity and history of back pain. *Can J Appl Physiol.* 2000;25:236-249.

53. Perkins J, Zipple JT. Nonspecific low back pain. In: Ehrman JK, Gordon PM, Visich PS, Keteyian SJ, eds. *Clinical Exercise Physiology.* Champaign, IL: Human Kinetics; 2003:483-502.

54. Pollock ML, Leggett SH, Graves JE, Jones A, Fulton MA, Circulli J. Effect of resistance training on lumbar extension strength. *Am J Sports Med.* 1989;17:624-629.

55. Proper KI, Heymans MW, Paw MJ, van Sluijs EM, van Poppel MN, van Mechelen W. Promoting physical activity with people in different places: A Dutch perspective. *J Sci Med Sport.* 2006;9:371-377.

56. Radebold A, Cholewicki, J, Polzhofer G, Greene H. Impaired postural control of the lumbar spine is associated with delayed muscle response times in patients with chronic idiopathic low back pain. *Spine.* 2001;26:724-730.

57. Reddell CR, Congleton JJ, Dale-Huchingson R, Montgomery JF. An evaluation of weight-lifting belt and back injury prevention training for airline baggage handlers *Appl Ergon.* 1992;23:319-329.

58. Renfro GL, Ebben WP. A review of the use of lifting belts. *Strength Cond J.* 2006;28:68-74.

59. Reyna JR, Leggett SH, Kenney K, Holmes B, Mooney V. The effect of lumbar belts on isolated lumbar muscle. Strength and dynamic capacity. *Spine.* 1995;20:68-73.

60. Risser WL, Risser JM, Preston D. Weight-training injuries in adolescents. *Am J Dis Child.* 1990;144:1015-1017.

61. Roberson RJ. *Perceived exertion for practitioners.* Champaign, IL: Human Kinetics; 2004.

62. Robertson RJ, Goss FL, Andreacci L, et al. Validation of the Children's OMNI-Resistance Exercise Scale of perceived exertion. *Med Sci Sports Exerc.* 2005;37:819-826.

63. Rogers RG. Research-based rehabilitation of the lower back. *Strength Cond J.* 2006;28:30-35.

64. Stevenson J, Swank AM. Core training: Designing a program for anyone. *Strength Cond J* 2004;26:34-37.

65. Thomas JS, Lavender SA, Corcos DM, Andersson GB. Effect of lifting belts on trunk muscle activation during a suddenly applied load. *Hum Factors.* 1999;41:670-676.

66. Tucci JT, Carpenter DM, Pollack ML, Graves JE, Leggett SH. Effect of reduced frequency of training and detraining on lumbar extension strength. *Spine.* 1992;17:1497-1501.

67. Twomey LT, Taylor JR, ed. *Physical Therapy of the Low Back.* New York: Churchill Livingstone; 1994.

68. Verna JL, Mayer JM, Mooney V, Pierra EA, Roberson VL, Graves JE. Back extension endurance and strength: The effect of variable angle Roman chair exercise training. *Spine.* 2002;27:1772-1777.

69. Waddell G, Feder G, Lewis M. Systematic review of bed rest and advice to stay active for acute low back pain. *Br J Gen Pract.* 1997;47:647-652.

70. Wathen NL. The Rule of 20 for setting resistance training intensity in patient populations. Paper presented at: NSCA National Convention; July, 2003; Minneapolis, MN.

71. Wilson E, Payton O, Donegan-Shoaf L, Dec K. Muscle energy techniques in patients with acute low back pain: A pilot clinical trial. *J Orthop Sports Phys Ther.* 2003;33:502-512.

72. Winett RA, Carpinelli RN. Potential health-related benefits of resistance training. *Prev Med.* 2001;33:503-513.

73. Zusman M. Structure-oriented beliefs and disability due to back pain. *Australian J Physiother.* 1998;44:13-20.

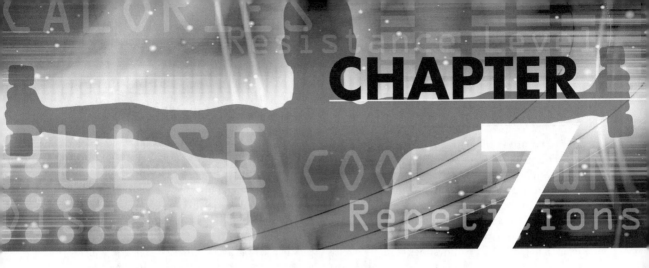

CHAPTER 7

RESISTANCE-TRAINING STRATEGIES FOR INDIVIDUALS WITH CHRONIC HEART FAILURE

Objectives

Upon completion of this chapter, the reader should be able to:

○ State the prevalence of heart failure in the United States and the associated economic costs of this condition

○ Describe the current state and limitations of the research evaluating the impact of resistance training on heart failure

○ Describe the role of resistance training in the treatment of heart failure

○ Discuss the specific factors to consider related to preexercise screening, exercise testing, and exercise prescription when designing a resistance-training program for individuals with heart failure

○ Explain the underlying rationale for designing a resistance-training program that incorporates muscular strength, endurance, and power for individuals with heart failure

INTRODUCTION

Heart failure is the pathological state in which an abnormality of cardiac function is responsible for failure of the heart to pump blood at a rate commensurate with the requirements of the metabolizing tissues, or to do so only from an elevated filling pressure (12). **Chronic heart failure (CHF)** is a multisystem syndrome with a variety of pathological abnormalities that reduce exercise tolerance and contribute to the symptoms of functional disability.

A common characteristic of CHF is **exercise intolerance,** which is the inability to sustain a submaximal level of exercise or activity. Because of both a reduced exercise capacity and concerns that the stress of exercise would further aggravate heart function, the enrollment of people with CHF in exercise training programs was uncommon until the early 1990s (16). Even after cardiac rehabilitation programs began to include CHF patients, the emphasis was on aerobic exercise, and resistance exercise was still assumed to be too stressful or dangerous.

Recent evidence indicates that the exercise intolerance experienced by individuals with CHF also involves a skeletal muscle pathology that is not sufficiently addressed by aerobic exercise alone. Ease and comfort when performing activities of daily living affect independence and quality of life, and these activities rely on muscular strength, endurance, and power in addition to aerobic-type training. These observations have led to a paradigm shift in exercise programming for patients with CHF to include muscular strength and endurance training. This chapter addresses resistance training for the individual with CHF due to **systolic dysfunction,** or reduced pumping capacity. Heart failure due to isolated **diastolic dysfunction,** or reduced ability of the heart to fill, is common but is not addressed in this chapter due to the absence of research detailing the effects of resistance training for this patient population.

PUBLIC HEALTH IMPACT: PREVALENCE AND ECONOMIC IMPACT

CHF is a major and growing public health problem in the United States, affecting approximately 5 million individuals, with more than 550,000 new diagnoses of heart failure each year (1). The prevalence of heart failure rises from 2 to 3 percent at age 65 to more than 80 percent in people over 80 years of age. CHF affects 1 in 100 individuals over the age of 65 years and is the most common cause of hospitalization for this age group. Heart failure patients have a poor quality of life that is related to exercise intolerance and frequent hospitalizations. As the disease progresses, patients become more incapacitated and deconditioned. Often, they are unable to perform simple daily tasks without **dyspnea,** or shortness of breath, or fatigue limiting such activities. The total direct cost of treating patients with CHF is estimated to be approximately $30 billion annually—more than what is spent on any other diagnosis (1, 2).

ETIOLOGY OF DISEASE

Although the mechanisms underlying CHF are not entirely clear, both central cardiovascular and peripheral muscular dysfunction contribute to the symptoms of heart failure. Muscle weakness, dyspnea on exertion, and general fatigue are common symptoms for individuals with heart failure. Etiologic factors for heart failure include ischemic heart disease—the underlying factor in approximately 60 percent of all cases—hypertensive heart disease, valvular heart disease, and a variety of metabolic, infectious, and toxic agents.

The **muscle hypothesis** outlined in Figure 7-1 provides a theoretical connection between cardiovascular and skeletal muscle dysfunction that contributes to the symptoms of heart failure (22). Etiological factors

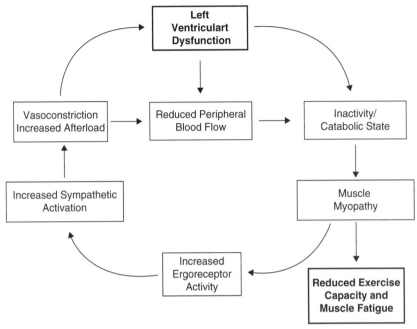

Figure 7-1 The Muscle Hypothesis.
Adapted from Monchamp and Frishman(23)

associated with skeletal muscle dysfunction include inactivity, malnutrition, constant or repeated episodes of inadequate nutritive blood flow, and prolonged exposure to altered neural-hormonal stimuli, including catecholamines and cytokines.

As presented in Figure 7-1, left ventricular dysfunction results in poor perfusion of peripheral muscles and, in combination with local endothelial dysfunction, elevated circulating and tissue cytokines lead to the skeletal muscle abnormalities common with this disease. The skeletal muscle myopathy that follows from reduced cardiac function has been associated with reduced ability to perform daily activities, which contributes to a reduced quality of life in heart failure patients. During exertion, the skeletal muscle myopathy results in an accumulation of metabolic byproducts, causing muscle fatigue and activation of ergoreceptors, chemoreceptors, and mechanoreceptors in the skeletal muscle. These

receptors are afferent nerve endings that transmit signals to the central nervous system, resulting in increased ventilation and sympathetic nervous system stimulation, which in turn causes increased dyspnea and peripheral resistance, respectively. The long-term negative consequence of the increase in sympathetic nervous system activity is an increase in vasoconstriction and afterload, both of which perpetuate the cycle of worsening heart failure and overactivation of the sympathetic nervous system (23).

EFFECTS OF CHF ON SKELETAL MUSCLE

Over the past 20 years, many studies have examined the mechanisms responsible for the exercise intolerance seen in individuals with CHF due to systolic dysfunction (6, 14, 15, 20, 21, 22, 26, 27).

Cardiopulmonary factors such as ejection fraction, reduced cardiac output, and reduced pulmonary capillary pressure were believed to be the primary limiting factors for individuals with CHF. However, these factors do not fully explain or correlate with the exercise intolerance and dyspnea noted in this population. The lack of correlation between decreased function and other cardiopulmonary factors has led investigators to search for other explanations for muscle fatigue and other symptoms observed with CHF. Research findings suggest that peripheral factors such as diminished blood flow, intrinsic skeletal muscle abnormalities, and neurohormonal alterations are also responsible for poor exercise tolerance (6, 14, 15, 20, 21, 22, 26, 27).

In healthy individuals, blood flow is elevated during exercise due to increases in cardiac output and arteriole vasodilation. However, reductions in blood flow, increases in blood lactate levels during exercise, and greater rates of fatigue have been documented in the working muscle of the individual with heart failure. Furthermore, structural alterations in the peripheral vasculature have also been reported (6, 15, 20, 21). A reduction in blood flow leads to inadequate oxygen delivery during exercise and contributes to increased glycolysis and fatigue, as well as increased neurohormonal responses, which lead to increased sympathetic nervous system activity. Reductions in endothelial nitric oxide and vascular function have been shown to be the primary mechanism responsible for the decrease in blood flow for individuals with heart failure (6, 15, 20, 21).

Within the skeletal muscle, a reduction in slow-twitch oxidative (Type I) fibers and an increase in fast glycolytic (Type IIb) fibers has also been documented in heart failure patients. In addition, mitochondrial function is reduced in individuals with heart failure and represents yet another mechanism contributing to reduced muscle function and increased muscle fatigue. Structural analysis of the muscle indicates a reduction in mitochondrial volume density and a reduced surface area in heart failure patients compared to healthy controls (27). These decreases in oxidative capacity are closely correlated to a reduction in exercise capacity. Finally,

increases in inducible nitric oxide synthase (iNOS) and nitric oxide in the skeletal muscle, likely due to a heart-failure related increase in tissue cytokines, are associated with down-regulation of mitochondrial creatine kinase expression (14). Viewed in sum, the above findings suggest that the functional aerobic and anaerobic capacity of patients with CHF is limited not only by the central oxygen transport system but also by the oxidative capacity of the mitochondria in the skeletal muscle.

Muscle atrophy and loss of muscle strength and endurance are also exhibited in individuals with CHF and partly explain the exercise intolerance and decreased ability to perform activities of daily living. Muscle atrophy and loss of muscle endurance are related to increased fatigue independent of muscle metabolic properties. This increase in fatigue has been attributed to a greater amount of atrophy in the slow-twitch (Type I) fibers, an increased recruitment of motor units, and a higher frequency of excitation required when performing a given motor task (21, 22).

BENEFITS OF RESISTANCE TRAINING FOR INDIVIDUALS WITH CHF

Resistance training positively impacts skeletal muscle and endothelial function and thus has the potential to interrupt or lessen the negative effects associated with the muscle hypothesis. Resistance training has been shown to positively impact some physical and psychosocial factors (31, 32, 33, 34) of CHF. Fatigue may be reduced, emotional effects may be ameliorated (24), and an increase in functional ability is often observed (18, 21, 22). Resistance training has also been found to improve peripheral blood flow in people with CHF (13, 18, 28). In addition, individuals with CHF have shown decreases in sympathetic nervous system activation and improved heart rate variability following exercise training (26, 28). Resistance training may also improve autonomic nervous system function

(19, 31), a possibly important finding in that heightened sympathetic nervous system activity is associated with a more adverse long-term prognosis.

Resistance training has been found to increase muscle mitochondrion size (27) and to improve muscle strength and endurance (4, 5, 25, 28). These improvements in strength allow the individual with heart failure to perform routine lifting tasks with a lower circulatory response and at a lower percentage of their maximal strength level, allowing for greater overall efficiency when performing activities of daily living. These findings underline the importance of a resistance-training program for improving muscle function for the individual with CHF.

Functional outcome in people with CHF has primarily been measured by performance on a 6-minute walking test, with resistance training being associated with an increase in the distance covered in 6-minutes (18, 21, 22). The results from these studies, related to functional outcomes

(18, 21, 22), are applicable to activities of daily life and provide strong support that an exercise-training program involving both aerobic training and resistance training can result in improvements in function for individuals with CHF.

Review of Research Supporting Resistance Training for CHF

Table 7-1 lists studies that have evaluated the impact of resistance training, either alone or in combination with aerobic conditioning, for individuals with heart failure. As stated earlier, the cumulative results of the impact of resistance training for individuals with CHF indicate increases in muscular strength, muscular endurance, quality of life, and functional measures. However, many of the resistance-training studies are limited, because they have studied subjects who are at a low to moderate

Table 7-1 Research on the Effects of Resistance Training in Chronic Heart Failure

Author	Number	Age/EF	Program Length	Intensity	Strength Gains
Falconer(10) (pre–post)	7 males	54.0 yrs 22%	1x/week for 6 weeks	60%	30.5%
Barnard(5) (randomized: 14 endurance training and strength training, 7 endurance training alone)	21 males	60.3 yrs 25%	2x/week for 8 weeks	60–80%	26.2%
Maiorana(18) (prospective, randomized cross-over)	13 males	60.0 yrs 26%	3x/week for 8 weeks	55–65%	17.9%
Selig(28) (pre–post)	33 males, 6 females	65.0 yrs 28%	3x/week for 12 weeks	not available	21.2% (continued)

Table 7-1 Research on the Effects of Resistance Training in Chronic Heart Failure (continued)

Author	Number	Age/EF	Program Length	Intensity	Strength Gains
Delargardelle(8) (randomized: 10 endurance training and strength training, 10 endurance training alone)	20 males	55.0 yrs	3x/week for 12 weeks	60%	not available
Delagardelle(7) (pre–post)	11 males, 3 females	57.0 yrs 29%	3x/week for 24 weeks	60%–80%	14%
Minotti(20) (pre–post)	5 males	60.0 yrs 27%	28-day wrist flexor training	not available	not available
Pu(25) (randomized: 40 progressive resistance training and 40 stretching exercise)	16 females	80.0 yrs	3x/week for 10 weeks	80%	43.4%
Tyni-Lenne(31) (pre–post)	24 females	60.0 yrs 29%	3x/week for 8 weeks two-leg knee extensions	65–75%	42% males, 61% females
Tyni-Lenne(32) (pre–post)	16 females	62.0 yrs 28%	3x/week for 16 weeks knee extensions only	65–75%	not available
Santoro(27) (pre–post)	5 males, 1 female	73.0 yrs 27%	2x/week for 16 weeks	40–60%	not available
Levinger(17) (randomized, controlled	15 males	57.0 yrs 34%	3x/week for 8 weeks	40–90%	18%

risk (ejection fractions >40 percent), are relatively young (40 to 60 years of age), and have been limited for the most part to male subjects. Furthermore, the resistance-training program design for several of the research studies is not practical for long-term care for several reasons: First, many are not reproducible due to insufficient detail regarding the progression of the training program (18, 28). Second, the length of the program is typically 12 weeks or less, which may not be sufficient to impact both neural and muscular adaptations. Third, many of the studies used localized muscle-training techniques, such as wrist flexion or knee extension, to investigate the mechanistic muscle changes that occur with resistance training (22, 31, 32, 33, 34). These localized training strategies are not ideal for long-term compliance.

Six studies utilized full-body training strategies, and these studies form the basis of our recommended 24-week program (5, 7, 8, 17, 25, 27). These six studies utilized both male and female subjects. The investigators used progressive resistance-training strategies with intensities ranging from 40 to 90 percent of the one-repetition maximum (1RM), frequencies of 2 to 3 days per week, and a training duration from 8 to 24 weeks. Full-body exercises were performed in the resistance-training program and included squats, leg presses, bench presses, military presses, biceps curls, and triceps extensions. Average strength gains ranged from 14 to 43.4 percent with a wide range of gains that most likely reflected the initial fitness status of the subjects.

DESIGNING RESISTANCE-TRAINING PROGRAMS FOR INDIVIDUALS WITH CHF

Individuals with CHF have greater overall morbidity and mortality rates than healthy people and individuals with most other forms of heart disease. Thus, current practice guidelines stratify individuals with CHF to the highest level of risk (2, 3). An extensive medical history and physical activity history should be performed prior to initiating any exercise regimen (3). In addition, there is a need to consider other comorbidities such as diabetes, which affects nearly 35 percent of patients with CHF, or advanced age, because most people who suffer from CHF are elderly. Degree of severity of heart failure is classified from A through D using a categorization system established by the American Heart Association (AHA) and the American College of Cardiology (ACC) (1, 2). Using this system, all individuals with left ventricular dysfunction are considered, regardless

of symptoms. Individuals at risk for developing heart failure are classified as Stage A; those who are asymptomatic and free of structural abnormalities as Stage B; individuals with structural abnormalities, with or without mild to moderate symptoms, as Stage C; and individuals with advanced structural concerns and quite limiting symptoms as Stage D. In addition, clinicians often use the New York Heart Association (NYHA) classification system to qualify to what extent symptoms limit a person's physical and daily activity (2, 3). In this system, Class I is a level of exertion that would elicit symptoms for a normal person, Class II is representative of symptoms that would be seen with ordinary exertion, Class III includes symptoms experienced during exertion somewhat less than ordinary exertion, and Class IV comprises symptoms that might occur at rest. Those individuals experiencing symptoms found in NYHA Classes II through IV would also fall within with AHA/ACC Stages C and D.

Drug regimens for treating heart failure are extensive and should be assessed so side effects can be considered before implementing any exercise program. Standard medical therapy includes **diuretics** to reduce blood volume and edema, **vasodilators** to reduce blood pressure and systemic vascular resistance, and **beta-adrenergic–receptor blockers** to interrupt the "toxic effects" of an overactive sympathetic nervous system (12). The use of digoxin for individuals with heart failure has been in practice for decades but with some controversy when recommended for individuals with heart failure accompanied by normal sinus rhythm. Other agents that may be used to treat individuals with heart failure attributable to systolic dysfunction include antiplatelet and anticoagulation therapies and an aldosterone antagonist to reduce blood pressure and systemic vascular resistance.

Exercise Testing Considerations

To determine eligibility and safety for exercise participation, individuals with CHF should undergo a medical screening consisting of a physical examination, a symptom-limited cardiopulmonary exercise test using the modified Naughton protocol, and a resting echocardiogram. Most individuals with CHF will stop the exercise test due to dyspnea or leg fatigue. A treadmill or cycle ergometer test will evaluate the safety of aerobic training; however, a recently developed exercise test consisting of 3 sets of 8RM leg presses (3 x 8 SST) may assist the clinician in determining whether resistance training is appropriate. Development of a specific protocol to evaluate the safety of resistance training for the individual with CHF is consistent with the need for the stress applied during an exercise test to reflect the unique combination of static and dynamic loads on the heart that occur during resistance training. Resistance training results in both pressure and volume loads on the heart related to the amount of weight lifted and phase of the lift; that is, whether the load is being raised or lowered. The echocardiographic stress test outlined in Table 7-2 was based on recommendations from Evans (9) and is intended to simulate a resistance-training regimen, 3 sets of 8RM in this case, leading up to progressive increases in work to exhaustion, which would be analogous to an incremental treadmill or cycle protocol. The leg press exercise should be used for this testing, as this exercise has been shown to elicit the highest blood pressure responses (19). The protocol consists of 3 sets of 8RM, simulating

a training session during which heart rate, blood pressure, end diastolic volume, end systolic volume, stroke volume, ejection fraction, and cardiac output are measured (30). Results for each variable are obtained at rest: during a warm-up set, following each set of resistance exercise, and during recovery. If all variables assessed are within normal limits, it is likely that resistance training would be safe for the individual. If resistance training is deemed to be safe, maximal strength testing is also recommended for evaluating baseline strength levels, establishing weight loads for training, and tracking changes in strength over time (3). Muscle strength should be measured using the 1RM method for all exercises to be included in the resistance-training program (11).

Absolute and relative contraindications to exercise testing and exercise training for heart failure are presented in the American College of Sports Medicine Guidelines (3). The most common problems specific to individuals with heart failure include postexercise hypotension, arrhythmias, and worsening heart failure symptoms (12). Signs or symptoms of worsening heart failure include weight gain of 1.5 to 2.0 kg over the previous 3 to 5 days, increased heart rate, increased dyspnea, and auscultatory findings of pulmonary edema. Any of these would

Table 7-2 Experimental Design for Echocardiogram-Guided Resistance-Training Stress Test

5 min	2 min	24 sec	2 min	24 sec	2 min	24 sec	2 min	24 sec	2 min
Weight and height recorded; positioned on leg press	Resting	Warm-up Set ~60 % 1RM	Recovery	Set 1 – 80% 1RM	Recovery	Set 2 – 80% 1RM	Recovery	Set 3 – 80% 1RM	After Exercise

Heart rate and blood pressure were obtained during rest and recovery and immediately following each stage of exercise.
Echocardiograms were obtained at rest following each exercise set and during recovery. Variables measured and/or calculated from echocardiogram include end diastolic and end systolic volumes, stroke volume, ejection fraction and cardiac output (30).

require cessation of exercise training (12). Some patients with heart failure experience a temporary increase in fluid accumulation 2 to 6 weeks after starting exercise, which may represent an increase in circulating plasma volume but typically does not preclude exercise training (29). Alterations in autonomic nervous system function and changes in medications may affect reflex response to positional changes, so care should be taken during lifting exercises that involve postural changes.

Resistance-Training Program Components

Individuals with heart failure have modest reductions in muscular strength relative to the healthy, age-matched population, but people with heart failure experience a substantial reduction in muscular endurance. The loss of muscular endurance is responsible for up to 40 percent of exercise intolerance in people with heart failure (20, 21). The resistance-training program design must take this factor into consideration and must also be based on previous studies conducted with a heart failure population using a full-body program (5, 7, 8, 17, 25, 27). The first 12 weeks of the resistance-training program will be performed as a circuit-training protocol. The 12-week program will be divided into two cycles: the first 8 weeks will include only machine-based exercises, and the last 4 weeks will substitute free-weight exercises for several of the machine-based exercises. The recommended program will consist of a series of resistance-training exercises performed in sequence with minimal rest (30-60 seconds) between exercises. The exercise professional should focus on shorter rest intervals, as muscular endurance is the factor most related to activities of daily living and most limiting for the individual with CHF. Approximately 8 to 12 repetitions of each exercise should be performed per circuit at a relative intensity of 50 to 80 percent of 1RM. Individuals will gradually progress to 3 sets of 8 repetitions at 80 percent of 1RM. Cardiac rehabilitation will likely be the best starting point for a resistance-training program tailored to an individual with CHF, because such a program will provide both education and supervision. Circuit weight-training programs can be efficiently performed in a rehabilitation setting. The second 12-weeks of the 24 week program can be divided into two 6-week cycles, with the first cycle performed in a health club setting and the second at both the health club and home settings. The health club environment will support continued supervision and education by exercise professionals.

The resistance-training program should be a full-body, progressive resistance-training program. An example of progression for the program is outlined in Table 7-3. Adequate rest and recovery are critical to optimal training outcomes. With the proposed regimen, more intense and less intense training periods are planned throughout the program so that stress does not accumulate to the point of adversity (11). Planned differences in intensity of training have been shown to prevent training plateaus often exhibited with progressive-overload programs (4, 5, 11). During the program, 1RM testing is performed frequently with the additional recommendation of beginning at low intensity (50 percent of 1RM) immediately after 1RM testing and progressing to 80 percent of 1RM prior to the next testing. Exercise training should be conducted under constant supervision and diligent spotting. Individuals should be properly oriented to the correct performance of each exercise and to each piece of equipment. Intermittent monitoring of heart rate and blood pressure should take place to ensure subject safety.

SAMPLE 24-WEEK PROGRAM

Weeks 1 through 8

Intensity will be set at 50 to 80 percent of 1RM, consistent with recommendations for beginning exercisers and their ability to attain optimal results consistent with the literature review provided in this chapter. Repetitions will range from 8 to 12, depending on the intensity; that is lower repetitions will be used at the higher intensities, and higher repetitions will be used at the lower intensities. The client should perform the prescribed sets and

Table 7-3 Periodized Progressive Resistance Training Program

Week	Monday (%RM, Sets x Repetitions)	Friday (%RM, Sets x Repetitions)
1	Baseline 1RM testing	50%, 2 x 12
2	50%, 2 x 12	1RM testing to revise intensity
3	50%, 2 x 12	50%, 2 x 12
4	60%, 2 x 10	70%, 2 x 10
5	80%, 1 x 8	80% 1 x 8
6	80%, 2 x 8	80%, 2 x 8
7	80%, 3 x 8	80% 3 x 8
8	80%, 3 x 8	1RM testing to revise intensity
9	50% 2 x 12	50% 2 x 12
10	60%, 2 x 10	70%, 2 x 10
11	80%, 1 x 8	80%, 2 x 8
12	80%, 3 x 8	1RM testing to revise intensity
13	50%, 2 x 12	50%, 2 x 12
14	50%, 2 x 12	50%, 2 x 12
15	60%, 2 x 10	70% 2 x 10
16	80%, 1 x 8	80%, 2 x 8
17	80%, 3 x 8	80%, 3 x 8
18	80%, 3 x 8	1RM testing to revise intensity
19	50% 2 x 12	50% 2 x 12
20	60% 2 x 10	70% 2 x 10
21	80%, 1 x 8	80%, 2 x 8
22	80%, 3 x 8	80%, 3 x 8
23	80%, 3 x 8	80%, 3 x 8
24	80%, 3 x 8	1RM testing to revise intensity

Weeks 1 through 8: machine based program in cardiac rehabilitation setting

Weeks 9 through 12: substitute dumbbell exercises for three of the machine based training

Weeks 13 through 18: machine based in a club setting

Weeks 19 through 24: machine and dumbbell exercises in both home and club setting repetitions for each exercise before moving to the next exercise. A brief 1-minute rest between sets should be allowed, and the estimated time to complete all the exercises should be approximately 20 minutes. The frequency of resistance training will be 2 days per week with 2 days in between training days as part of the cardiac rehabilitation program. Exercises will consist of leg presses, squats, shoulder presses, leg extensions, lat pulldowns, and cable biceps curls for weeks 1 through 8.

Weeks 9 through 12

At week 9, dumbbell lunges, dumbbell shoulder presses, and dumbbell curls will be substituted for the leg extensions, the machine shoulder presses, and cable biceps curls, respectively. The addition of the dynamic free-weight program at week 9 is beneficial for several reasons. First, it has been shown that the neuromuscular system is optimally challenged by activities that affect activities of daily living. Second, the free-weight program is reproducible outside of the clinic and thus provides resistance-training techniques that can be performed independently after completion of supervised exercise. Lastly, the dynamic free-weight program mimics the balance and strength requirements of activities such as walking and climbing stairs, facilitating the transfer of muscular strength gains to activities of daily life. In addition, 1RM testing is performed at frequent intervals during the training to appropriately adjust the exercise intensity.

Weeks 13 through 18

Upon graduation from cardiac rehabilitation, it is recommended that an individual with CHF spend 6 weeks in a club-based program to gain confidence and continue with education in an environment outside of a rehabilitation setting. The collaboration of the client with a personal trainer educated in working with individuals with heart conditions is also recommended. The recommended program will be similar with respect to recommended exercises in the first 8 weeks of cardiac rehabilitation, with intensity set at 50 to 80 percent of 1RM, and repetitions will range from 8 to 12 depending on

the intensity. The frequency of resistance training will be 2 days per week with a 2-day rest interval in between. Exercises will comprise the leg press, squat, shoulder press, leg extension, lat pulldown, and cable biceps curl exercises for weeks 12 through 18. Trainers in the rehabilitation setting may add or replace these exercises with any exercise that will work the same muscle groups, and such variation of the exercise routine may aid in encouraging adherence to the exercise program.

Weeks 19 through 24

At week 19, the dumbbell lunges, dumbbell shoulder presses, and dumbbell curls learned in cardiac rehabilitation can be performed in the home environment. The client may exercise in both the home setting and the health club setting, depending on personal preferences.

CASE STUDY

Ms. R is a 54-year-old woman, weighing 67.7 kg with a height of 163 cm. She had an anteroseptal myocardial infarction (MI) in 1996 that was treated with angioplasty and stent placement. Medications prescribed upon discharge from the hospital included a beta-blocker, an ACE inhibitor, and a cholesterol-lowering agent. Risk factors for the subject included a family history of heart disease: both Ms. R's mother and father died of an MI. Ms. R had been a smoker for most of her life, but quit immediately after her MI and has been smoke-free ever since. Her blood pressure has remained below 120 over 80, most likely due to her current medical therapy including the beta-blocker and ACE inhibitor.

Ms. R was asymptomatic for 4 years when she noted episodes of chest discomfort and shortness of breath during walking and cutting the grass. The occurrence of her chest pain was random, in that pain was present during an activity on one occasion but not the next. Her cardiologist suggested she undergo a cardiac catheterization to evaluate possible progression of the disease. Results of the catheterization procedure showed akinesis of anterolateral, anteroapical, and inferoapical walls; anterobasal hypokinesis; an ejection fraction of 30 percent; and a 60 to 70 percent in-stent restenosis of the mid-left anterior descending artery. Medical management was the treatment her cardiologist decided was best for her, and her ACE inhibitor was increased to 20 mg. Since then, Ms. R has not complained of any chest discomfort. Her physician increased her ACE inhibitor to 40 mg daily to achieve the maximum benefit, and Ms. R continues to do well with medical management.

Two years later, Ms. R enrolled in a research study and was randomized to a high-intensity, progressive strength and aerobic training group. Her aerobic power, expressed as peak oxygen consumption, was measured on a treadmill using the modified Naughton protocol. Ventricular function was measured with echocardiography performed during a standardized lifting test, which consisted of a warm-up set performed at 50 percent of a predetermined 1RM, followed by 3 sets performed at 70 percent of 1RM. Echocardiograms were performed at rest, during the last repetition for each of 3 sets of leg presses, and at the end of recovery. Ejection fraction was calculated using the formula (EDV-ESV)/ EDV. No detrimental changes in ventricular function were observed, as indicated by the ejection fraction results for the standard lifting task. Muscle strength was measured by the 1RM method for leg press, squat, shoulder press, leg extension, lat pulldown, and biceps curl exercises. All strength measurements were made with identical equipment positioning and technique before and following training.

Ms. R's exercise-training program consisted of cardiovascular training 3 days a week and resistance training 2 days a week for 36 sessions. She trained 15 minutes on both the treadmill and air-dyne bike at 60 to 80 percent of her heart rate reserve following a 5-minute warm-up at 50 percent of heart rate reserve. Exercise intensity was increased 0.5 Metabolic Equivalents of Task METs per week, consistent with patient tolerance. The exercises used for resistance training included the leg press, shoulder press, leg extension, lat pulldown, cable biceps curl, and horizontal squat, starting at

Table 7-4 Resistance-Training Results Measured in Kg at Baseline and after 12 and 24 Weeks of Training

Variable	Baseline	12 Weeks	24 Weeks
Leg press	69.7	110.6	130.8
Leg extension	41.8	62.7	–
Lat pull down	37.6	50.2	54.2
Squat	18.2	34.5	–
Dumbbell squat		36.4	40.7
Dumbbell lunges		26.3	31.4
Shoulder press	27.8	27.8	–
Dumbbell press		6.8	11.3
Cable bicep curl	29.3	37.6	
Dumbbell bicep curl		6.8	13.6

60 percent of 1RM and progressing to 80 percent as outlined in the first 12 weeks of Table 7-3. Ms. R demonstrated substantial gains in strength over the course of the training program (Table 7-4).

At the end of the training program, both systolic and diastolic blood pressure at rest were lower than at the beginning of the program (128/82 before training versus 108/72 after). Cardiopulmonary testing revealed improvements in VO₂ peak, an increase of 7 ml per kilogram per minute; METs increased by 2; peak workload reflected an increase from 3.0 mph at a 12.5 percent grade to 3.4 mph at a 14 percent grade; and Ms. R stated she was asymptomatic during the test. An echocardiography stress test showed that over the 24 weeks of training, baseline ejection fraction had increased from 19 to 40, and peak ejection fraction during the third set increased from 39 to 53. Likewise, 1RM strength had increased in most of the exercises (see Table 7-4).

Summary

Common characteristics of patients with heart failure are fatigue and exercise intolerance related to both cardiovascular and muscular dysfunction. Both aerobic training and resistance training are necessary for decreasing the symptoms associated with CHF and returning the individual to a high quality of life. Numerous research studies have shown that regular aerobic and resistance-training exercise improve not only exercise capacity but also muscle function. With appropriate screening and testing, most individuals with CHF can participate in high-intensity resistance training with no problems or exacerbation of symptoms or disease. Exercise professionals can safely work with these clients in cardiac rehabilitation settings as well as in the health club environment.

Key Terms

Beta-adrenergic–receptor blockers
Chronic heart failure
Diastolic dysfunction
Diuretics
Dyspnea
Exercise intolerance
Heart failure
Muscle hypothesis
Systolic dysfunction
Vasodilators

Study Questions

1. State the prevalence of heart failure in the United States and the associated economic costs of this condition.

2. Describe the current state of research and limitations of the research evaluating the impact of resistance training on heart failure.

3. Describe the role of resistance training in the treatment of heart failure.

4. Explain the specific factors to consider related to preexercise screening, exercise testing, and exercise prescription when designing a resistance-training program for individuals with heart failure.

5. Explain the underlying rationale for designing a resistance-training program that incorporates muscular strength, endurance, and power for individuals with heart failure.

References

1. Thom T, Hasse N, Rosamond W, et al and the AHA statistics committee. Heart disease and stroke statistics—2006 update: A report from the American Heart Association statistics committee and stroke statistics subcommittee. *Circulation.* 2006;113:e85-151.

2. ACC/AHA 2005 guidelines update for the diagnosis and management of chronic heart failure in the adult: A report of the American College of Cardiology/American Heart Association task force on practice guidelines. American College of Cardiology Web Site. Available at: http://www.acc.org/clinical/guidelines/failure//index.pdf.

3. ACSM. *ACSM's Guidelines for Exercise Testing and Prescription.* 6th ed. Philadelphia: Lippincott, Williams and Wilkins; 2000.

4. Adams KJ, Barnard, KL, Swank, AM, Mann, E, Kushnick, MR, DM Denny. Combined high-intensity strength and aerobic training in diverse phase II cardiac rehabilitation patients. *J. Cardiopulm Rehabil.* 1999;19:209-215.

5. Barnard, KL, Adams, KJ, Swank, AM, Kaelin, M, Kushnik, MR, Denny DM. Combined high-intensity strength and aerobic training in patients with congestive heart failure. *Journal of Strength and Conditioning Research.* 2000;14(4):383-388.

6. Coats AJ, Adamopoulus S, Radaelli A, et al. Controlled trial of physical training in chronic heart failure. Exercise performance, hemodynamics, ventilation and autonomic function. *Circulation.* 1992;85:2119-2131.

7. Delagardelle C, Feiereisen P, Autier P, Shita R, Krecke R, Beissel J. Strength/endurance training versus endurance training in congestive heart failure. *Med Sci Sport Exerc.* 2002;34(12):1868-1872.

8. Delagardelle, C, Feiereisen, P, Krecke, R, Essamri, B, Beissel, J. Objective effects of a 6-months endurance and strength training program in outpatients with congestive heart failure. *Med Sci Sport Exerc.* 1999;31:1102-1107.

9. Evans WJ. Reversing sarcopenia: How weight training can build strength and vitality. *Geriatrics.* 1996;51:46-53.

10. Falconer, TM, Logan, TL, Stone, JA, Haennel, RG. The safety and efficacy of resistance training in stable heart failure patients [abstract]. *J. Cardiopulmonary Rehabil.* 1998;18:351.

11. Fleck SJ, Kraemer WJ. *Designing Resistance Training Programs.* 2nd ed. Champaign, IL: Human Kinetics; 1997.

12. Hanson P. Exercise testing and training in patients with chronic heart failure. *Med. Sci Sports Exerc.* 1994;26:527-537.

13. Hare DL, Ryan TM, Selig SE, Pellizzer AM, Wrigley TV, Krum H. Resistance exercise training increases muscle strength, endurance and blood flow in patients with chronic heart failure. *Am J Cardiol.* 1999;83:1674-1677.

14. Hambrecht R, Adams V, Gielen S, et al. Exercise intolerance in patients with chronic heart failure and increased expression of inducible nitric oxide synthase in the skeletal muscle. *J Am Coll Cardiol.* 1999;33:174-179.

15. Harrington D, Anker SD, Coats AJ. Preservation of exercise capacity and lack of peripheral changes in asymptomatic patients with severely impaired left ventricular function. *Eur Heart J.* 1998;19:O29-034.

16. Keteyian SJ, Brawner CA, Schairer JR. Exercise testing and training of patients with heart failure due to left ventricular dysfunction. *J Cardiopulmonaryl Rehabil.* 1997;17:19-28.

17. Levinger I, Bronks R, Cody DV, Linton I, Davie A. The effect of resistance training on left ventricular function and structure of patients with chronic heart failure. *Int J Cardiol.* 2005;105:159-163.

18. Maiorana A, O'Driscoll G, Cheetham C, et al. Combined aerobic and resistance exercise training improves functional capacity and strength in CHF. *J Appl Physiol.* 2000;88:1565-1570.

19. McKelvie RS, McCartney N, Tomlinson C, Bauer R, MacDougall JD. Comparison of hemodynamic responses to cycling and resistance exercise in congestive heart failure secondary to ischemic cardiomyopathy. *Am J Cardiol.* 1995;76:977-979.

20. Minotti, JR, Johnson, EC, Hudson, TL, et al. Skeletal muscle response to exercise training in congestive heart failure. *J Clin Invest.* 1990;86:751-758.

21. Minotti JR, Christoph I, Oka, R, Weiner MW, Wells, L, Massie BM. Impaired skeletal muscle function in patients with congestive heart failure: Relationship to systemic exercise performance. *J Clin Invest.* 1991;88:2077-2082.

22. Minotti JR, Pillay P, Chang L, Wells, L, Massie BM. Neurophysiological assessment of skeletal muscle fatigue in patients with congestive heart failure. *Circulation.* 1992;86:903-908.

23. Monchamp T, Frishman WH. Exercise as a treatment modality for congestive heart failure. *Heart Dis.* 2002;4:110-116.

24. Oka RK, DeMarco T, Haskell WL, et al. Impact of a home-based walking and resistance training program on quality of life in patients with heart failure. *Am J Cardiol.* 2000;85:365-369.

25. Pu CT, Johnson MT, Forman DE, et al. Randomized trial of progressive resistance training to counteract the myopathy of chronic heart failure. *J Appl Physiol.* 2001;90:2341-2350.

26. Roveda F, Middlekauff HR, Rondon M, et al. The effects of exercise training on sympathetic neural activation in advanced heart failure. *J Am Coll Cardiol.* 2003;42:854-860.

27. Santoro C, Cosmas A, Forman D, et al. Exercise training alters skeletal muscle mitochondrial

morphometry in heart failure patients. *J Cardiovasc Risk.* 2002;9:377-381.

28. Selig SE, Carey MF, Menzies DG, et al. Moderate-intensity resistance exercise training in patients with chronic heart failure improves strength, endurance, heart rate variability and forearm blood flow. *J Card Fail.* 2004;10(1):21-30.

29. Sullivan J. Exercise training in heart failure: An intervention whose time has come. *J Card Fail.* 1997;3:13-15.

30. Swank AM, Funk D, Manire JT, Degruccio L, Dimitriadis CK, Denny DM. Echocardiographic evaluation of stress test for determining safety of participation in strength training. *J Strength Cond Res.* 2005;19:389-393.

31. Tyni-Lenne R, Dencker K, Gordon A, Jansson E, Sylven C. Comprehensive local muscle training increases aerobic working capacity and quality of life and decreases neurohormonal activation in patients with chronic heart failure. *Eur J Heart Fail.* 2001;3:47-52.

32. Tyni-Lenne R, Gordon A, Sylven C. Improved quality of life in chronic heart failure patients following local endurance training with leg muscles. *J Card Fail.* 1996;2(2):111-117.

33. Tyni-Lenne R, Gordon A, Europe E, Jansson E, Sylven C. Exercise-based rehabilitation improves skeletal muscle capacity, exercise tolerance and quality of life in both women and men with chronic heart failure. *J Card Fail.* 1998;4:9-17.

34. Tyni-Lenne R, Gordon A, Jansson E, Bermann G, Sylven C. Skeletal muscle endurance training improves peripheral oxidative capacity, exercise tolerance, and health-related quality of life in women with chronic congestive heart failure secondary to either ischemic cardiomyopathy or idiopathic dilated cardiomyopathy. *Am J Cardiol.* 1997;80:1025-1029.

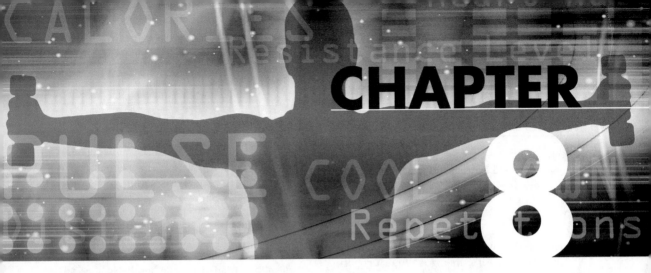

CHAPTER 8

RESISTANCE-TRAINING STRATEGIES FOR ADULT OBESITY

Objectives

Upon completion of this chapter, the reader should be able to:

- Identify the prevalence of obesity in the United States and the associated economic costs
- Explain the utility and limitations of using body mass index (BMI) to define obesity
- Describe the role of resistance training in the treatment of obesity
- Explain the factors to consider when designing a resistance-training program for obese individuals
- Provide the underlying rationale for designing a resistance-training program that incorporates muscular strength, endurance, and power for obese individuals
- Describe appropriate exercise progression and exercise choices for individuals who are obese

INTRODUCTION

Obesity is one of the most prevalent conditions among adults and is commonly defined using **body mass index (BMI),** which is a ratio of the weight of body in kilograms to the square of its height in meters. Obesity is associated with the onset of significant health problems, and it has risen to epidemic levels in the United States over the past few decades (19). This finding is of great concern, because obesity is a precursor to numerous major health problems including cardiovascular disease, non–insulin-dependent diabetes mellitus, hypertension, sleep apnea, dyslipidemia, osteoarthritis, and many cancers (29). Therefore, it is important to better understand behavioral patterns, nutritional strategies, and exercise modalities that contribute to the development of obesity and to examine the contribution of each in the treatment of obesity.

PREVALENCE AND ECONOMIC COST OF ADULT OBESITY

The prevalence of adult obesity has reached epidemic proportions in the United States. An estimated 66.3 percent of adults in the United States are overweight, with greater than 32.2 percent classified as obese (38). These trends are occurring at even higher rates in non-Hispanic black and Mexican American populations, with the rates of obesity in these ethnicities at 76.1 percent and 75.8 percent, respectively (38). Unfortunately, these trends have been increasing over the last few decades. Parikh and colleagues reported in 2007 that incidence rates of overweight increased twofold, and obesity more than threefold, over the previous five decades (40). These results suggest that this increase is not a recent phenomenon, but rather a persistent pattern throughout the last few decades.

Data from the Framingham Heart Study found that over a 10- to 30-year period, the long-term risks for white men and women of becoming obese

were greater than 25 percent (44). The average percentage of body fat for U.S. males is approximately 15 to 18 percent, for females it is approximately 22 to 25 percent. Body-fat levels greater than 22 to 25 percent and 35 to 38 percent are considered obese for males and females, respectively (20).

The economic cost of obesity can be defined in terms of both direct and indirect costs. Direct costs include those to the health care system for diagnosis, treatment, physician visits, and hospitalizations for the comorbidities associated with obesity. Indirect costs include lost worker productivity and lost income due to disability caused by obesity. The indirect costs are harder to estimate and may be underestimated, because additional costs associated with increases in body weight, such as impaired physical functioning and increased risk of infertility, are not typically included in these estimates. Obesity has been associated with a greater annual medical expenditure and more burden on health care resources compared to normal-weight individuals. In 1995 the indirect obesity-attributable costs were estimated to be $48 billion. In 2003, the direct costs of obesity in the United States were estimated to be $75 billion—an increase of 56 percent over the previous 8 years, with approximately 50 percent of those expenditures covered by Medicare and Medicaid (13).

ETIOLOGY OF ADULT OBESITY

Factors influencing body-weight regulation are complex and include a number of genetic, hormonal, metabolic, dietary, and environmental influences (31, 34, 35, 46, 50). For most individuals, the cause of obesity is primarily related to imbalances between energy intake and energy expenditure. **Energy balance** is achieved when the level of energy intake equals the level of energy expenditure, and it is most accurately calculated over a number of days or weeks rather than day to day. In the case of adult obesity, individuals are in a state of positive energy balance, meaning they consume more energy than they are expending. Conversely, a negative energy balance indicates greater energy expenditure than intake, which results in weight loss. Energy expenditure is affected by resting metabolic rate, the thermic effect of digestion, and exercise (42, 56). Although positive energy balance for an individual with adult obesity is created due to decreases in energy expenditure and increases in energy intake, this problem is not always controllable. Individual factors such as genetic predisposition and hypothalamic alterations may impact the energy balance equation by lowering energy expenditure through impaired resting metabolism (4, 6). Thus, it is important to recognize that increases in body weight or lack of weight loss can be caused by a multitude of factors and are not necessarily associated with a sedentary lifestyle, lack of motivation, or noncompliance with diet and exercise recommendations.

BODY MASS INDEX (BMI)

Body mass index (BMI) is a simple and relatively straightforward way to classify individuals based on anthropometrics. BMI is calculated by dividing weight in kilograms by height in meters squared. Table 8-1 provides a simple way to determine BMI using weight in pounds and height in inches. Recommendations for an ideal BMI range are made by government bodies and the World Health Organization based on epidemiological studies that have assessed the relationship between weight and chronic disease (11, 15, 54, 55). In most cases, lower BMI is related to a lower risk for cardiovascular disease, hypertension, diabetes, several types of cancer (kidney, colon, breast, and endometrial), and associated comorbidities (15, 36, 52, 54, 55). Table 8-2 lists the current BMI classifications and corresponding disease risks.

Using BMI to identify obese individuals is not without its limitations. BMI does not distinguish the quality of body weight; that is, it cannot distinguish between fat and fat-free body mass, bone, or protein. Thus, it is possible that an individual can be classified as obese based on the BMI and still have a relatively low level of excess body fat. This finding is often the case with body builders, power lifters, and professional football players, who tend to have a high amount of lean body mass relative to total body size. A study by Harp and Hecht (18) reported on the prevalence of overweight and obesity in professional football players in the National Football League (NFL) during 2003 and 2004. They found that 97 percent of football players in the league were classified as overweight, 56 percent met criteria for Class I obesity, 26 percent met the criteria for Class II obesity, and 3 percent met the criteria for Class III obesity. In contrast, a study conducted on the body size and composition of NFL football players found BMI to be a poor indicator of an athlete's health status, because it failed to consider body composition (26). Despite meeting BMI criteria for overweight or obesity, most NFL football players had body composition values that were classified as "healthy" or "good." Only offensive linemen, whose performance is often related to total overall mass and size, had body composition that was considered to be "poor." Therefore, when defining obesity, the exercise professional must not only consider overall body mass but also the quality of the body mass.

BODY FAT DISTRIBUTION

In addition to discerning total body composition, knowing where body fat is carried is important. **Central adiposity**, also known as **android obesity**, is found in individuals who carry excess amounts of body fat in the abdominal area and trunk. **Gynoid obesity** is characterized by excess amounts of body fat in the lower-body region, in the hips and thighs. Central adiposity is identified through a simple waist measurement: men with a waist circumference greater than 40 inches and women with a waist circumference greater than 35 inches are at greater risk for cardiovascular disease, diabetes, stroke, and certain cancers (8, 32, 36, 52). For individuals with a high amount of central adiposity, increases in energy expenditure and decreases in caloric intake are recommended to decrease body weight (24).

Table 8-1 Body Mass Index Chart

Weight in Pounds

		Healthy Weight						Overweight							Obese									
58in	91	96	100	105	110	115	119	124	129	134	138	143	148	153	158	162	167
59in	94	99	104	109	114	119	124	128	133	138	143	148	153	158	163	168	173
60in	97	102	107	112	118	123	128	133	138	143	148	153	158	163	158	174	179
61in	100	106	111	116	122	127	132	137	143	148	153	158	164	169	174	180	185
62in	104	109	115	120	126	131	136	142	147	153	158	164	169	175	180	186	191
63in	107	113	118	124	130	135	141	146	152	158	163	169	175	180	186	191	197
64in	110	116	122	128	134	140	145	151	157	163	169	174	180	186	192	197	204
65in	114	120	126	132	138	144	150	156	162	168	174	180	186	192	198	204	210
66in	118	124	130	136	142	148	155	161	167	173	179	186	192	198	204	210	216
67in	121	127	134	140	146	153	159	166	172	178	185	191	198	204	211	217	223
68in	125	131	138	144	151	158	164	171	177	184	190	197	203	210	216	223	230
69in	128	135	142	149	155	162	169	176	182	189	196	203	209	216	223	230	236
70in	132	139	146	153	160	167	174	181	188	195	202	209	216	222	229	236	243
71in	136	143	150	157	165	172	179	186	193	200	208	215	222	229	236	243	250
72in	140	147	154	162	169	177	184	191	199	206	213	221	228	235	242	250	258
73in	144	151	159	166	174	182	189	197	204	212	219	227	235	242	250	257	265
74in	148	155	163	171	179	186	194	202	210	218	225	233	241	249	256	264	272
75in	152	160	168	176	184	192	200	208	216	224	232	240	248	256	264	272	279
BMI	19	20	21	22	23	24	25	26	27	28	29	30	31	32	33	34	35

adults who are moderately active and who have no known risk factors will have a greater capacity to engage in resistance training than the morbidly obese and bed ridden. Programs should be designed according to the functional capacity of the individual, keeping in mind the limitations regarding weight-bearing versus non–weight-bearing exercise, orthopedic problems, range of motion, and flexibility as well as the goals for the primary outcome of the training program, which should include improved functional ability, muscular endurance, strength, and improvements in body composition. These parameters will dictate the lower and upper limits of the training program. For example, an individual may have a functional capacity of 4 metabolic equivalents of task (METs) and may not be able to perform weight-bearing resistance activity for more than 5 minutes. Parameters such as these should be factored into the program design.

Exercise Testing Considerations

When working with obese individuals, it is important to conduct appropriate screening procedures to ensure the safety of engaging in a resistance-training program. Specific screening tests for obese adults should include the following:

- ○ Medical history
- ○ Current medication use
- ○ Weight history
- ○ Body composition

Medical history is the most important screening consideration before starting any resistance-training program in any at-risk population. Obtain medical clearance from a primary care physician to identify possible contraindications to exercise or considerations for supervision. In addition, exercise testing is imperative to determine the level of training to prescribe for the individual. Exercise testing will not only act as a safety measure, it will also provide the exercise professional with limitations to the program design for each individual.

Along with a medical history, obtain a list of medications that the individual is currently taking.

Adult obesity is associated with a number of comorbid conditions such as hypertension, diabetes, cardiovascular disease, and osteoarthritis, and therefore some medications may have been prescribed. Thus, identifying medications the client is currently taking, including the dosage, frequency, and reason for the prescription, to determine any potential influence the medication may have on resistance-training responses, is essential. Two medications, sibutramine, sold by prescription under the brand name Meridia, and orlistat, sold by prescription under the brand name Xenical and over the counter as Alli, are commonly prescribed for the long-term treatment of obesity. Sibutramine is a serotonin-norepinephrine reuptake inhibitor, and the primary mechanism of action is to reduce food intake by increasing feelings of satiety. It has been shown to have a stimulatory effect on both heart rate and blood pressure (7, 48). Studies comparing sibutramine to a placebo found increases of 4 to 5 beats per minute in heart rate and 1 to 3 mmHg in systolic and diastolic blood pressure in subjects taking sibutramine (7). Furthermore, acute increases in blood pressure responses have been reported during resistance training (33, 37), so caution should be taken to monitor blood pressure responses before, during, and after resistance training to ensure client safety. Orlistat is an inhibitor of lipases, and the primary mechanism of action is to increase fecal fat loss. Unlike sibutramine, orlistat does not have an impact on cardiovascular responses during exercise, but side effects associated with orlistat include fecal incontinence, oily spotting, and flatus with discharge (12). Although orlistat is generally well tolerated, clients should be cautioned that gastrointestinal side effects may be experienced during resistance training, so timing of meals may become an important consideration to reduce these negative effects.

Weight history, the history of average body weight including weight gains and losses during adulthood, is an important consideration with individuals engaging in a weight-loss program. Discussing weight history can help the exercise professional ascertain a client's level of motivation for changing eating and exercise behaviors, and it may also provide information about the potential barriers and the likelihood of success. For example, an individual who has struggled with weight management and physical inactivity since childhood may have additional barriers to overcome compared to someone who became obese as an adult. Discussing whether they have struggled with body weight in the past, and also identifying those factors that may have negatively impacted previous attempts at weight loss and exercise participation, can provide further insight. Additionally, the individual should be queried as to how those same factors may impact current attempts at weight loss and physical activity.

Body composition, the combination of fat mass and fat-free mass, can be an important tool for assessing fat distribution and health risk in obese adults. Numerous anthropometric methods to evaluate body composition and fat distribution are available, and each method has its strengths and weaknesses. A few of the more common methods to assess body composition are outlined in Table 8-4.

Overweight and obese individuals have an increased risk for a number of diseases, which often increases their risk for complications during exercise testing and training. After obtaining medical clearance, a number of factors should be weighed before deciding upon appropriate exercise testing. Exercise testing is a highly recommended and useful consideration prior to designing a resistance-training program. Resistance-exercise testing, however, may not be appropriate for all individuals, therefore it is important to determine which participants may be at greatest risk for experiencing an adverse event while engaging in resistance exercise, based on information contained in the medical history and obtained through consultation with clients.

Resistance-exercise testing that relies on using 1RM and other testing protocols, such as multiple-RM tests, have proven to be safe for a variety of populations including cardiac patients, elderly, and children (20, 49). The most accurate method of prescribing resistance-training intensity is to administer 1RM tests to determine maximal strength. These tests can be administered using either free weights or weight machines. Although a 1RM effort is considered the "gold standard"

for exercise testing, both 1RM and multiple-RM (e.g. 6RM, 10RM) protocols can be used to determine a baseline value for prescribing exercise intensity.

Training Program Components

As with all resistance-training programs, progressive overload should be incorporated so that adaptations and increases in muscular endurance, strength, and power occur in a gradual and safe manner. The degree of progressive overload will also depend on the initial functional capacity, as well as the frequency, intensity, and volume of training. For a bed-ridden individual who is unable to perform weight-bearing exercise, overload can be achieved by having them stand out of bed periodically throughout the day. On the other hand, for the individual who is targeting muscular strength, overload would most likely come from increasing the amount of resistance. Regardless of the type of overload, consistently increase the amount of work being performed once adaptations have occurred. Some evidence suggests that novice weight lifters do not self-select exercise intensities that promote muscular strength and hypertrophy. A study examining weight-lifting exercise intensities for a variety of upper- and lower-body exercises by previously untrained men and women found that both men and women lifted a resistance equal to 42 to 57 percent of 1RM (17). Although increases in muscular endurance may be possible with these intensities and with sufficient volume, this training stimulus would not be sufficient for individuals who are interested in muscular strength and power. Thus, providing novice weight lifters with appropriate instruction, supervision, and feedback is essential to ensure an appropriate training stimulus and overload schedule that matches the client's individual needs and goals.

Use of RPE to determine subjective exercise intensity is an effective method of prescribing exercise intensity in obese adults. Although the Borg 15-point categoryRPE scale and CR-10 ratio scales continue to remain popular in clinical and health fitness settings, more recent scales have been developed that make use of both pictorial and verbal descriptors to

Table 8-4 Methods of Assessing Body Composition

Measure	Rationale	Utility in Overweight and Obese Populations
Waist–hip ratio (WHR)	Identify individuals who are predominantly upper- versus lower-body fat carriers.	WHR has been associated with disease risk and mortality. It is an inexpensive tool that can be used with clients in conjunction with other methods, to provide an overall estimate of health risk.
Waist circumference (WC)	Studies have shown a close relationship between WC and cardiovascular disease.	Studies have suggested that WC is a better marker of visceral fat than WHR, meaning it may better estimate health risk. Using this tool in conjunction with other measurements will provide a better assessment than relying solely on one tool.
Abdominal sagittal diameter	Studies have shown sagittal diameter to be more predictive of metabolic risk factors than WHR or WC.	Although it may be a better predictor of risk factors, correlation between this measure and the simpler waist circumference is relatively high. Waist circumference is easier to assess and may therefore be a more appropriate screening tool.
Skinfold thicknesses	Inexpensive measurement; portable and reliable in specific populations	Less precise in overweight and obese populations compared to circumference measurements. If too much adipose tissue is present, the calipers may not expand enough to obtain an accurate measurement.
Bioelectrical impedance (BIA)	Fast, noninvasive, and relatively inexpensive measure of body composition; less obtrusive for clients than skinfold measures or hydrostatic weighing	BIA may be affected by factors such as eating, drinking, and exercise, which affect hydration status. Ideally suited for determining change in body composition over time and during periods of weight loss.
Hydrostatic Weighing	Considered the gold standard for assessment of total body adiposity	Hydrostatic weighing is available in some research, laboratory, and hospital facilities but is not generally available to the public. In addition, obese individuals with an extremely high amount of body fat may be too buoyant to obtain a measure of total body fat.
Air displacement plethysmography ("Bod Pod")	Convenient, fast assessment of total body adiposity; requires minimal technician skill	The "Bod Pod" is relatively expensive and may not be available in all areas. However, it is a highly convenient, fast, and reliable measure of total body adiposity. Research has shown the Bod Pod to be highly correlated to measures of body fat from hydrostatic weighing.
Computed tomography (CT) scan	Considered the gold standard for measuring adipose tissue compartments and sometimes total body adiposity	This method is not practical to use during as an everyday assessment, even though it is valid and reliable. It is very useful to differentiate between different compartments that may have fatty tissue, such as subcutaneous and visceral adipose tissue.

assist individuals monitoring exercise intensity. The OMNI RPE scale (Figure 8-1) is applicable to a wide range of individuals and physical abilities (45). The OMNI RPE scale designed for resistance training can be used to prescribe resistance-exercise intensity by having individuals select an exercise intensity that corresponds to the preferred training program outcome. To use this scale, individuals would take the following steps:

- Select an initial training goal, such as endurance, hypertrophy, or power.
- Have the client use trial and error to select an initial weight that corresponds to the OMNI training zone. For example, if an individual were interested in training for muscular hypertrophy, a weight would be selected that corresponded to an intensity of 6 on the OMNI scale, if that felt somewhat hard following completion of the first repetition. Keep in mind that initially it may take

several trials before the individual identifies a weight that feels like a 6, but over time, this process will become easier.

- The individual should complete as many repetitions as necessary until an RPE of 10 had been reached for the exercise set. If the individual completed more than 6 repetitions, the weight was too light, so a heavier weight should be selected for the next set. If the individual completed fewer than 3 repetitions, the weight was too heavy, and a lighter weight should be selected for the next set.

The OMNI RPE scale for resistance training does not use a predetermined number of repetitions per set. Rather, the individual completes as many repetitions as necessary until an RPE of 10 is reached. A benefit of prescribing resistance training in this manner is that clients naturally make adjustments in the amount of weight lifted by always choosing a weight that corresponds

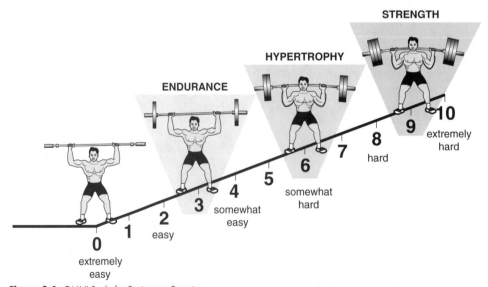

Figure 8-1 OMNI Scale for Resistance Exercise.
Reprinted with permission from Robertson RJ. *Perceived Exertion for Practitioners*. Champaign, IL: Human Kinetics; 2004.

with the starting RPE on the scale. Over time, as strength increases, a weight that previously felt like a 6 will begin to feel like a lower number, so the amount of weight used will increase. Thus, clients are always working at an optimal training intensity to maximize program goals.

The American College of Sports Medicine (ACSM) recommends 1 set of 8 to 12 repetitions of 8 to 10 exercises that utilize major muscle groups (arms, shoulders, chest, abdomen, back, hips, and legs) 2 or 3 days a week for enhanced strength, muscular endurance, and maintenance of fat-free mass (1). Although a repetition range lower than 8 to 12 may better optimize strength and power (14), the training goal for an at-risk person, such as those who are obese and untrained, should focus on improvements in functional capacity, neuromuscular development, strength, and endurance. Emphasizing this goal will increase mobility, facilitate activities of daily living, and lead to decreased pain during activities to allow the individual to progressively increase energy expenditure. Therefore, increase the number of repetitions to 10 to 15 per set, lower the load, and increase the number of sets per exercise to 2 or 3 for safety purposes when first implementing a resistance-training program with someone who is obese.

Both muscular strength and endurance can be enhanced by overloading the system with external resistance in the form of static and dynamic exercises. Static or isometric activities are less functional due to their limited ability to mimic everyday activities, and they may actually be unsafe because of their resultant acute increase in blood pressure. Therefore, use dynamic activities for the obese individual, allowing for a greater range of motion, and encourage slower, controlled rhythmical movements with a normal breathing pattern during lifting. Exercise selection should include multiple-joint activities such as body-weight squats, seated chest presses, and lat pulldowns. These movements will not only utilize more overall muscle mass, thereby increasing energy expenditure, they are also more functional movements and have a greater carryover to activities of daily living. Movements should mimic those that an individual would do on

a regular basis, such as sitting and standing, lifting groceries or other materials from overhead, or bending down to pick objects up from the floor.

A variety of exercise equipment is available to choose from when designing a resistance-training program for the obese individual. Each type of equipment has both advantages and limitations that are determined by the skill of the individual, the cost of the equipment, and access to exercise facilities. Resistance-training machines are often recommended for the purpose of safety and comfort, because they eliminate uncertainty about the movement and usually do not require a spotter (20). However, machines are not typically designed for obese individuals, and the client simply may not fit into the seat of a resistance-training machine. In this case, equipment modifications are required to prevent discomfort, promote safety, and reduce embarrassment. Moreover, resistance-training machines have less carryover to activities of daily living compared to free weights, because machines only allow the body to move in one plane, and everyday activities do not have this set movement pattern.

An alternative to weight machines is free weights. Free weights require more training, both for safety and to understand specific movement patterns. A spotter is also encouraged to ensure safety during resistance training with free weights, which can be beneficial to increase motivation and adherence. The balance and stability required during free-weight exercises is beneficial and may have a carryover into everyday activities. Free-weight routines do not have to include traditional dumbbells or barbells; simple weighted objects such as milk jugs, laundry detergent containers, or soup cans are just as effective and may be most appropriate for home-based deconditioned individuals. Other equipment that may be useful includes resistance tubing, stability balls, and medicine balls. Each of these devices may provide variation in training programs, potentially enhancing adherence and motivation because of the variety. A selection of sample exercises with examples of progression based on training level is provided in Table 8-5.

Table 8-5 Sample of Exercises According to Training Level

Beginner	Intermediate	Advanced
Legs: A) Standing and sitting from a chair B) Body weight lunge holding on to bench for stability	A) Body-weight wall squats with back against a stability ball to allow for squatting motion B) Body-weight lunge with hands on hips	A) Squats, holding dumbbells at sides of the body B) Standing lunge, holding dumbbells in hands
Chest: A) Standing wall push-up so body is nearly parallel to wall at arms distance B) Seated chest press	A) Standing wall push-up at a 45-degree angle from wall B) Supine barbell press	A) Floor push-up with knees on ground B) Supine dumbbell press
Back: A) Seated row B) Superman back extensions on hands and knees	A) Dumbbell row B) Prone back extensions	A) Lat pulldown B) Dumbbell deadlift
Shoulders: A) Dumbbell lateral raise	A) Seated dumbbell military press	A) Standing military press
Arms: A) Seated dumbbell biceps curl B) Triceps pushdown	A) Standing dumbbell biceps curl B) Overhead dumbbell triceps extension	A) Barbell biceps curl B) Seated dips

Behavioral Considerations

Compliance to exercise programs is problematic for all individuals but particularly with sedentary and deconditioned individuals. Obese individuals often elect to participate in an exercise regimen for reasons other than personal choice. Often these motivations include recommendations from physicians, suggestions from family and friends, or guilt or worry over material they read in a newspaper or magazine or saw on television. Therefore it is important to recognize that not all individuals will be willing to adopt and maintain an exercise program.

Motivational Readiness for Change refers to the readiness to adopt and engage in regular, structured physical activity. Measuring motivational readiness for change can help the exercise professional determine the likelihood that an individual will successfully adopt an exercise program. A sample of questions and a flow chart for determining an individual's motivational readiness for change is provided in Figure 8-2. An individual who is in *precontemplation* is not considering changing behaviors and is very unlikely to adopt an exercise program. Someone who is in *contemplation* is considering changing behaviors but has yet to take the necessary steps to begin a physical activity program. Individuals in *preparation* have begun to take steps to become more active but may be inconsistent with physical activity behavior. Finally, individuals who are in *action* or *maintenance*

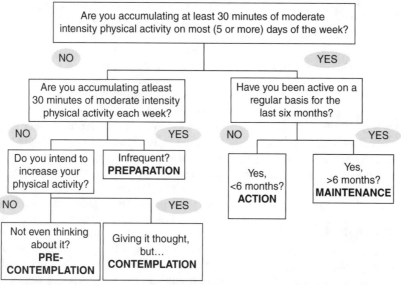

Figure 8-2 Motivational Readiness to Change.

Reprinted with permission from Blair SN, et al. *Active Living Every Day.* Champaign, IL: Human Kinetics; 2001.

have adopted a physical activity program. Individuals in action, however, have adopted this behavior for less than 6 months, whereas those in maintenance have been participating in physical activity for 6 months or longer.

SAMPLE 24-WEEK PROGRAM

This sample 24-week program is intended to start an untrained, obese individual on a resistance-training regimen using the guidelines outlined in this chapter. The untrained individual should start a program with beginner-level exercises to grow accustomed to the movements and feelings of how muscles work. Training to failure is unnecessary and can put an untrained individual at risk for cardiovascular complications. The first 8 weeks of the 24-week program begin with 2 sets per exercise, progressing to 3 sets of 10 to 15 repetitions. At the end of 8 weeks, the intermediate exercises are implemented, and sets decrease to 2 to ensure proper

form, because the client may be fatigued earlier with changing exercises. As individuals grow accustomed to the exercises, the number of sets increases to 3 for the final 4 weeks of the phase. Finally, during the last 8 weeks of the 24-week program, the individual should understand his or her body, how to contract different muscles, and how various movements affect the muscles. Therefore the advanced versions of each of the exercises are implemented, but the sets decrease to 2 for the first 4 weeks and increase to 3 for the final 4 weeks. The exercises selected are primarily multiple-joint exercises to increase the energy expenditure with activity and utilize the larger muscle groups in the body during movement. Advanced trainees may utilize different training splits for body parts and may incorporate more exercises per body part.

Weeks 1 through 4

Perform exercises 3 days per week with 1 day of rest between sessions. Complete 2 sets of 10 to 15 repetitions for each of the beginning exercises listed in Table 8-5.

Weeks 5 through 8

Perform exercises 3 days per week with 1 day of rest between sessions. Complete 3 sets of 10 to 15 repetitions for each of the beginning exercises listed in Table 8-5.

Weeks 9 through 12

Perform exercises 3 days per week with 1 day of rest between sessions. Complete 2 sets of 10 to 15 repetitions for each of the intermediate exercises listed in Table 8-5.

Weeks 13 through 16

Perform exercises 3 days per week with 1 day of rest between sessions. Complete 3 sets of 10 to 15 repetitions for each of the intermediate exercises listed in Table 8-5.

Weeks 17 through 20

Perform exercises 3 days per week with 1 day of rest between sessions. Complete 2 sets of 10 to 15 repetitions for each of the advanced exercises listed in Table 8-5.

Weeks 21 through 24

Perform exercises 3 days per week with 1 day of rest between sessions. Complete 3 sets of 10 to 15 repetitions for each of the advanced exercises listed in Table 8-5.

CASE STUDY

Mr. L, a 54-year-old man with Class I obesity (BMI = 32.3 kg/m^2) is interested in participating in a resistance-training program to increase functional ability, decrease body fat, and to improve overall muscle tone, strength, and endurance. After completing his medical history, you learn that he has type 2 diabetes and is on a number of medications to control his blood glucose levels. Other than obesity and diabetes, he has no known disease or anything else in his medical history that precludes him from beginning a sound diet and exercise regimen.

Because Mr. L is a sedentary individual with some previous exercise experience, a program of 2 sets of 10 to 15 repetitions per exercise is prescribed. He is set up with a program that uses multiple-joint exercises to enhance the energy expenditure of the movements during his weight-loss efforts. He is also instructed to test his blood glucose before, during, and after training to determine what effect resistance and aerobic training are having on his blood glucose levels. The resistance is monitored closely to ensure that he increases the intensity when training and also to ensure he is using proper form during his exercises. His cardiovascular exercise started at 20 minutes per day, 5 days per week. Each subsequent week, 5 minutes were added per day until a maximum of 60 minutes per day was reached by week 8.

After 8 weeks with an improved diet, resistance training, and regular cardiovascular exercise, Mr. L had lost approximately 16 pounds. In addition, his body fat levels decreased 4 percent, measured using bioelectrical impedance, and he maintained his previous level of lean body mass and felt as though he had increased his coordination, balance, and ability to feel more comfortable with activities of daily living. He has since been taken off his medications for diabetes and now has the energy to play with his grandchildren without getting out of breath.

Summary

Prevalence of overweight and obesity has risen to epidemic levels: in the United States, 66.3 percent of the adult population is overweight, and approximately 32.2 percent are obese. Adopting a healthy diet and a sound exercise regimen that includes regular cardiovascular exercise, along with resistance exercise, is optimal. Research has suggested that cardiovascular exercise is most important for overall energy expenditure during weight loss and for weight maintenance. Resistance exercise can also play an important role in weight loss by improving functional capacity, muscular endurance, and neuromuscular development, which enhances mobility, activities of daily living, and lessens pain, straining, and discomfort during activities. Resistance training can and should be a part of the exercise prescription during weight loss to assist with functional capacity and allow for greater mobility with cardiovascular activities. These two modes of exercise, combined with a sound decrease in energy intake, is the optimal way to successfully decrease body fat and maintain weight loss.

Key Terms

Android obesity
Body composition
Body mass index (BMI)
Central adiposity
Energy balance
Gynoid obesity
Motivational Readiness for Change
Obesity
Weight history

Study Questions

1. Define the prevalence of overweight and obesity, and list five comorbidities associated with these conditions.

2. Discuss the benefits and limitations of the body mass index (BMI) in defining obesity.

3. What is the role of resistance training in a weight-loss or weight-maintenance program?

4. What are three considerations for resistance-exercise testing and training of overweight and obese individuals?

References

1. American College of Sports Medicine position stand. The recommended quantity and quality of exercise for developing and maintaining cardiorespiratory and muscular fitness and flexibility in healthy adults . *Med Sci Sports Exerc.* 1998;30:975-991.

2. Ballor DL, Harvey-Berino JR, Ades PA, Cryan J, Calles-Escandon J. Contrasting effects of resistance and aerobic training on body composition and metabolism after diet-induced weight loss. *Metabolism.* 1996;45(2):179-183.

3. Ballor DL, Katch VL, Becque MD, Marks CR. Resistance weight training during caloric restriction enhances lean body weight maintenance. *Am J Clin Nutr.* 1998;47(1):19-25.

4. Bogardus C, Lillioja S, Ravussin E, et al. Familial dependence of the resting metabolic rate. *N Engl J Med.* 1986;315(2):96-100.

5. Borg P, Kukkonen-Harjula K, Fogelholm M, Pasanen M. Effects of walking or resistance training on weight loss maintenance in obese, middle-aged men: A randomized trial. Int J Obes Relat Metab Disord. 2002;26(5):676-683.

6. Bouchard C, Tremblay A, Nadeau A, et al. Genetic effect in resting and exercise metabolic rates. *Metabolism.* 1989;38(4):364-370.

7. Bray GA, Greenway FL. Current and potential drugs for treatment of obesity. *Endocr Rev.* 1999;20(6):805-875.

8. Bray GA, Jablonski KA, Fujimoto WY, et al. and Diabetes Prevention Program Research Group. Relation of central adiposity and body mass index to the development of diabetes in the Diabetes Prevention Program. *Am J Clin Nutr.* 2008;87(5):1212-1218.

9. Bryner RW, Ullrich IH, Sauers J, et al. Effects of resistance vs. aerobic training combined with an 800 calorie liquid diet on lean body mass and resting metabolic rate. *J Am Coll Nutr.* 1999;18(2):115-121.

10. Donnelly JE, Sharp T, Houmard J, et al. Muscle hypertrophy with large-scale weight loss and resistance training. *Am J Clin Nutr.* 1993;58:561-565.

11. Ezzati M, Lopez AD, Rodgers A, Vander Hoorn S, Murray CJ, and Comparative Risk Assessment Collaborating Group. Selected major risk factors and global and regional burden of disease. *Lancet.* 2002;360(9343):1347-1360.

12. Filippatos TD, Derdemezis CS, Gazi IF, Nakou ES, Mikhailidis DP, Elisaf MS.

Orlistat-associated adverse effects and drug interactions: A critical review. *Drug Saf.* 2008;31(1):53-65.

13. Finkelstein EA, Fiebelkorn IC, Wang, G. State-level estimates of annual medical expenditures attributable to obesity. *Obes Res.* 2004;12(1):18-24.

14. Fleck SJ, Kraemer WJ. *Designing Resistance Training Programs 3rd Ed..* Champaign, IL. Human Kinetics; 2004.

15. Flegal KM, Graubard BI, Williamson DF, Gail MH. Excess deaths associated with underweight, overweight and obesity. *JAMA.* 2005;293(15):1861-1867.

16. Geliebter A, Maher MM, Gerace L, Gutin B, Heymsfield SB, Hashim SA. Effects of strength or aerobic training on body composition, resting metabolic rate and peak oxygen consumption in obese dieting subjects. *Am J Clin Nutr.* 1997;66(3):557-563.

17. Glass SC, Stanton DR. Self-selected resistance training intensity in novice weight lifters. *J Strength Cond Res.* 2004;18:324-327.

18. Harp JB, Hecht L. Obesity in the National Football League. *JAMA.* 2005;293:1061-1062.

19. Hedley AA, Ogden CL, Johnson CL, Carroll MD, Curtin LR, Flegal KM. Prevalence of overweight and obesity among US children, adolescents and adults, 1999-2002. *JAMA.* 2004;291(23):2847-2850.

20. Heyward VH. *Advanced Fitness Assessment and Exercise Prescription.* Champaign, IL. Human Kinetics; 2006.

21. Hunter GR, Byrne NM, Sirikul B, et al. Resistance training conserves fat-free mass and resting energy expenditure following weight loss. *Obesity.* 2008;(5):1045-1051.

22. Ibanez J, Izquierdo M, Arguelles I, et al. Twice-weekly progressive resistance training decreases abdominal fat and improves insulin sensitivity in older men with type 2 diabetes. *Diabetes Care.* 2005;28(3):662-667.

23. Jakicic JM. The role of physical activity in prevention and treatment of body weight gain in adults. *J Nutr.* 2002;(12):3826S-3829S.

24. Jakicic JM, Clark K, Coleman E, et al, and American College of Sports Medicine. American College of Sports Medicine position stand. Appropriate intervention strategies for weight loss and prevention of weight regain for adults . *Med Sci Sports Exerc.* 2001;33(12): 2145-2156.

25. Jakicic JM, Marcus BH, Gallagher KI, Napolitano M, Lang W. Effect of exercise duration and intensity on weight loss in overweight, sedentary women: A randomized trial. *JAMA.* 2003;290(10):1323-1330.

26. Kraemer WJ, Torine JC, Silvestre R, et al. Body size and composition of National Football League players. *J Strength Cond Res.* 2005;19(3):485-489.

27. Kraemer WJ, Volek JS, Clark KL, et al. Physiological adaptations to a weight-loss dietary regimen and exercise programs in women. *J Appl Physiol.* 1997;83(1):270-279.

28. Kraemer WJ, Volek JS, Clark KL, et al. Influence of exercise training on physiological and performance changes with weight loss in men. *Med Sci Sports Exerc.* 1999;31(9):1320-1329.

29. Kopelman PG. Obesity as a medical problem. *Nature.* 2000;404(6778):635-43.

30. Kukkonen-Harjula KT, Borg PT, Nenonen AM, Fogelholm MG. Effects of a weight maintenance program with or without exercise on the metabolic syndrome: A randomized trial in obese men. *Prev Med.* 2005;41(3-4):784-790.

31. Leibel RL, Rosenbaum M, Hirsch J. Changes in energy expenditure resulting from altered body weight. *N Engl J Med.* 1995;332(10):621-628.

32. Lemieux S, Prud'homme D, Bouchard C, Tremblay A, Després JP. A single threshold value of waist girth identifies normal-weight and overweight subjects with excess visceral adipose tissue. *Am J Clin Nutr.* 1996;64(5):685-693.

33. Lentini AC, McKelvie RS, McCartney N, Tomlinson CW, MacDougall JD. Left ventricular response in healthy young men during heavy-intensity weight-lifting exercise. *J Appl Physiol.* 1993;75(6):2703-2710.

34. Martínez-Hernández A, Enríquez L, Moreno-Moreno MJ, Martí A. Genetics of obesity. *Public Health Nutr.* 2007;10:1138-1144.

35. McPherson R. Genetic contributors to obesity. *Can J Cardiol.* 2007;23(Suppl A):23A-27A.

36. National Cholesterol Education Program. Second report of the expert panel on the detection, evaluation and treatment of high blood cholesterol in adults (Adult Treatment Panel II). *Circulation.* 1994;90:1333-1345.

37. Narloch JA, Brandstater ME. Influence of breathing technique on arterial blood pressure during heavy weight lifting. *Arch Phys Med Rehabil.* 1995;76(5):457-462.

38. Ogden CL, Carroll MD, Curtin LR, McDowell MA, Tabak CJ, Flegal KM. Prevalence of overweight and obesity in the United States: 1999-2004. *JAMA.* 2006;295(13):1549-1555.

39. Ohrvall M, Berglund L, Vessby B. Sagittal abdominal diameter compared with other anthropometric measurements in relation to cardiovascular risk. *Int J Obes.* 2000;24(4):497-501.

40. Parikh NI, Pencina MJ, Wang TJ, et al. Increasing trends in incidence of overweight and obesity over 5 decades. Am J Med. 2007;120(3):242-50.

41. Pavlou KN, Krey S, Steffee WP. Exercise as an adjunct to weight loss and maintenance in moderately obese subjects. *Am J Clin Nutr.* 1989;49(suppl 5):1115-1123.

42. Pratley R, Nicklas B, Rubin M, et al. Strength training increases resting metabolic rate and norepinephrine levels in healthy 50- to 65-year-old men. *J Appl Physiol.* 1994;76(1):133-137.

43. Pronk NP, Donnelly JE, Pronk SJ. Strength changes induced by extreme dieting and exercise in severely obese females. *J Am Coll Nutr.* 1992;11(2):152-158.

44. Ramachandran SV, Pencina MJ, Cobain M, Freiberg MS, D'Agostino, RB. Estimated risks for developing obesity in the Framingham Heart Study. *Ann Intern Med.* 2005;143(7):473-480.

45. Robertson RJ. *Perceived Exertion for Practitioners.* Champaign, IL: Human Kinetics; 2004.

46. Romao I, Roth J. Genetic and environmental interactions in obesity and type 2 diabetes. *J Am Diet Assoc.* 2008;108(4 suppl 1):S24-S28.

47. Ross R, Pedwell H, Rissanen J. Response of total and regional lean tissue and skeletal muscle to a program of energy restriction and resistance exercise. *Int J Obes.* 1995;19(11):781-787.

48. Rotstein A, Inbar O, Vaisman N. The effect of sibutramine intake on resting and exercise physiological responses. *Ann Nutr Metab.* 2008;52(1):17-23.

49. Salem JG, Wang MY, Sigward S. Measuring lower extremity strength in older adults: The stability of isokinetic versus 1RM measures. *J of Aging and Physical Activity.* 2002;10:489-503.

50. Saris WH. Sugars, energy metabolism and body weight control. *Am J Clin Nutr.* 2003;78(4):850S-857S.

51. Shaw I, Shaw BS. Consequence of resistance training on body composition and coronary artery disease risk. *Cardiovasc J S Afr.* 2006;17(3):111-116.

52. The sixth report of the joint national committee on prevention, detection, evaluation, and treatment of high blood pressure. *Arch Intern Med.* 1997;157(21):2413-2446.

53. Wajchenberg BL. Subcutaneous and visceral adipose tissue: Their relation to the metabolic syndrome. *Endocr Rev.* 2000;21(6):697-738.

54. World Health Organization. Obesity: Preventing and Managing the Global Epidemic. Report of a WHO consultation. *World Health Organ Tech Rep Ser.* 2000;894:1-253

55. World Health Organization. Physical status: The use and interpretation of anthropometry. Report of a WHO Expert Committee. *World Health Organ Tech Rep Ser.* 1995;854:1-452

56. Zahorska-Markiewicz B. Thermic effect of food and exercise in obesity. *Eur J Appl Physiol Occup Physiol.* 1980;44(3):231-235.

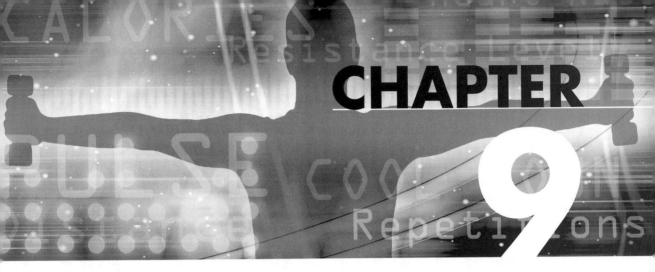

CHAPTER 9

RESISTANCE-TRAINING STRATEGIES FOR OBESE YOUTHS

Objectives

Upon completion of this chapter, the reader should be able to:

- ○ Discuss the public health implications of pediatric obesity
- ○ Describe the etiology of pediatric obesity
- ○ Identify research supporting the safety and efficacy of youths resistance training
- ○ Discuss the role of resistance training in treating pediatric obesity
- ○ Describe different methods of resistance training and understand special considerations to enhance participant safety during exercise testing and training
- ○ Describe program variables used to design resistance-training programs for youths, and discuss the relationship between the number of repetitions, training intensity, number of sets, training velocity, rest periods between sets, and training frequency
- ○ Explain the concept of periodization and its application to the design of youths resistance-training programs
- ○ Design safe, effective, and progressive resistance-training programs for obese children and adolescents

INTRODUCTION

The prevalence of obesity in children and adolescents is increasing at an alarming rate and has become front-page news across the country. This unabated epidemic is occurring in boys and girls across all socioeconomic strata, and the likelihood that an obese child will become an obese adult is both real and alarming (62, 66, 106). If current trends continue, pediatric obesity will likely pose an unprecedented burden on youths, their families, and our health care system. Understanding the etiology of pediatric obesity is important. Learning how sensible lifestyle choices such as regular physical activity and proper nutrition can improve the body composition and enhance the health and well-being of children and adolescents is a growing area of interest among researchers, health care providers, school teachers, and government officials.

For the purpose of this chapter, the term *obese* refers to a body mass index (BMI) equal to or greater than the 95th percentile of the age- and gender-specific BMI. The term *overweight* refers to a BMI between the 85th and 94th percentile (9). Although others use the term "overweight" to describe youths with a BMI equal to or greater than the age- and gender-specific 95th percentiles (2, 106), the Institute of Medicine of the National Academies and an expert committee representing national health care organizations contend that the term "obese" more accurately reflects the serious nature of this medical concern (9, 66). The term **childhood** refers to the period of life before the development of secondary sex characteristics, such as pubic hair and reproductive organs (approximately age 11 in girls and 13 in boys). The term **adolescence** refers to the period between childhood and adulthood and includes girls 12 to 18 years and boys 14 to 18 years. The terms **youths** and **pediatric** are broadly defined to include children and adolescents.

PREVALENCE AND ECONOMIC IMPACT OF YOUTHS OBESITY

Over the past three decades, the prevalence of pediatric obesity has more than doubled for adolescents, and it has more than tripled for children (9, 63, 83). Among American youths aged 2 to 19 years, data from a national survey, using BMI as a main outcome measure, indicate that 31.9 percent of youths are overweight, and 16.3 percent are obese (83). Approximately 9 million American children over 6 years of age are considered obese (66). Unfortunately, this number may increase, because 24.4 percent of American children aged 2 to 5 years are overweight, and 12.4 percent are already obese (83). While the number of obese youths in other nations is also increasing, the prevalence of childhood obesity is greatest among American youths (76, 106, 108). Today, pediatric obesity, with its associated comorbid conditions and likelihood of persistence into adulthood, is considered a critical public health threat for the 21st century (62, 66, 110).

As the prevalence of pediatric obesity continues to increase, weight-related respiratory, cardiovascular, and endocrine problems will likely be seen at an increased rate in children and adolescents. Furthermore, it is probable that comorbidities present during childhood and adolescence will persist into adulthood (25, 81, 114). Based on current trends, it is estimated that 20 percent of overweight 4 year olds, and as many as 80 percent of overweight adolescents, will become obese adults (26, 60).

The direct economic burden of this epidemic is staggering. Obesity-associated hospital costs for youths have more than tripled over a two-decade period (109), with the Surgeon General's "call to action" on obesity indicating that $117 billion annually in health care costs could be attributed to obesity and obesity-related complications (106). This estimate consumes 6 percent of our national health care dollars due to increased physician visits, lost productivity, and treatment of secondary conditions that include diabetes and coronary artery disease (56).

Aside from health care costs and psychosocial consequences, the epidemic of pediatric obesity will have a direct impact on the welfare of our military. At present, nearly 80 percent of new recruits who exceed the U.S. military weight-for-height standards leave the military before they complete their first term of enlistment (67). Unless interventions specifically designed to reduce obesity in children and adolescents are successfully implemented, the readiness of the military may be at risk, future health care costs will continue to increase, and youths with a BMI greater than the age- and gender-specific 95th percentiles will be considered "normal."

ETIOLOGY OF PEDIATRIC OBESITY

Complex interactions between familial, psychological, sociocultural, economic, and environmental factors likely play a role in the development of pediatric obesity (2). While genetic conditions such as Prader-Willi syndrome cause low muscle tone, cognitive disabilities, and a chronic feeling of hunger that can predispose a child or adolescent to fat accumulation, no evidence suggests that genetics alone are responsible for the large increase in obesity among youths over the past 10 to 20 years. Thus other influences, particularly environmental factors, need to be closely examined. **Environmental risk factors** that include family dynamics, such as parental food choices and degree of parental adiposity, and the lack of safe places for physical activity, lack of consistent access to healthful food choices, increased consumption of energy-dense fried foods and carbonated beverages, changes in the availability of physical education, and increased access to television, videos, and computer games all play a potential role in the epidemic of obesity among children and adolescents (2, 25). Moreover, some parents do not perceive overweight to be a health issue for their children (68).

Clinicians have recognized that very small changes in the **energy balance** equation repeated day after day can result in weight loss or weight gain in the long term. For example, if the excess daily energy intake over energy needs for a child is 120 kilocalories (kcal), the equivalent of a 12-ounce soda, the child will gain over 5 kilograms (kg) of fat in one year. Thus if this child consumes an extra 120 kcal every day starting in first grade, he may be 60 kg overweight by the time he graduates high school. Minor changes in energy balance are hardly noticeable in the short term and are difficult to detect by available analytical techniques, but they can clearly result in obesity in the long term. While there are indications that the total energy intake of adolescents has increased over the years (30), no significant increased trends in energy intake have been reported in children (29). Nonetheless, children and adolescents are not consuming the recommended servings of fruits and vegetables daily (4), and energy-dense foods high in fat and sugar are now sold in many schools (57).

The increasing prevalence of pediatric obesity is primarily due to a reduction in total daily energy expenditure. Even though the energy cost of any given movement increases as a child becomes obese, societal changes during the last several decades have reduced the need to be physically active. Only 28 percent of high school students attend physical education class daily (22), and children's motorized transportation to and from school has increased (21, 23). Children spend more time with electronic media, such as video games and computers, and on a typical day, 33 percent of children watch television for more than 3 hours (89). Increased urbanization has resulted in a lack of safe play areas, as well as a reduction in the need to perform daily physical activities such as yard work.

Since obese youths may lack the motor skills and confidence to be physically active, they may actually perceive physical activity to be discomforting and embarrassing. National survey data of children aged 9 to 13 years revealed that 61 percent do not participate in any organized physical activity during nonschool hours, and 23 percent do not participate in any free-time physical activity (22). Data from the National Health and Nutrition Examination Survey identified low fitness, estimated from a submaximal treadmill test, in 33.6 percent of American adolescents (20). Sadly, this decline in physical activity may start during the preschool years in obese children (54).

Additional Medical Concerns from Youths Obesity

The epidemic of pediatric obesity has significant ramifications for the present and future health of children and adolescents. Current trends in obesity have led some observers to predict that the overall adult life expectancy will decrease due to the increased prevalence of obesity-related comorbidities, such as type 2 diabetes, cardiovascular disease, and cancer (82). The increasing incidence of type 2 diabetes in youths, which was formerly called *adult onset diabetes,* is particularly troubling, because conditions related to diabetes—kidney failure, amputation and blindness—will occur earlier in life. Once a disease of middle age and the elderly, type 2 diabetes now accounts for up to 45 percent of all new cases of diabetes in children and adolescents who, in most cases, are virtually always obese (15). For American children born in the year 2000, the lifetime risk of being diagnosed with diabetes is estimated to be 30 percent for boys and 40 percent for girls (82).

Another serious complication of childhood obesity is **metabolic syndrome**, which is a clustering of traits that include hyperinsulinemia, obesity, hypertension, and hyperlipidemia (2, 24, 100). Recent findings indicate that metabolic syndrome is present in 30 percent of U.S. adolescents who are obese (24). Even in obese youths who do not have diabetes, metabolic syndrome has a profound effect on their cardiovascular health. Research has demonstrated that obese youths have elevated blood levels of inflammation markers and impaired endothelial function (53). In the landmark

Bogalusa study, a higher BMI in adolescents and young adults was associated with more extensive fatty streaks and raised atheromas in coronary arteries (13).

Other important medical complications associated with pediatric obesity include asthma, sleep problems, gastrointestinal problems, and orthopedic disorders (2, 9, 26). In addition, obesity can exacerbate a common female hormonal disorder known as *polycystic ovary syndrome* (6). The onset of this syndrome is often around the time of menarche and is typically associated with excess weight gain. All of these conditions are becoming more common in obese children and adolescents and can have serious consequences for health and well-being.

In addition to metabolic, orthopedic, respiratory, and cardiovascular consequences, the development of obesity during childhood and adolescence may also be related to psychiatric disorders, including depression and low self-esteem. Research has shown that adults who had been diagnosed with major depression during their youths had a greater BMI than adults who did not suffer from depression during their youths (85). Others observed that in a sample of over 9000 children, depression scores were highest in children with the greatest increase in BMI over the course of 1 year (55) Obese youths have fewer friends, miss more school days, and are often ostracized and teased about their weight (56, 102). Schwimmer and colleagues (92) observed that obese children and adolescents have a lower health-related quality of life than youths who are healthy—and they report having a similar quality of life as those diagnosed with cancer. Psychological stress imposed on obese youths is associated with an increase in suicidal ideations and suicide attempts (28).

BENEFITS OF RESISTANCE TRAINING FOR OBESE YOUTHS

Along with dietary changes and behavior modification, regular physical activity is a cornerstone of treatment for obese youths. Although both normal-weight and obese children and adolescents have traditionally been encouraged to participate in aerobic activities such as walking and swimming, they have not always been encouraged to participate in resistance training. Unfounded concerns regarding the potential effects of strength-building exercise on the growth and development of young weight lifters has sometimes limited their participation in this type of exercise.

However, over the past two decades, a compelling body of evidence has accumulated to indicate that resistance training can be a safe, effective, and beneficial method of conditioning for all youths, regardless of body size (14, 31, 49, 61, 107). Research into the effects of resistance training on normal-weight and obese children and adolescents has increased over the years, and the qualified acceptance of youths resistance training by medical and fitness organizations has become almost universal. The American Academy of Pediatrics (1), the American College of Sports Medicine (3), the British Association of Sports and Exercise Science (17), the Canadian Society for Exercise Physiology (10), and the National Strength and Conditioning Association (34) all support participation in youths resistance-training activities, provided the program is appropriately designed and competently supervised.

In addition to enhancing muscular strength and local muscular endurance, appropriately prescribed and competently supervised resistance-training programs may also offer observable health benefits for boys and girls. Regular participation in resistance-training activities has been shown to positively influence bone mineral density (80), cardiorespiratory fitness (36, 112), blood lipids (101, 113), and psychosocial well-being (65). In terms of youths sports participation, a growing body of evidence suggests that preparatory conditioning that includes resistance training may reduce the incidence of sports-related injuries (43, 64). This finding may be particularly important for inactive youths whose musculoskeletal systems may not be prepared for the demands of regular sports practice and competition. Some observers suggest

that the risk of sports-related injuries could be reduced by as much as 50 percent if aspiring young athletes were better prepared for sports participation prior to practice and competition (72, 79, 96).

Due to the epidemic of pediatric obesity, the effect of resistance training on body composition has received increased attention (45, 105, 111). Although aerobic exercise is typically prescribed for decreasing body fat, several youths resistance-training studies have reported a decrease in fatness among normal-weight participants (48, 75, 95) as well as overweight or obese children and adolescents (12, 94, 97, 98, 104). Watts and colleagues (110) found that circuit-resistance training, which included cycle ergometry and resistance training, not only improved the body composition of obese adolescents, it also normalized vascular dysfunction in these subjects. Other researchers found that participation in a resistance-training program significantly decreased body fat and increased insulin sensitivity in overweight adolescent males (94). These important findings highlight the potential clinical relevance of resistance training in overweight and obese youths.

Obese youths are less willing, and often unable, to participate in prolonged periods of moderate to vigorous aerobic exercise without rest. Excess body weight not only hinders the performance of weight-bearing physical activity, such as jogging, but the risk of musculoskeletal overuse injuries should also be considered. However, most obese children and adolescents find resistance-training activities enjoyable, because this type of exercise is not aerobically taxing, and it provides an opportunity for all youths—regardless of body size—to experience success and feel good about their performance. Thus the first step in encouraging obese children and adolescents to exercise may be to increase confidence in their ability to be physically active, which in turn may lead to an increase in regular physical activity, an improvement in body composition, and exposure to a form of exercise that we hope will be carried over into adulthood. The potential benefits of resistance training for obese youths are summarized in Table 9-1.

Table 9-1 Potential Benefits of Youths Resistance Training

- Increase muscle strength and power
- Increase local muscular endurance
- Increase bone mineral density
- Increase cardiorespiratory fitness
- Improve blood lipid profile
- Improve body composition
- Improve motor performance skills
- Enhance sports performance
- Increase resistance to injury
- Enhance mental health and well-being
- Stimulate a more positive attitude toward lifetime physical activity

Literature Review of Research Supporting Resistance Training for Obese Youths

The results from several investigations illustrate that exercise programs that include resistance training can improve the health and body composition of both normal-weight and obese youths (5, 12, 47, 93, 94, 97, 98, 110, 116). Sothern and colleagues studied the safety and feasibility of a moderate-intensity resistance-training program (1 set of 8 to 12 repetitions at 60 percent 1RM) in a group of obese children during a multidisciplinary outpatient treatment program (98). There were no reported injuries or accidents, and favorable changes in body composition were observed following 10 weeks of resistance training. Similar findings were reported by Benson and colleagues, who noted significant improvements in central and whole-body adiposity in normal-weight and overweight children after 8 weeks of resistance training (2 sets of 8 repetitions at 80 percent of 1RM) (12). Conversely, Treuth and colleagues reported significant increases in fat mass and subcutaneous abdominal adipose tissue following 5 months of resistance training (2 sets of 12 to 15 repetitions at ≥ 50 percent of 1RM) in obese girls (104). Although intra-abdominal adipose tissue remained stable following the training period in this study (104), it is likely that a higher

training intensity and training volume might have more favorable effects on body composition.

Shabi and colleagues examined the effects of 16 weeks of resistance training (1 to 3 sets of 3 to 15 repetitions at 62 to 97 percent of 1RM) on insulin sensitivity and body composition in overweight adolescent males (94). Participation in this program significantly decreased body fat and increased insulin sensitivity. Compliance with this intervention was impressive: 96 percent of the participants completed the resistance-training program. Since the increase in insulin sensitivity remained significant after adjustment for changes in total fat mass and total lean mass, training-induced qualitative changes in skeletal muscle appear to have contributed to enhanced insulin action. Others identified muscular strength as an independent and powerful predictor of better insulin sensitivity in youths aged 10 to 15 years (11). Table 9-2 summarizes studies examining the effects of resistance training on obese children and adolescents.

DESIGNING RESISTANCE-TRAINING PROGRAMS FOR OBESE YOUTHS

The findings from research studies, as well as observations from health care professionals and physical education teachers, provide compelling evidence that resistance training can be safe, effective, and worthwhile for children and adolescents (31, 49, 61, 107). A variety of training modalities and different combinations of sets and repetitions have provided an adequate stimulus for strength enhancement and favorable changes in body composition in both normal-weight and overweight youths. However, youths resistance-training programs need to be carefully prescribed, because unsupervised or poorly performed strength testing and resistance training may be injurious. Risser and colleagues (87) noted several examples in which children and adolescents suffered serious musculoskeletal

Table 9-2 Effects of Resistance Training on Body Composition and Weight in Overweight and Obese Youths

Study Author	Age of Subjects	Study Design	Exercise Program	Main Findings
Benson et al(12)	12.3 ± 1.3 yrs	RT (n = 32); CNT (n = 38)	8 wks, 2x/wk, 2×8 reps at 80% 1RM, 11 exercises	RT improved FFM, BMI, %BF
Schwingshandt et al(93)	11.0 ± 2.5 yrs (RT & Diet) 12.2 ± 2.7 yrs (Diet)	RT & Diet (n = 14); Diet (n = 16)	12 wks, 2x/wk, $2{-}4 \times 10$ reps at 50–100% 10RM, 12 exercises, w/1 yr follow-up	RT & Diet ↑ FFM; After 1 yr. Δ in BW was inversely correlated with Δ FFM
Shabi et al(94)	15.1 ± 0.5 (RT) 15.6 ± 0.5 (CNT)	RT (n = 11); CNT (n = 11)	16 wks, 2x/wk, $1{-}3 \times 3{-}15$ reps at 62–97% 1RM, 5 exercises	RT ↓ % BF, ↑ IS
Sothern et al(98)	7-12 yrs	RT & Diet (n = 15) CV & Diet (n = 17)	10 wks, 3x/wk, $1 \times 8{-}12$ reps at 60% 1RM, 12 exercises, w/1 yr follow-up	RT & Diet ↓ % BF; Both groups ↓ BW, % IBW, BMI. RT & Diet maint. % BF after 1 yr
Treuth et al(104)	7-10 yrs	RT (n = 11) Control (n = 11)	5 months, 3x/wk, $2 \times 12{-}15$ reps at ≥50% 1RM; 7 exercises	RT ↑ BW, FFM, FM, & SAAT; RT ↓ IAAT
Watts et al(110)	14.3 ± 1.5 yrs (CWT); 14.9 ± 2.7 yrs (CNT)	CWT (n = 19) CNT (n = 20)	8 wks, 3x/wk; CWT: RT: 55–70% of 1RM, 7 exercises; CV = 65–85% HR max on cycle.	↓ in trunk and abdominal fat; normalized FMD
Yu et al(116)	10.5 ± 1.0 yrs	CWT & Diet (n = 41); Diet (n = 41)	6 wk; 3x/wk; CWT: RT: $1 \times 10{-}30$ reps, 9 EX; CV 60-70% HR max	Both groups ↓ BMI; CWT & Diet ↑ FFM > Diet.

↑ = increase; ↓ = decrease; Δ = change; > = more than; BF = body fat; BMI = body mass index, BW = body weight; CNT = control group; CV = cardiovascular; CWT = circuit weight training; FFM = fat-free mass; FM = fat mass; FMD = flow-mediated dilation; HR = heart rate; IAAT = intra-abdominal adipose tissue; IBW = ideal body weight; IS = insulin sensitivity; reps = repetitions; RM = repetition maximum; RT = resistance training; SAAT = subcutaneous abdominal adipose tissue; wk = week; yr = year injuries—including ruptured intervertebral discs, spondylolysis, and spondylolisthesis—while lifting weights with inadequate supervision and instruction, inappropriate training loads, and incorrect exercise technique. An increased risk of injury exists for children and adolescents who use exercise equipment at home without qualified supervision and safe equipment (69).

One traditional concern associated with youths resistance training involves the potential for injury to the epiphyseal plate or growth cartilage. Although epiphyseal plate fractures have been reported in adolescent weight trainers (59, 74, 91), these reports were case studies and typically involved improper lifting techniques or the lifting of heavy loads with inadequate supervision. Some clinicians believe that the risk of an epiphyseal plate fracture in children may be less than in adolescents, because the epiphyseal plates of children are stronger and more resistant to shearing-type forces (78). To date, an injury to the growth cartilage has not been reported in any prospective youths resistance-training study that was competently supervised and appropriately designed. The greatest concern for children and adolescents who perform resistance training is the risk for overuse soft tissue injuries (16, 87). Although the incidence of this type of injury is difficult to determine because it does not always result in a visit to a physician, limited data suggest that the risk of developing this type of injury is noteworthy (16, 18, 87). In one report involving adolescent athletes, 50 percent of the 98 reported injuries were to the lower back (18). Although these competitive athletes presumably trained with maximal or near maximal loads, similar injuries could occur in obese youths who do not follow sensible exercise guidelines.

Although no minimal age requirement has been set for participation in a resistance-training program, all children should understand the potential risks and benefits associated with training. All training sessions should be conducted by qualified exercise professionals who understand the fundamental principles of resistance exercise, appreciate the uniqueness of childhood and adolescence, take the time to listen to each child's concerns, and closely monitor each participant's ability to tolerate the exercise. These characteristics are particularly important for overweight and obese youths, who typically have limited experience participating in a structured exercise program. Close supervision, age-appropriate instruction, and a safe exercise environment are paramount. In short, it is always better to underestimate the physical abilities of participants rather than overestimate them and risk negative consequences such as dropout or injury. Obese children and adolescents should be seen by their physician or health care provider before they begin this or any other exercise program. In addition, youths with preexisting medical conditions, such as hypertension or seizure disorders, should be withheld from resistance training until medical clearance is obtained (2).

When working with obese children and adolescents, it is important to remember that the goal of the program should not be limited to increasing muscle strength and improving body composition. Teaching youths about their bodies, promoting safe training procedures, and providing a stimulating program that gives participants a more positive attitude toward resistance training and physical activity are equally important.

Exercise Testing Considerations

Assessing muscular strength and local muscular endurance with traditional fitness tests such as the push-up, chin-up, and abdominal curl-up is common practice in most physical education classes and youths fitness programs. Standardized testing procedures have been developed for youths, and normative data for children and teenagers are available (8) However, excess body fat can hinder the performance of obese youths in weight-bearing physical activities. In fact, in many instances obese youths are unable to perform even one repetition of a push-up or chin-up. Conversely, obese youths can perform repetition-maximum (RM) strength testing using weight machines and free weights. Despite previous concerns that RM testing may cause structural damage to children and adolescents, no injuries have been reported in prospective studies involving normal-weight and obese youths who performed 1RM or 10RM strength tests under qualified supervision (12, 41, 86, 94, 101, 106, 116).

When strength testing obese youths who have limited or no experience, providing each participant with an opportunity to practice proper exercise technique on several occasions before the testing session is important. Qualified exercise professionals should demonstrate the proper performance of each exercise and offer guidance and instruction. Although strength-testing guidelines for adults suggest that a predetermined RM (e.g., 1RM or 10RM) should be arrived at within 5 sets (7), observations indicate that additional sets may be necessary to accurately determine the 1RM in youths who have no experience (41). Interestingly, a young lifter's perception of a given weight as light, medium, or heavy may waiver during the first 3 to 5 testing sets. That is, as the weight increases, some youths may perceive the weight to be easier than the previous set. In one report involving normal-weight youths, 68 percent of the subjects—65 out of 96 subjects—who could not lift a weight during their first 1RM attempt successfully completed the lift on their second attempt (41). When strength testing obese youths, a gradual increase in the weight used for testing, combined with additional testing sets and a second attempt if necessary, may aid in the accuracy of strength testing.

The type of warm-up performed before a strength test is important. Over the past few years, long-held beliefs regarding the routine practice of static stretching before an event have been questioned (70, 103, 115). Recently, there has been rising interest in warm-up procedures that involve the performance of dynamic movements—hops, skips, jumps, and movement-based exercises for the upper and lower body—designed to elevate core body temperature, enhance motor unit excitability, improve kinesthetic awareness, and maximize active ranges of motion (35, 88). Findings from several studies suggest that low-intensity aerobic exercise and static stretching before physical activity may be suboptimal for preparing youths for strength and power testing (32, 33, 77). Static stretching should not be eliminated from a child's physical activity program, but rather instructors, coaches, and health care providers should consider the potential impact of static stretching beforehand on strength and power testing. A reasonable suggestion is to perform dynamic activities during the warm-up and static stretching during the cooldown.

The assessment of any physical fitness measure in an obese child, who may already have preconceived notions about his or her physical abilities, requires competent and caring instruction. Professionals should develop a friendly rapport with each child, and the exercise area should be nonthreatening. Since most obese youths have limited experience performing strength tests, professionals should reassure children that they can safely perform at a high level of exertion. When assessing youths, it is also important to avoid the "pass or fail" mentality that may discourage some boys and girls from participating. Instead, consider referring to the strength test as a "challenge" in which all participants can feel good about their performance and get excited about monitoring their progress. Positive encouragement and posters of children performing different exercises can serve as useful motivational tools. Following the strength assessment, it is important to cool down afterwards with gentle calisthenics and stretching exercises.

Training Program Components

Despite various claims about the best resistance-training program for children and adolescents, there does not appear to be an optimal combination of sets, repetitions, and exercises that will promote favorable adaptations in muscular strength and body composition for all youths. Rather, many program variables need be altered over time to achieve desirable outcomes. Resistance-training programs for obese youths need to be individualized and based on each participant's health history, training experience, personal goals, and time available for exercise. Table 9-3 summarizes resistance-training guidelines for children and adolescents.

Table 9-3 General Youths Resistance Training Guidelines

- Provide qualified instruction and supervision.
- Make sure the exercise environment is safe and free of hazards.
- Teach youths the benefits and concerns associated with resistance training.
- Begin each session with a 5- to 10-minute warm-up period.
- Start with 1 or 2 sets of 10 to 15 repetitions with a light load and a variety of exercises.
- Progress to 2 or 3 sets of 6 to 15 repetitions depending on individual needs and goals.
- Increase the resistance gradually as strength improves.
- Focus on the correct exercise technique instead of the amount of weight lifted.
- Strength train two to three times per week on nonconsecutive days.
- Use individualized workout logs to monitor progress.

Choice and Order of Exercise

Although a limitless number of exercises can be used to enhance muscular fitness, it is important to select exercises appropriate for an obese child's body size, fitness level, and exercise technique experience. The choice of exercises should promote muscle balance across multiple joints and between opposing muscle groups, for example, quadriceps and hamstrings. Weight machines, both child sized and adult sized, as well as free weights, elastic bands, and medicine balls have been used by normal-weight and obese youths in clinical- and school-based exercise programs (5, 36, 37, 44, 47, 86, 94, 95, 98). If an obese child cannot fit on a child-sized weight machine, adult-sized machines may be a viable option for selected exercises. With most weight-machine exercises, the path of movement is fixed, and therefore the movement is stabilized and easier to perform. Moreover, since most weight-machine exercises are performed in the sitting position, excess body weight does not hinder the performance of obese individuals. This consideration is important when choosing exercises for obese youths who have limited experience resistance training. In most cases, it may be reasonable to start resistance training on weight machines and gradually progress to free weights and medicine-ball exercises, which generally require more coordination and skill to perform correctly. Regardless of the mode of exercise, the concentric and eccentric phases of each lift should be performed in a controlled manner with proper exercise technique.

The sequence of exercises may be arranged in many ways in a resistance-training session. Most obese youths will perform total-body workouts several times per week, involving multiple exercises that stress all major muscle groups each session. Large muscle group exercises should be performed before smaller muscle group exercises, and multiple-joint exercises should be performed before single-joint exercises. Following this exercise order will allow heavier weights to be used on the multiple-joint exercises, because fatigue will be less of a factor. Performing more challenging exercises earlier in the workout, when the neuromuscular system is less fatigued, is beneficial for this population. For example, a barbell squat should be performed early in the training session, so that the child can practice the exercise without undue fatigue.

Training Intensity

The use of RM loads is a relatively simple method to prescribe resistance-training intensity. Studies involving adults suggest that RM loads of 6 or less have the greatest effect on developing muscle strength, whereas RM loads of 20 or more have the greatest impact on developing local muscular endurance (19). However, most studies involving youths suggest that lighter loads and higher repetitions (e.g., 10-15 RM) are most beneficial for enhancing muscular strength during the initial adaptation period (40,47,48). Since different combinations of sets and repetitions may be needed to promote long-term gains in muscular fitness, the best approach for an obese child may be to start resistance training with a single set of 10 to 15 repetitions on a variety of exercises, and then systematically perform additional sets, and vary the training intensity to avoid training plateaus and optimize training adaptations.

A percentage of a child's 1RM also can be used to determine the training intensity. Beginners can use a training resistance of approximately 60 to 70 percent of 1RM, because strength gains are primarily due to neuromuscular adaptations during this phase of training (84, 86). As children and adolescents get stronger and gain training experience, heavier resistances of up to 70 to 80 percent of 1RM may be needed to make continual gains in muscular strength and performance. This method of prescribing resistance exercise requires the evaluation of the 1RM on all exercises used in the training program. In many cases this testing is not realistic because of the time required to perform 1RM testing correctly on 8 to 10 different exercises. Furthermore, maximal resistance testing for small muscle group assistance exercises (e.g., biceps curls and lying triceps extensions) typically is not performed.

Exercise professionals who work with obese youths should also be knowledgeable of the relationship between the percentage of the 1RM and the number of repetitions that can be performed. In general, most youths can perform about 10 repetitions using 75 percent of their 1RM. However, the number of repetitions that can be performed at a given percentage of 1RM varies with the amount of muscle mass required to perform the exercise. For example, at a given percentage of the 1RM (e.g., 50 percent), normal-weight children can perform more repetitions on a large muscle group exercise, such as the leg press, compared with a smaller muscle group exercise such as the chest press (46). Therefore, prescribing a resistance-training intensity of 70 percent of 1RM on all exercises may not be appropriate. At this intensity a child may be able to perform 20 or more repetitions on a large muscle group exercise, and this volume may not be ideal for enhancing muscle strength.

Falk and colleagues (50) observed that the level of adiposity was a strong negative predictor of the resistance-training effect of the lower limbs following 3 school years of resistance training (1 to 4 sets, 5 to 30 repetitions at 50 to 60 percent of 1 RM, 2 to 3 days per week). Greater strength gains in normal-weight children—those with 14.5 to 16.7 percent body fat—compared with the so-called nonresponders with 23.5 to 32.8 percent body fat were found over the 3-year study period, suggesting that a training intensity appropriate to increase strength in normal-weight children may be insufficient in children who have excess body fat. These researchers suggested that obese youths may need a higher relative intensity or higher percent training intensity to produce the desired result. This finding may be particularly important for lower-extremity exercises, because the lower body in obese youths is relatively strong, because it is trained on a daily basis to carry excess body weight.

When prescribing an appropriate training intensity for youths, it seems reasonable to first establish a repetition range and then adjust the training load to maintain the desired training intensity. Recently, a child-specific, perceived-exertion rating scale has been used to assess the perception of exertion of children during resistance training (38). The **perceived exertion for children scale** contains verbal expressions, along with a numerical response range of 0 to 10, and five pictorial descriptors that represent a child at varying levels of exertion doing resistance training (Figure 9-1). Subjective information from this scale, combined with information on training experience and training goals, can be used to assist in the prescription of safe and effective youths resistance-training programs. For example, findings suggest that an effort rating of 6 or 7 on the perceived exertion for children scale is consistent with a training intensity of approximately 75 percent of the one-repetition maximum, which is a desirable training intensity for most youths (38).

Training Volume

The National Strength and Conditioning Association Guidelines recommend that children and adolescents perform 1 to 3 sets on each exercise

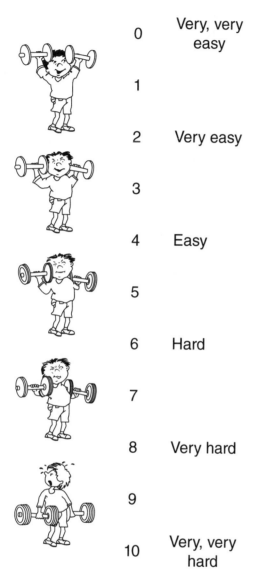

0	Very, very easy
1	
2	Very easy
3	
4	Easy
5	
6	Hard
7	
8	Very hard
9	
10	Very, very hard

Figure 9-1 Perceived Exertion for Children (PEC) scale.

Faigenbaum A, Milliken L, Cloutier G, Westcott W. Perceived exertion during resistance exercise in children. *Percept Mot Skills.* 2004;98:627-637

to achieve muscular fitness goals (34). In general, 1-, 2-, and 3-set protocols will be effective for normal-weight and obese youths during the first few months of resistance training, provided that reasonable training loads are used. However, studies involving adults suggest that multiple set, periodized programs result in superior gains in muscle strength and performance in individuals with training experience (71). Although long-term training studies (>6 months) are needed to explore the effects of different training programs on muscular strength and body composition in normal-weight and obese youths, a multiple-set training protocol is likely to be more effective than a single-set protocol for maximizing training adaptations and maintaining exercise adherence in youths over the long term.

Obese children and adolescents should start with a single-set program and gradually increase the number of sets, depending on personal goals and time available for training. A single-set protocol reduces training time and provides a practical approach for participants who do not train regularly. However, it is also possible that a multiple-set protocol can be a time-efficient method of training. For example, instead of performing 1 set of 12 different exercises during every workout, children can perform 2 sets of 6 exercises or 3 sets of 4 exercises. With a careful selection of multiple-joint exercises, all muscle groups can be trained each exercise session, regardless of the number of sets or exercises performed. By periodically varying the sets, repetitions, and number of exercises—that is, by varying the training volume—the training stimulus will remain effective, and therefore the adaptations to the training program will be maximized.

Rest Intervals

In general, the length of the rest interval between sets and exercises will influence energy recovery and the training adaptations that take place. Training intensity, training goals, and fitness level will influence the rest interval. Although few data examining the effects of rest interval length on strength performance in younger populations are available, it appears that children and adolescents can resist fatigue to a greater extent than adults during several repeated sets of resistance exercise (42, 117). Thus, a shorter rest interval may suffice in children and adolescents when performing a moderate-intensity resistance-exercise protocol, although the likelihood that adolescents may fatigue more rapidly than children should be considered. In general, a rest period of 1 to 2 minutes between sets is appropriate for most beginners. Short rest periods—that is, less than 30 seconds between sets—need to be carefully prescribed because of the muscular discomfort associated with this type of training. However, over time, the rest periods can be reduced gradually to provide ample opportunity for the body to tolerate circuit training.

Repetition Velocity

The velocity or cadence at which an exercise is performed can affect adaptations to training (51). Since beginners need to learn how to perform each exercise correctly, it is recommended that untrained youths perform exercises in a controlled manner at a moderate velocity. As youths gain experience, different training velocities may be used depending on the choice of exercise and program goals. For example, selected medicine-ball exercises can be performed at a higher velocity than traditional strength-building exercises with weight machines and free weights. Although additional research is needed, it is likely that the performance of different training velocities within a training program may provide the most effective training stimulus.

Training Frequency

Training frequency typically refers to the number of training sessions per week. A training frequency of two to three times per week on nonconsecutive days is recommended for children and adolescents (2, 34). Limited evidence indicates that 1 day per week of resistance training may be suboptimal for enhancing muscular strength in normal-weight children (39). Following 8 weeks of progressive resistance training with 1 set of 10 to 15 repetitions of 12 exercises, normal-weight children who performed resistance training once per week achieved 67 percent of the 1RM strength of children who strength trained twice per week (39). A training frequency of 2 to 3 days per week on nonconsecutive days allows adequate recovery between sessions and will be effective for enhancing muscle strength and performance. Factors such as the training volume,

training intensity, exercise selection, and nutritional intake should also be considered when prescribing a training frequency for an obese youths, as these factors may influence the child's ability to recover from and adapt to the training program.

Periodization for Youths Resistance Training

While the concept of periodization, or program variation, has been part of resistance-training program design for adults for many years (71, 73, 99), our understanding of the benefits of periodized training compared with nonperiodized programs for normal-weight and obese children and adolescents has not been studied. Since periodized training programs have proven to be more effective than nonperiodized programs in adults (71), it is intuitively attractive to assume that periodization may benefit obese children and adolescents who need to enhance their health and fitness.

Obese children and adolescents who participate in well-designed periodized resistance-training programs and continue to improve their health and fitness may be more likely to adhere to an exercise program into adulthood. For example, if a child's lower-body routine consists of leg extension and leg curl exercises, performing the leg press and dumbbell squat exercises on alternate days will likely reduce the potential for staleness and boredom with the routine. Furthermore, varying the training weights, number of sets, or rest interval between sets can help to prevent training plateaus, which are not uncommon after the first 8 to 12 weeks of resistance training. Program variation with adequate recovery will allow obese youths to make even greater gains, because the body will be challenged to adapt to greater demands.

By alternating training intensities, obese youths can minimize the risk of overtraining and maximize the potential for maintaining training-induced strength gains (52). In addition, professionals should consider school vacation schedules or travel plans when incorporating periods of active rest—that is, recreational activities or low-intensity, low-volume exercises—into a long-term training schedule. Periods of active rest will allow for physical and psychological recovery from resistance training and will help to promote long-term adherence to an exercise program (71).

SAMPLE 24-WEEK PROGRAM

Resistance training should be recommended to obese children and adolescents as one part of a multicomponent physical activity program that also includes games and activities designed to enhance cardiorespiratory fitness. The 24-week progressive resistance-training program discussed in this section consists of three 8-week mesocycles designed to promote gains in muscular fitness, maximize energy expenditure, and provide a safe and enjoyable experience for obese children and adolescents who have no experience with resistance training. The program begins with a single set of 10 to 15 repetitions of weight-machine exercises and progresses to 2 to 3 sets with heavier loads on more complex free-weight exercises. When obese youths begin resistance training, performing a single set of 10 to 15 repetitions per exercise two to three times per week will not only allow for positive changes in muscle function, it will also provide an opportunity for participants to gain confidence in their abilities before progressing to more advanced levels. Over time, continual gains can be made by adding new exercises or by gradually increasing the resistance, the number of repetitions, or the number of sets. On average, a 5 to 10 percent increase in training load, typically 2 to 10 pounds, is appropriate for most exercises. Not every training session needs to be more intense than the previous one, but over time, the demand placed upon a child's body should be gradually increased.

Weeks 1 through 8

After physician clearance is obtained, initial testing and evaluation are conducted, and beginning intensities are prescribed. Resistance training will take place on 3 nonconsecutive days of the week. Begin with a 5-minute dynamic warm-up, and then complete a single set of 10 to 15 repetitions, with 1 to 2 minutes rest between sets, of the leg press, leg extension, leg curl, chest press, seated row, shoulder press, biceps curl, triceps pushdown, lower-back extension, and abdominal curl exercises. Finish training by performing 5 minutes of static stretching.

The child should be taught how to record his progress on a workout log, and an instructor should provide guidance regarding appropriate starting weights, when to progress, and training tips on proper lifting technique to encourage controlled movements. In general, if the child can perform 15 repetitions on an exercise with proper form, the child should increase the weight by about 5 to 10 percent and reduce the repetitions to 10. Since the last repetition of each set should represent momentary muscular fatigue, exercising within the prescribed repetition-maximum training zone of 10 to 15 repetitions will automatically provide progressive overload, because as the child gets stronger, the weight required to stay in the prescribed training zone increases.

Weeks 9 through 16

During this second phase, the program will include 10 minutes of moderate-intensity dynamic warm-up activities prior to resistance training. This warm-up will involve movement-based exercises with light-weight (1 kg) medicine balls for the upper and lower body. The warm-up activities and choice of exercises during this phase are designed to enhance energy expenditure while maximizing fitness gains.

Training will include 1 to 2 sets of 8 to 15 repetitions, and new free-weight exercises, which require more balance and coordination, will be introduced. During this phase, the concept of periodization of training to optimize gains, provide variety to the program, and reduce the risk of overtraining is taught. The training intensity will vary throughout the week by performing each exercise for 8 to 10 repetitions with a moderate to heavy weight on Monday and Friday, for example; allow 1 to 2 minutes rest between sets, then do 12 to 15 repetitions with a relatively light weight on Wednesday, allowing less than 1 minute of rest between sets. Although the last repetition of each set should represent momentary muscular fatigue, the focus of each training session should remain on the quality of the movement, not the amount of weight lifted.

Exercises for Monday and Friday sessions will include 1 to 2 sets of 8 to 10 repetitions of the back squat, leg extension, leg curl, bench press, front lat pulldown, shoulder press, barbell curl, and triceps extension. Exercises for Wednesday sessions will include 1 to 2 sets of 12 to 15 repetitions of the leg press, leg extension, chest press, seated row, dumbbell lateral raise, dumbbell hammer curl, and triceps pushdown. Additionally, 2 sets of 10 to 15 repetitions of the lower-back extension and abdominal curl should be performed on Monday and Friday; and 2 sets of 10 to 15 repetitions of the kneeling trunk extension and abdominal curl should be performed on Wednesdays. Each session should conclude with 5 minutes of static stretching.

Weeks 17 through 24

During the third phase of the program, the dynamic warm-up activities will include 15 minutes of higher intensity movement-based exercises with light-weight (1 to 2 kg) medicine balls. To optimize training adaptations, the resistance-training sessions will include 1 to 3 sets of 8 to 15 repetitions of a variety of weight-machine and free-weight exercises that will vary throughout the week. All training sessions are followed by 5 minutes of static stretching.

On Mondays, perform 2 to 3 sets of 8 to 10 repetitions with a relatively heavy weights and 1 to 2 minutes rest between sets and exercises. Exercises will include the back squat, body-weight lunge, calf raise, bench press, dumbbell incline chest press, dumbbell row, front lat pulldown, dumbbell shoulder press, dumbbell biceps curl, and triceps pushdown. In addition, complete 3 sets of 10 to 15 repetitions of the kneeling trunk extension and abdominal curl.

Wednesday's training will involve 1 to 2 sets of 12 to 15 repetitions with a relatively light weights and rest periods shorter than 1 minute between sets and exercises. Exercises will include the back squat, body-weight lunge, calf raise, bench press, dumbbell

fly, dumbbell row, assisted chin-up, dumbbell lateral raise, dumbbell hammer curl, and assisted dip. Also complete 3 sets of 10 to 15 repetitions of the lower-back extension and twisting abdominal curl.

Friday's training will include 2 to 3 sets of 10 to 12 repetitions with a relatively moderate weight and a 1 minute rest period between sets and exercises. Exercises will include the back squat, body-weight lunge, calf raise, bench press, dumbbell incline chest press, dumbbell row, front lat pulldown, dumbbell shoulder press, dumbbell biceps curl, and triceps pushdown. Also complete 3 sets of 10 to 15 repetitions of the kneeling trunk extension and abdominal curl.

CASE STUDY

The parents of a 15-year old boy, J, weighing 95 kg with a height of 172 cm (BMI 32 kg/m^2) expressed concern about their child's body weight and lack of interest in any type of physical activity. J does not regularly participate in any type of physical activity and spends most of his free time surfing the Internet and playing video games. His parents encouraged him to join an after-school children's workout program at a local YMCA. Other than obesity, J has no other medical conditions that preclude participation in a sensibly prescribed fitness program that includes resistance training. While J and his family need guidance from a registered dietitian to improve their eating habits, the focus of this case study is on resistance training.

The short-term goal is for J to gain confidence in his abilities to be physically active while participating regularly in an enjoyable form of exercise. Since it is unlikely that he will be able or willing to perform prolonged periods of aerobic exercise, resistance training characterized by brief periods of work—10 to 15 repetitions followed by adequate rest between sets—would be appropriate for J during the initial adaptation phase of training. Regular participation in resistance training will result in noticeable gains in muscular fitness and will provide an opportunity for J to feel good about his accomplishments. Furthermore, since obese youths are relatively strong, they often receive unsolicited positive feedback from nonobese peers in the training area, who are often impressed by how much weight they can lift.

Because J was untrained, he participated in low-intensity warm-up activities that included walking and calisthenics, followed by a general resistance-training program as illustrated in the 24-Week Program. J's program consisted of exercises that emphasized the major muscle groups and progressed towards more advanced movements as he gained confidence in his abilities to resistance train. Throughout the program, J was encouraged to keep track of his progress on a workout log and to ask questions. Each class had an educational component, so J could understand the concept of fitness and gain the knowledge, skills, and self-motivation to regularly engage in physical activity.

Over the 24-week period, J had the opportunity to choose exercises and modify the program to suit his needs, goals, and abilities. He made remarkable gains in muscle strength and noticeable improvements in his aerobic capacity. Furthermore, midway through the resistance-training program, at about week 12, J started to participate in a recreational swim program at the YMCA twice per week. Because normal-weight and obese youths participated in the same resistance-training program, he made friends with lots of other boys and girls who were impressed with his muscle strength. Although his body weight did not change after the first 8 weeks of the program, favorable changes in body composition were observed by week 24. This change was due, at least in part, to his regular participation in resistance training and recreational swimming, as well as the efforts of his parents to improve his eating habits at home and at school. This case highlights the value of resistance training for obese youths and underscores the importance of parental support and encouragement.

Summary

Regular participation in resistance training, along with other types of physical activity, gives obese children and adolescents yet another opportunity to improve their health, fitness, and quality of life. Scientific evidence and clinical observations indicate that youths resistance-training programs are no more risky than other sports and activities in which children and adolescents regularly participate, and they may offer observable health benefits to boys and girls. However, resistance training is a specialized method of conditioning that needs to be carefully prescribed. When conducted by competent exercise professionals who possess a sound understanding of resistance-training principles and genuinely appreciate the physical and psychosocial uniqueness of childhood and adolescence, regular resistance training can offer many benefits and may often lead to a lifelong interest in an enjoyable type of physical activity.

Key Terms

Adolescence
Childhood
Energy balance
Environmental risk factors
Metabolic syndrome
Pediatric
Perceived exertion for children scale
Youths

Study Questions

1. What are the physical and psychosocial consequences of childhood obesity, and what impact will the current epidemic of childhood obesity have on our health care system in the future?

2. What environmental factors contribute to the epidemic of pediatric obesity, and what can be done to increase total daily energy expenditure in children and adolescents?

3. Discuss the potential health and fitness value of youths resistance training, and explain why resistance training may be particularly beneficial for an obese child.

4. Outline program variables that need to be considered when designing a youths resistance-training program, and discuss special considerations for training and testing obese youths.

References

1. American Academy of Pediatrics. Strength training by children and adolescents. Pediatrics. 2008;121:835-840.

2. American Academy of Pediatrics. Prevention of pediatric overweight and obesity. Pediatrics. 2003;112:424-430.

3. American College of Sports Medicine. ACSM's Guidelines for Exercise Testing and Prescription. 7th ed. Baltimore: Lippincott, Williams & Wilkins; 2006.

4. American Dietetic Association. Position of the American Dietetic Association: Dietary guidance for healthy children ages 2-11 years. J Am Diet Assoc. 2004;104(4):660-677.

5. Annesi JJ, Westcott WL, Faigenbaum AD, Unruh JL. Effects of a 12-week physical activity protocol delivered by YMCA after-school counselors (Youth Fit for Life) on fitness and self-efficacy changes in 5 to 12 year old boys and girls. Res Quart Exerc Sport. 2005;76:468-476,

6. Asuncion M, Calvo R, San Millan J, Sancho J, Avila S, Escobar-Morreale H. A prospective study of the prevalence of the polycystic ovary syndrome in unselected Caucasian women from Spain. J Clin Endocrinol Metab. 2000;85:2434-2438.

7. Baechle T, Earle R, Wathen D. Resistance training. In: Baechle T, Earle R, eds. Essentials of Strength Training and Conditioning. 2nd ed. Champaign, IL: Human Kinetics; 2000:395-426.

8. Bar-Or O, Rowland T. Pediatric Exercise Science. Champaign, IL: Human Kinetics; 2004.

9. Barlow S. Expert committee recommendations regarding the prevention, assessment, and treatment of child and adolescent overweight and obesity: Summary report. Pediatrics. 2007;120:S164-S192.

10. Behm DG, Faigenbaum AD, Falk B, Klentrou P. Canadian Society for Exercise Physiology position paper: Resistance training in children and adolescents. J Appl Physiol Nutr Metab. 2008;33:547-561.

11. Benson A, Torade M, Singh M. Muscular strength and cardiorespiratory fitness is associated with higher insulin sensitivity in children and adolescents. Int J Pediatr Obes. 2006;1:222-231.

12. Benson A, Torade M, Fiatarone-Singh M. The effect of high-intensity progressive resistance training on adiposity in children: A randomized controlled trial. Int J Obes. 2008;32(6): 1-12.

13. Berenson GS, Srinivan SR, Bao W, Newman WP, Tracy RE, Wattigney WA. Association between multiple cardiovascular risk factors and atherosclerosis in children and young adults: The Bogalusa Heart Study. New Engl J Med. 1998;338(23):1650-1656.

14. Blimkie C, Bar-Or O. Muscle strength, endurance and power: trainability during childhood. In: The Young Athlete. Hebestreit H, Bar-Or O, eds. Malden, MA: Blackwell Publishing; 2008:65-83.

15. Botero D, Wolfsdorf J. Diabetes mellitus in children and adolescents. Arch Med Res. 2005;36:281-290.

16. Brady T, Cahill B, Bodnar L. Weight-training related injuries in the high school athlete. Am J Sports Med. 1982;10:1-5.

17. British Association of Exercise and Sport Sciences. BASES position statement on guidelines for resistance exercise in young people. J Sports Sci. 2004;22:383-390.

18. Brown E, R Kimball. Medical history associated with adolescent power lifting. Pediatrics. 1983;72:636-644.

19. Campos G, Luecke T, Wendeln H, et al. Muscular adaptations in response to three different resistance training regimens: Specificity of repetition maximum training zones. Eur J Appl Physiol. 2002;88:50-60.

20. Carnethon M, Gulati M, Greenland P. Prevalence and cardiovascular disease correlates of low

cardiorespiratory fitness in adolescents and adults. *JAMA*. 2005;294:2981-2988.

21. Centers for Disease Control and Prevention. Barriers to children walking and biking to school - United States, 1999. *Morb Mort Wkly Rep*. 2002;51(32):701-704.

22. Centers for Disease Control and Prevention. Physical activity levels among children aged 9 to 13 years: United States, 2002, *Morbidity and Mortality Weekly Report*. 2003;52(33):785-788.

23. Centers for Disease Control and Prevention. Participation in high school physical education: United States, 1991–2003. *Journal of School Health*. 2005;75(2):47-49.

24. Cook S, Weitzman, M, Auinger P, Nguyen M, Dietz W. Prevalance of a metabolic syndrome phenotype in adolescents: Findings from the third National Health and Nutrition Examination Survey, 1988-1994. *Arch Pediatr Adol Med*. 2003;157(8):821-827.

25. Daniels S, Arnett D, Eckel R, et al. Overweight in children and adolescents: Pathophysiology, consequences, prevention and treatment. *Circulation*. 2005;111:1999-2012.

26. Dietz A. Health consequences of obesity in youth: Childhood predictors of adult disease. *Pediatrics*. 1988;101(3):518-525.

27. Dietz W. Overweight in childhood and adolescence. *N Engl J Med*. 2004;350:855-857.

28. Eisenberg ME, Neumark-Sztainer D, Story M. Associations of weight-based teasing and emotional well-being among adolescents. *Arch Pediatr Adolesc Med*. 2003;157:733-738.

29. Enns CW, Mickle SJ, Goldman JD. Trends in food and nutrient intakes by children in the United States. *Fam Econ Nutr Rev*. 2002;14(2):56-68.

30. Enns CW, Mickle SJ, Goldman JD. Trends in food and nutrient intakes by adolescents in the United States. *Fam Econ Nutr Rev*. 2003;15(2):15-27.

31. Faigenbaum A. Resistance training for children and adolescents: Are there health outcomes? *Am J Lifestyle Med*. 2007;1:190-200.

32. Faigenbaum A, Bellucci M, Bernieri A, Bakker B, Hoorens K. Acute effects of different warm-up protocols on fitness performance in children. *J Strength Cond Res*. 2005;19:376-381.

33. Faigenbaum A, Kang J, McFarland J, et al. Acute effects of different warm-up protocols on anaerobic performance in teenage athletes. *Ped Exerc Sci*. 2006;17:64-75.

34. Faigenbaum A, Kraemer W, Cahill B, et al. Youth resistance training: Position statement paper and literature review. *Strength and Conditioning*. 1996;18(6):62-75.

35. Faigenbaum A, McFarland J. Guidelines for implementing a dynamic warm-up for physical education. *J Phys Ed Rec Dance*. 2007;78:25-28.

36. Faigenbaum A, McFarland J, Johnson L, et al. Preliminary evaluation of an after-school resistance training program. *Percept Mot Skills*. 2007;104:407-415.

37. Faigenbaum A, Mediate P. The effects of medicine ball training on physical fitness in high school physical education students. *The Physical Educator*. 2006;63(3):161-168.

38. Faigenbaum A, Milliken L, Cloutier G, Westcott W. Perceived exertion during resistance exercise in children. *Percept Mot Skills*. 2004;98:627-637.

39. Faigenbaum A, Milliken L, LaRosa-Loud R, Burak B, Doherty C, Westcott W. Comparison of 1 and 2 days per week of strength training in children. *Res Quart Exerc Sport*. 2002;73:416-424.

40. Faigenbaum A, Milliken L, Moulton L, Westcott W. Early muscular fitness adaptations in children in response to two different resistance training regimens. *Pediatr Exerc Sci*. 2005;17:237-248.

41. Faigenbaum A, Milliken L, Westcott W. Maximal strength testing in healthy children. *J Strength Cond Res.* 2003;17(1):162-166.

42. Faigenbaum A, Ratamess N, McFarland J, Kaczmarek J, Coraggio M, Kang J, Hoffman J. Effect of rest interval length on bench press performance in boys, teens and men. *Pediatr Exerc Sci.* In press.

43. Faigenbaum A, Schram J. Can resistance training reduce injuries in youth sports? *Strength and Conditioning Journal.* 2004;26(3):16-21.

44. Faigenbaum A, Westcott W. *Strength and Power for Young Athletes.* Champaign, IL: Human Kinetics; 2000

45. Faigenbaum A, Westcott W. Resistance training for obese children and adolescents. *Pres Coun Phys Fit Sports Res Digest.* 2007;8:1-8.

46. Faigenbaum A, Westcott WL, Long C, Loud R, Delmonico M, Micheli L. Relationship between repetitions and selected percentages of the one repetition maximum in healthy children. *Pediatr Phys Ther.* 1998;10:110-113.

47. Faigenbaum A, Westcott W, Loud R, Long C. The effects of different resistance training protocols on muscular strength and endurance development in children. *Pediatrics.* 1999;104:e5.

48. Faigenbaum A, Zaichkowsky L, Westcott W, Micheli L, Fehlandt A. The effects of a twice per week strength training program on children. *Pediatr Exerc Sci.* 1993;5:339-346.

49. Falk B, Tenenbaum G. The effectiveness of resistance training in children. A meta-analysis. *Sports Med.* 1996;22:176-186.

50. Falk B, Sadres E, Constantini N, Zigel L, Lidor R, Eliakim A. The association between adiposity and the response to resistance training among pre- and early-pubertal boys. *J Pediatr Endocrinol Metab.* 2002;15:597-606.

51. Fleck S, Kraemer W. *Designing resistance training programs.* 3rd ed. Champaign, IL: Human Kinetics; 2004.

52. Fry A, Kraemer W. Resistance exercise overtraining and overreaching. *Sports Med.* 1997;23(2):106-129.

53. Gielen S, Hambrecht R. The childhood obesity epidemic. Impact on endothelial function. *Circulation.* 2004;109:1911-1911.

54. Gillis LJ, Kennedy LC, Bar-Or O. Overweight children reduce their activity levels earlier in life than healthy weight children. *Clin J Sport Med.* 2006;16(1):51-55.

55. Goodman E, Whitaker R. A prospective study of the role of depression in the development and persistence of adolescent obesity. *Pediatrics.* 2002;110:497-504.

56. Gortmaker SL, Must A, Perrin J, Sobel A, Dietz W. Social and economic consequences of overweight in adolescence and young adulthood. *N Engl J Med.* 1993;329: 1008-1012.

57. Gregor N, Edwin C. Obesity: A pediatric epidemic. *Pediatr Ann.* 2001;30(11):694-700.

58. Greves HM, Rivara FP. Report card on school snack food policies among the United States' largest school districts in 2004-2005: Room for improvement. *Int J Behav Nutr Phys Act.* 2006;3(1):1.

59. Gumbs V, Segal D, Halligan J, Lower G. Bilateral distal radius and ulnar fractures in adolescent weight lifters. *Am J Sports Med.* 1982;10:375-379.

60. Guo SS, Chumlea WC. Tracking of body mass index in children in relation to overweight in adulthood. *Am J Clin Nutr.* 1999;70(suppl):145S-148S.

61. Guy J, Micheli L. Strength training for children and adolescents. *J Am Acad Ortho Surg.* 2001;9:29-36.

62. USDHH. *Healthy People 2010.* 2nd ed. Washington, DC: US Department of Health and Human Services; 2000.

63. Hedley A, Ogden C, Johnson C, Carroll M, Curtin L, Flegal K. Prevalence of overweight

and obesity among US children, adolescents and adults, 1999-2002. *JAMA*. 2004;291: 2847-2850.

64. Hewett T, Myer G, Ford K. Reducing knee and anterior cruciate ligament injuries among female athletes. *J Knee Surg*. 2005;18:82-88.

65. Holloway J, Beuter A, Duda J. Self-efficacy and training in adolescent girls. *J Appl Soc Psychol*. 1988;18:699-719.

66. Institute of Medicine of the National Academies. *Preventing Childhood Obesity: Health in the Balance*. Washington, DC: The National Academies Press; 2005.

67. Institute of Medicine. *Weight Management: State of the Science and Opportunities for Military Programs*. Washington, DC: National Academy Press; 2003.

68. Jain A, Sherman SN, Chamberlin DL, Carter Y, Powers SW, Whitaker RC. Why don't low-income mothers worry about their preschoolers being overweight? *Pediatrics*. 2001;107(5):1138-1146.

69. Jones C, Christensen C, Young M. Weight training injury trends. *Phys Sports Med*. 2000;28:61-72.

70. Knudson D, Magnusson P, McHugh, M. Current issues in flexibility fitness. *Pres Coun Phys Fitness Sports Res Digest*. 2000;3(10):1-8.

71. Kraemer W, Adams K, Cafarelli E, et al. Progression models in resistance training for healthy adults. *Med Sci Sports Exerc*. 2002;34:364-380.

72. Kraemer W, Fleck S. *Strength Training for Young Athletes*. 2nd ed. Champaign, IL: Human Kinetics; 2005.

73. Kraemer W, Ratamess N. Fundamentals of resistance training: Progression and exercise prescription. *Med Sci Sports Exerc*. 2004;36:674-688.

74. Kuczmarski RJ, Ogden CL, Grummer-Strawn LM, et al. 2000 CDC growth charts: United States. *Adv Data*. 2000;314:1-27.

75. Lillegard W, Brown E, Wilson D, Henderson R, Lewis E. Efficacy of strength training in prepubescent to early postpubescent males and females: Effects of gender and maturity. *Pediatr Rehabil*. 1997;1:147-157.

76. Lissau I, Overpeck MD, Ruan WJ, Due P, Hulstein B, Hediger M. Body mass index and overweight in adolescents in 13 European countries, Israel and the United States. *Arch Pediatr Adolesc Med*. 2004;158:27-33.

77. McNeal J, Sands W. Acute static stretching reduces lower extremity power in trained children. *Pediatr Exerc Sci*. 2003;15:139-145.

78. Micheli L. Strength training in the young athlete. In: Brown E, Branta C, eds. *Competitive sports for children and youth*. Champaign, IL: Human Kinetics; 1988:99-105.

79. Micheli L. Preventing injuries in sports: What the team physician needs to know. In: *F.I.M.S. Team Physician Manual*. 2nd ed. Chan K, Micheli L, Smith A, et al, eds. Hong Kong: CD Concept; 2006:555-572.

80. Morris F, Naughton G, Gibbs J, Carlson J, Wark J. Prospective ten-month exercise intervention in premenarcheal girls: Positive effects on bone and lean mass. *J Bone Min Res*. 1997;12:1453-1462.

81. Must A, Jacques PF, Dallal GE, Bajema CJ, Dietz WH. Long-term morbidity and mortality of overweight adolescents. A follow-up of the Harvard Growth Study of 1922 to 1935. *N Engl J Med*. 1992;327:1350-1355.

82. Narayan KM, Boyle JP, Thompson TJ, Sorensen SW, Williamson DF. Lifetime risk for diabetes mellitus in the United States. *J Am Med Assoc*. 2003;290(14):1884-1890.

83. Ogden CL, Carrol LR, Flegal KF. High body mass index for age among US children and adolescents. *JAMA*. 2008;299:2401-2405.

84. Ozmun J, Mikesky A, Surburg P. Neuromuscular adaptations following prepubescent strength training. *Med Sci Sports Exerc*. 1994;26:510-514.

85. Pine DS, Goldstein RB, Wolk S, Weissman MM. The association between childhood depression and adult body mass index. *Pediatrics.* 2001;107(5):1049-1056.

86. Ramsay J, Blimkie C, Smith K, Garner S, MacDougall J, Sale D. Strength training effects in prepubescent boys. *Med Sci Sports Exerc.* 1990;22:605-614.

87. Risser W. Weight training injuries in children and adolescents. *Am Fam Physician.* 1991; 44:2104-2110.

88. Robbins D. Postactivation potentiation and its practical application: A brief review. *J Strength Cond Res.* 2005;19:453-458.

89. Roberts D, Foehr U, Rideout V, Brodie M. *Kids and Media @ the New Millennium.* Menlo Park, CA: Henry J. Kaiser Family Foundation; 1999.

90. Rutledge I, Faccioni A. Dynamic warm-ups. *Sports Coach.* 2001;24(1):20-22.

91. Ryan J, Salciccioli G. Fracture of the distal radial epiphysis in adolescent weight lifters. *Am J Sports Med.* 1976;4:26-27.

92. Schwimmer J, Burwinkle T, Varni J. Health-related quality of life of severely obese children and adolescents. *JAMA.* 2003;289:1813-1819.

93. Schwingshandl J, Sudi K, Eibi B, Wallner S, Borkenstein M. Effect of an individualized training programme during weight reduction on body composition: A randomized trial. *Arch Dis Child.* 1999;81:426-428.

94. Shabi G, Cruz M, Ball G, et al. Effects of resistance exercise on insulin sensitivity in overweight Latino adolescent males. *Med Sci Sports Exerc.* 2006;38:1208-1215.

95. Siegal J, Camaione D, Manfredi T. The effects of upper-body resistance training in prepubescent children. *Pediatr Exerc Sci.* 1989;1:145-154.

96. Smith A, Andrish J, Micheli L. The prevention of sports injuries of children and adolescents. *Med Sci Sports Exerc.* 1993;25(suppl 8):1-7.

97. Sothern M. Exercise as a modality in the treatment of childhood obesity. *Pediatr Clin North Am.* 2001;48:995-1015.

98. Sothern M, Loftin J, Udall J, et al. Safety, feasibility and efficacy of a resistance training program in preadolescent obese youth. *Am J Med Sci.* 2000;319(6):370-375.

99. Stone MH, O'Bryant H, Garhammer J. A hypothetical model for strength training. *J Sports Med.* 1981;21:342-351.

100. Sun SS, Liang R, Huang T, et al. Childhood obesity predicts adult metabolic syndrome: The Fels longitudinal study. *J Pediatr.* 2008;152:191-200.

101. Sung R, Yu C, Chang S, Mo S, Woo K, Lam C. Effects of dietary intervention and strength training on blood lipid level in obese children. *Arch Dis Child.* 2002;86:407-410.

102. Taras H, Potts-Datema W. Obesity and student performance at school. *J School Health.* 2005;75:291-295.

103. Thacker S, Gilchrist J, Stroup D, Kimsey C. The impact of stretching on sports injury risk: A systematic review of the literature. *Med Sci Sports Exerc.* 2004;36:371-378.

104. Treuth M, Hunter G, Figueroa-Colon R, Goran M. Effects of strength training on intra-abdominal adipose tissue in obese prepubertal girls. *Med Sci Sports Exerc.* 1998;30:1738-1743.

105. Treuth M, Hunter G, Pichon C, Figueroa-Colon R, Goran M. Fitness and energy expenditure after strength training in obese prepubertal girls. *Med Sci Sports Exerc.* 1998;30:1130-1136.

106. USDHHS. *The Surgeon General's call to action to prevent and decrease overweight and obesity.* Rockville, MD: U.S. Department of Health and Human Services, Public Health Service, Office of the Surgeon General; 2001.

107. Vaughn J, Micheli L. Strength training recommendations for the young athlete. *Phys Med Rehabil Clin N Am.* 2008;19:235-245.

108. Vincent S, Pangrazi R, Raustorp A, Tomson L, Cuddihy T. Activity level and body mass index of children in the United States, Sweden and Australia. *Med Sci Sports Exerc.* 2003;35:1367-1373.

109. Wang G, Dietz W. Economic burden of obesity in youths aged 6 to 17 years: 1979–1999. *Pediatrics.* 2002;109(5):E81-E86.

110. Watts K, Beye P, Siafarikas A, et al. Exercise training normalizes vascular dysfunction and improves central adiposity in obese adolescents. *J Am Coll Cardiol.* 2004;43:1823-1827.

111. Watts K, Jones T, Davis E, Green D. Exercise training in obese children and adolescents. *Sports Med.* 2005;35:375-392.

112. Weltman A, Janney C, Rians C, et al. The effects of hydraulic resistance strength training in prepubertal males. *Med Sci Sports Exerc.* 1986;18:629-638.

113. Weltman A, Janney C, Rians C, Strand K, Katch F. Effects of hydraulic-resistance strength training on serum lipid levels in prepubertal boys. *Am J Dis Child.* 1987; 141:777-780.

114. Wisemandle W, Maynard L, Guo SS, Siervogel RM. Childhood weight, stature, and body mass index among never overweight, early onset overweight and late onset overweight groups. *Pediatrics.* 2000;106(1):e14.

115. Young W, Behm D. Should static stretching be used during a warm-up for strength and power activities? *Strength and Conditioning Journal.* 2002;24(6):33-37.

116. Yu C, Sung R, So R, et al. Effects of strength training on body composition and bone mineral content in children who are obese. *J Strength Cond Res.* 2005;19:667-672.

117. Zafeiridis A, Dalamitros A, Dipla K, Manou V, Galanis N, Kellis S. Recovery during high-intensity intermittent anaerobic exercise in boys, teens and men. *Med Sci Sports Exerc.* 2005;37:505-512.

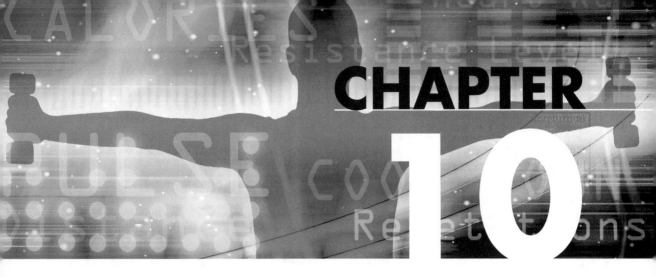

CHAPTER 10

RESISTANCE-TRAINING STRATEGIES FOR INDIVIDUALS WITH TYPE 1 DIABETES MELLITUS

Objectives

Upon completion of this chapter, the reader should be able to:

- Identify the prevalence and associated economic costs of type 1 diabetes mellitus (T1D), also known *as insulin-dependent diabetes mellitus (IDDM)* or *autoimmune diabetes*
- Describe the pathophysiology of T1D and possible relationships between T1D and coronary artery disease
- Describe the beneficial role of resistance training in individuals with T1D
- Explain the specific factors to consider related to preexercise screening, exercise testing, and exercise prescription when designing a resistance-training program for individuals with T1D

INTRODUCTION

Diabetes is a group of metabolic conditions generally resulting in **hyperglycemia,** defined as fasting blood glucose above 125 mg/dl or a random glucose level of 200 mg/dl or greater. Defects and abnormalities in both the secretion and action of insulin may be present, depending upon the specific form of diabetes. **Insulin** is a hormone produced in the pancreas that facilitates the entrance of glucose into the cell, and its production may be compromised in diabetes. **Insulin receptors,** specialized sites on a cell membrane where insulin acts, may be resistant to insulin, resulting in the associated hyperglycemia. Both type 1 diabetes mellitus (T1D) and type 2 diabetes mellitus (T2D) may be associated with hyperglycemia; **hypoglycemia,** defined as fasting blood glucose below 60 to 70 mg/dl with symptoms; and **hypoinsulinemia,** which describes abnormally low insulin blood levels; or **hyperinsulinemia,** which describes abnormally high levels. Which conditions are present depends on the exact clinical and physiological status, the type of diabetes, the age of onset, and the coexisting risk factors of the individual (8, 17, 26). Table 10-1 outlines disorders of hypoglycemia in diabetes mellitus.

Table 10-1 Disorders of Hypoglycemia

Types		Stages			
		Normoglycemia		Hyperglycemia	
	Normal glucose regulation	Impaired glucose tolerance or Impaired fasting glucose (Pre-diabetes)	Diabetes Mellitus		
			Does not require insulin	Insulin required for control	Insulin required for survival
Type 1*	←				→
Type 2	←			→	
Other types**	←			→	
Gestational diabetes**	←		→		

*Even after presenting in ketoacidosis, these patients can briefly return to normoglycemia without requiring continuous therapy; called a "honeymoon" remission.

**In rare instances, patients in these categories (e.g. Vacor toxicity, Type 1 diabetes presenting in pregnancy) may require insulin for survival.

Copyright© 2006 American Diabetes Association. From *Diabetes Care.* 2006;29:S43-S48. Reprinted with permission from The American Diabetes Association.

Table 10-2 Symptoms of Type 1 Diabetes Mellitus (40)

- Increased thirst and frequent urination
- Extreme hunger
- Weight loss or weight gain
- Fatigue
- Blurred vision
- Slow-healing sores or frequent infections
- Tingling in hands and feet
- Red, swollen, or tender gums

T1D is thought to be an immune-mediated disorder that selectively attacks and destroys the beta cells, or insulin-producing cells, of the pancreas, resulting in a deficiency of the production and release of insulin. The deficiency leads to hypoinsulinemia and resultant hyperglycemia. The presence of serologic markers such as islet cell and insulin autoantibodies at the time of diagnosis provides support for the autoimmune nature of T1D (16, 17). Classic signs and symptoms of T1D are presented in Table 10-2, and T1D usually afflicts individuals younger than age 30 years. Onset of T1D, however, can occur well into the fifth and sixth decades of life (16, 35).

PREVALENCE AND ECONOMIC IMPACT OF T1D

The prevalence of T1D is approximately 5 to 10 percent—1 to 2 million cases—of all diagnosed cases of diabetes in the United States (41). To survive, individuals with T1D must have exogenous insulin delivered either by injection or pump. About 16 percent of all diabetics are treated with insulin alone, virtually 100 percent of individuals with T1D, and another 14 percent are treated with insulin and an oral hypoglycemic agent (41). Non-Hispanic whites are more likely to have T1D than either Hispanic or non-Hispanic Blacks (41). In contrast to T1D, the

dramatic increase in the incidence of T2D in the last two decades is directly proportional to the increasing incidence of obesity in the U.S. population, leading some to describe this condition as "diabesity."

The total prevalence of T2D among individuals aged 20 years or older in the United States is estimated to be 23.6 million people, or approximately 10.7 percent of the population (13). Of the estimated 23.6 million cases of diabetes, 17.9 million are diagnosed, but 5.7 million cases remain undiagnosed (41). Approximately 186,300 individuals younger than 20 years of age have either T1D or T2D (41). Among adults, there are about 1.6 million new cases of diabetes diagnosed each year (41). Among individuals younger than 20 years of age, about 15,000 new cases of T1D and 3,700 new cases of T2D are diagnosed each year (41).

In 2006, diabetes was the seventh leading cause of death listed on U.S. death certificates (41). In addition, according to death certificates, diabetes contributed to a total of 233,619 deaths in 2005 (41). Diabetes is the leading cause of blindness among adults aged 20 to 74 years. Diabetes is also the leading cause of kidney failure, accounting for 44 percent of new cases in 2005, and for nontraumatic lower-limb amputations, accounting for more than 60 percent (41). In addition, 75 percent of adults with self-reported diabetes have hypertension, 84 percent of deaths among individuals with diabetes are due to cardiovascular disease, and 60 to 70 percent of individuals with diabetes have peripheral **neuropathy**, or nerve damage (41).

The total direct and indirect medical costs of diabetes in the United States are approximately $174 billion per year (41). Individuals with diagnosed diabetes incur average expenditures of $11,744 per year, of which $6,649 is attributed to diabetes. Individuals with diagnosed diabetes, on average, have medical expenditures that are approximately 2.3 times higher than expenditures in the absence of diabetes. Approximately one of every five health care dollars in the United States is spent caring for someone with diagnosed diabetes, and approximately one of every ten health care dollars is attributed directly to treating diabetes (41).

Mortality secondary to T1D prior to age 20 is low—less than 5 percent. Over 40 percent of those with T1D survive longer than 40 years after diagnosis (41). A positive genetic profile, good medical and self-care, and tight **glycemic control**—defined as managing **glycated hemoglobin**, in which the percentage of hemoglobin bound with glucose is less than 7.0 percent—appear to improve survival rates (31, 41). By the time individuals with T1D reach their 40s and 50s, both men and women demonstrate coronary artery calcification; and by age 55, coronary artery disease mortality reaches 35 percent, compared to less than 10 percent in populations without T1D. Premature mortality and morbidity from coronary artery disease approaches 10 percent in people with T1D (36).

ETIOLOGY OF T1D

T1D, also known as **insulin-dependent diabetes mellitus** or **autoimmune diabetes**, is caused by destruction of the beta cells of the pancreas, initially reducing and ultimately eliminating insulin production. At some point in the progression of the disease, individuals with T1D must use supplemental, exogenous insulin to maintain normal physiology and to prevent morbidity and mortality. The most common mechanism of beta-cell destruction in T1D is through a process called **apoptosis**, a "programmed" destruction of cells that occurs due to intracellular, rather than extracellular, processes. The etiology of the aberrant apoptosis that occurs in T1D is not completely understood but is likely due to the imposition of environmental variables such as enteroviruses and rotaviruses, rubella, and possibly exposure to other microbes and pathogens in genetically predisposed individuals (16).

Susceptibility to T1D varies genetically in individuals (27, 36, 44). Exposure to environmental factors such as viruses, toxins, medications, and other pathogens is thought to predispose some individuals to T1D. The genetic predisposition and exposure to one or more unknown environmental stimuli enhances or facilitates the onset of the autoimmune dysfunction and apoptosis of beta cells. Further, it appears that the actual onset of T1D involves the intersection of the right trigger and the right time (16). Traditionally, T1D was thought to be a disease of childhood and early adolescence, with few people diagnosed in adulthood. Data suggest that perhaps 50 to 60 percent of those diagnosed with T1D today are younger than 16 to 18 years of age, leaving a significant number of individuals to be diagnosed after 18 years of age (44).

The evolution of T1D involves increasingly impaired insulin production, decreased insulin secretion with accompanying hyperglycemia, and ultimately **ketoacidosis**—the accumulation of excessive keto acids in the blood stream—leading to dehydration, hyperglycemia, ketonuria, and increased levels of glucagon. Between 15 to 67 percent of individuals with T1D initially present with ketoacidosis (16). Early recognition of signs and symptoms may result in diagnosis and treatment prior to the first incidence of ketoacidosis.

C-peptide is a protein marker used to detect the destruction of beta cells, and it contributes to the diagnosis of T1D. Low c-peptide levels suggest the presence of islet cell antibodies, which are almost always found prior to the actual onset of T1D (16). In fact, in relatives of people with T1D, the presence of known, specific autoantibodies—for example, GADA and/or autoinsulin antibodies—prior to the onset of abnormally low levels of c-peptide predicts T1D with an accuracy greater than 90 percent (16). These tests are expensive and tedious to perform, thus availability and ease of access may be limited, leaving c-peptide as the primary marker of beta-cell destruction and T1D. The onset and progression of T1D can be highly variable, and some individuals may persist into adulthood with autoimmune dysfunction, beta-cell destruction, and increased antibody levels, despite being able to maintain glucose homeostasis (16, 36, 44).

Complications of T1D

T1D is pathophysiologically different from T2D but has similar accompanying microvascular and macrovascular complications (10, 14, 25, 45, 46).

These complications may result in organ damage and other clinical problems, making effective treatments complicated and multifactorial. Proteinuria, microalbuminuria, and **nephropathy**—that is, kidney disease—are often implicated in, and thought to be precursors of, risk for coronary artery disease in T1D, although the literature is controversial in clarifying this issue. In fact, it appears that the risk factors for these conditions and for coronary artery disease are similar and may develop in parallel with each other rather than serially (36). Thus, coronary artery disease may develop independently of proteinuria and nephropathy in T1D, giving added weight to the importance of lifestyle in the etiology of coronary artery disease in individuals with T1D (34, 36).

BENEFITS OF RESISTANCE TRAINING FOR INDIVIDUALS WITH T1D

The benefits of resistance training for individuals with T2D are well documented. Although the literature is both sparse and inconclusive regarding the health benefits of resistance training for those with T1D, the benefits are generally thought to parallel those observed in individuals with T2D. A comprehensive review and statement about resistance training for those with T2D has been published recently (24). And Table 10-3 outlines the known effects of resistance training on various physiological variables, and it discusses the use of resistance training for individuals with T2D in detail. Of relevance was the finding across many studies that resistance training enhances insulin sensitivity, and it increases daily energy expenditure and quality of life—important findings pertinent to individuals with T1D. The review points out the advantages of increased muscle mass and bone mineral density in terms of insulin receptors and sensitivity that have also been demonstrated after resistance training (24). The consistent beneficial outcomes associated with resistance training for individuals with T2D, and several other special populations (9), as well as the general contribution of resistance training to

health status seems to make these findings pertinent to individuals with T1D as well.

Both of the reviews mentioned above recommend the use of resistance training in the exercise regimens of individuals with diabetes. In addition, the American College of Sports Medicine (ACSM) recommends a moderate- to high-intensity resistance-training program defined as 70 to 85 percent of the one-repetition maximum (1RM) (1, 3). A review in a published position statement from the National Strength and Conditioning Association (NSCA) on "Health Aspects of Resistance Exercise Training" has also been published, but it does not specifically address T1D (15). It appears that moderate- to high-intensity resistance training that is associated with significant increases in fat-free muscle mass may in turn affect decreases in glycated hemoglobin, which can be used as a long-term measure of hyperglycemia. This change in glycated hemoglobin is likely secondary to the increased fat-free muscle mass, though the exact mechanism is not clear (24). Thus it is speculated that increased fat-free muscle mass is one reason that insulin sensitivity, glycemic control, and markers of glycemic control, such as glycated hemoglobin, improve.

As stated earlier in this discussion, the literature on resistance training in T1D is sparse and inconclusive. Two articles in the literature specifically studied patients with T1D, with resistance training as the independent treatment variable. Durak (22) used a randomized, crossover design—that is, without a control group—with resistance training in 8 males with T1D. Significant changes in muscular strength and endurance were associated with the training program. Both glycated hemoglobin and total cholesterol improved after 10 weeks of training. No additional changes were documented in lipid profile, body composition, insulin use, or diet (22). Ramalho and associates (43) studied the effects of resistance training versus aerobic training in 16 patients with T1D. The authors did not document changes in muscular strength or endurance secondary to resistance training, if these were even measured. Difficulties and deficiencies with design and outcome measurement make this study less than definitive and render any conclusions tenuous.

Table 10-3 Benefits of Resistance Training on Various Physiological Variables (9, 15, 24, 42)

Risk Factors	Effect		Note
	AH	**T1D**	
Glucose tolerance	NA	$\downarrow, \uparrow$	Reduction of acute response to graded treadmill test; decreased glycated hemoglobin; decreased use of insulin
Glycemic control, glycated hemoglobin	NA	$\downarrow, \uparrow, \pm$	Improved when hyperglycemia present (one study)
Insulin sensitivity	$\uparrow$	Unk	In hyperglycemia and glycemic clamps during hyperinsulinemia
Insulin dose	NA	$\downarrow$	Improved in both T1D studies
Hypertension	$\downarrow, \uparrow, \pm$	Unk	
Blood pressure	$\downarrow$	Unk	Significant but small decrease due to resistance training
Arterial stiffness	$\downarrow, \uparrow, \pm$	Unk	Mixed results from research
Endothelial function	$\uparrow$	Unk	One controlled study demonstrates increased FMD in overweight women
Obesity prevention	$\pm$	Unk	Rationale provides positive effects but is not yet confirmed
Obesity	$\downarrow, \pm$	Unk	Modest weight loss with increased muscle mass
Visceral adipose tissue	$\downarrow$	Unk	May be gender specific
Fat-free mass	$\pm$	$\uparrow$	
HDL	$\pm, \uparrow$	$\downarrow, \pm$	Changes with circuit training or aerobic training combined with resistance training
LDL	$\downarrow, \pm$	Unk	
Cardiovascular endurance fitness	$\uparrow$	$\pm$	Circuit training increases VO_2 Max significantly, but less than aerobic training

Key: AH = apparently healthy; T1D = Type 1 diabetes; T2D = Type 2 diabetes; $\downarrow$ = decrease; $\uparrow$ = increase or improved; $\pm$ = no effect; Unk = unknown

SPECIAL CONSIDER-ATIONS FOR EXERCISE TESTING AND TRAINING

Because the complications of T1D are many and varied and may not be associated with overt symptoms, a detailed medical examination by a physician should precede exercise testing before participation in any exercise program, including resistance training. All systems should be evaluated with special consideration for the common complications associated with T1D in cardiovascular, nervous, renal, and visual systems. Table 10-4 describes the clinical status when the physical exam should include an exercise test with either radionuclide, echocardiographic, and/or pharmacological exercise testing. These additional tests should be seriously considered in this population due to the prevalence of silent ischemia (4, 6).

Contraindications to both exercise training and exercise testing in T1D include poor glycemic control or blood glucose greater than 250 mg/dl with the presence of ketones, proliferative retinopathy, recent laser therapy for retinopathy, severe neuropathy, and renal disease (5). People with T1D should avoid high-intensity resistance training programs during periods of poor glycemic control or exacerbation of symptoms and complications, especially for example, after laser treatment for retinopathy.

Exercise Training Considerations

T1D is a disease in which there is metabolic dysfunction that includes abnormalities in glucose, insulin, and fat metabolism. Insulin is an anabolic hormone that is essential to protein synthesis, muscle growth, and development. Therefore before a safe and effective resistance-training program is initiated or progressed in individuals with T1D, it is essential that optimal medical management be achieved. In this case, "optimal medical management" means the best possible management, not only of blood glucose, but also of other clinical conditions and complications such as hypertension, dyslipidemia, atherosclerosis, peripheral arterial disease, retinopathy, and neuropathy that may effect mortality and morbidity in individuals with T1D. Additionally, exercise results in altered insulin and glucose regulation, thus several precautions are important. Table 10-5 outlines the recommendations for optimal medial management of T1D.

Through different physiological mechanisms, both insulin and exercise cause enhanced glucose transport, particularly into muscle cells. Since individuals with T1D do not produce significant amounts of insulin, they must rely on **exogenous insulin** from an injection or insulin pump to assure a proper balance between peripheral glucose utilization and hepatic glucose production, or *gluconeogenesis* (12). In addition, counterregulatory hormones such as glucagon may not respond in a normal manner. Therefore one of the most critical potential adverse responses to exercise is hypoglycemia. Table 10-6 outlines factors that may determine, alone or in combination, the acute effects of an exercise session on glucose metabolism in individuals with T1D.

The end result is that people with T1D must become experts in self-care. They must be very self-aware, and they must learn to be attentive to their own physiological situation to adhere to a long-term exercise program successfully.

Table 10-4 Graded Exercise Testing and T1D (4)

When considering initiation of an exercise program of moderate to high intensity, graded exercise testing is recommended for individuals who have an underlying risk for cardiovascular disease based on the following criteria:

- Age >35 years
- Age >25 years and T1D duration of >15 years
- Presence of additional risk factors for cardiovascular disease
- Presence of retinopathy or nephropathy with albuminuria or autonomic neuropathy
- Peripheral Vascular Disease

Table 10-5 Optimal Medical and Lifestyle Management for Type 1 Diabetes (4, 6)

Characteristics of Optimal Health Management

- Fasting blood glucose <100 mg/dl
- Random blood glucose <140 mg/dl
- Glycated hemoglobin (HbA1c) <6.5%
- Total cholesterol <200 mg/dl
- LDL cholesterol <100 mg/dl
- HDL cholesterol >40 mg/dl
- Triglycerides <150 mg/dl
- Total LDL/HDL ratio <4.0
- Blood pressure <130/85 mmHg
- BMI <25.0
- Waist-to-hip ratio <0.96 (males) or <0.85 (females)
- Minimum of 30 minutes of aerobic exercise every day
- Resistance training 2 to 3 days a week, 30 to 45 minutes, 8 to 10 exercises at 60 to 80% of 1RM, 2 to 3 sets, 8 to 12 repetitions
- 15 to 20 minutes of specific static stretching, 5 days a week
- Adherence to a high fiber, low fat, diet with consistent caloric content

Table 10-6 Factors Affecting Exercise-Related Hypoglycemia and Hyperglycemia

- Type and amount of insulin and how it is administered (injection, inhalation, insulin pump)
- The timing of the insulin administration prior to exercise
- Level of blood glucose prior to exercise and insulin administration
- Timing, quantity, and type of food ingested prior to exercise (carbs or protein)
- Intensity and duration of exercise
- Metabolic and other comorbidities, such as upper respiratory or urinary tract infections, influenza, or other acute medical conditions

Hypoglycemia is a constant risk for individuals with T1D, and precautions to prevent exercise-related hypoglycemia are essential to observe. Tight glycemic control has been shown to be associated with fewer diabetic complications as well as a later onset of such complications (18, 19, 20, 21). Since the Diabetes Control and Complications Trial (DCCT) confirmed the benefits of tight control for individuals with T1D, it is highly recommended that this control be achieved prior to initiating a vigorous resistance-training program (18, 19, 20, 21). Interestingly, tight glycemic control is also associated with increased risk and incidence of hypoglycemia (2, 17, 47). Exercise alters the response to circulating insulin. Hypoglycemia alters

glucose regulation during exercise, thus the risk of hypoglycemia during exercise for an individual with T1D is increased (11) Other risk factors for hypoglycemia in T1D include the presence of neuropathy; increased frequency of self-monitored blood glucose, presumably related to tight control of blood glucose; a threshold for hypoglycemic symptoms of blood glucose below 54 mg/dl, and an insulin dose greater than 0.1 unit per kilogram of body weight (2).

Finally, an increased risk of a late-onset postexercise hypoglycemia has been found in individuals with T1D (38). **Late-onset postexercise hypoglycemia** is defined as hypoglycemia that occurs from 6 to 24 hours after exercise or activity. This condition may be caused, or at least mediated, by the postexercise restoration of muscle and liver glycogen levels using blood glucose. Increased insulin sensitivity is one outcome of exercise, resulting in enhanced uptake of glucose in the postexercise state. Increased intensity, long-duration exercise seems to be more frequently associated with this type of hypoglycemia. Increased intake of carbohydrates in the postexercise period, along with modifications in the exercise regimen, can prevent this type of hypoglycemia (37).

Interestingly, and perhaps counterintuitively, it has been shown that high-intensity, intermittent cardiovascular exercise may offer some protection from hypoglycemia. In fact, this type of exercise has been shown to cause increases in blood glucose in the short term (29, 30). Guelfi compared high-intensity exercise (4-second sprints every 2 minutes for a total of 20 minutes) to no exercise in T1D and found that the risk of postexercise hypoglycemia was not increased (29). In a second study, Guelfi showed that the decline in blood glucose is greater during moderate intensity exercise than during high-intensity exercise in T1D (30). Bussau recommended adding a short bout of high-intensity exercise after a session of moderate exercise to reduce the risk of postexercise hypoglycemia (11).

Individuals with T1D should take precautions to minimize the risk of moderate to severe hypoglycemic episodes when initiating an exercise program. Special considerations with respect to meals and food intake prior to and after exercise training are part of the careful planning that should occur. Individuals with T1D often have much better control of blood glucose when they have relatively strict and repetitive routines for both insulin and food intake. For example, exercising before breakfast may bring on a hypoglycemic state simply because of the long fasting period since the previous meal. Similarly, exercise preceding any meal will likely mean exercising at a time when blood glucose may be declining or at a low. This situation can be moderated by a preexercise snack, preferably one that includes protein rather than a snack high in simple carbohydrates. A ratio of about 3 to 4 grams of carbohydrates per gram of protein and about 150 to 200 kilocalories is recommended. Reducing the insulin dosage prior to planned exercise may also be necessary, but any change in dosage of insulin needs to be in collaboration with the client's physician. Planning for safe exercise and prevention of hypoglycemia for the individual with T1D must take place with

Table 10-7 Guidelines for Regulating Glycemic Response to Exercise (7)

1. Metabolic control before physical activity:
   - Avoid physical activity if fasting glucose levels are >250 mg/dl and ketosis is present. Use caution if glucose levels are >300 mg/dl and ketosis is not present.
   - Ingest additional carbohydrates if glucose levels are <100 mg/dl.

2. Blood glucose monitoring before and after physical activity:
   - Identify when changes in insulin or food intake are necessary.
   - Learn the glycemic response to different physical activity conditions.

3. Food intake:
   - Consume additional carbohydrates as needed to avoid hypoglycemia.
   - Carbohydrate-based foods should be readily available during and after physical activity.

ongoing knowledge of blood glucose patterns and the current health status of the individual (see Table 10-7).

Knowledge of the action and timing of both long-acting and short-acting insulin are important for the person with T1D and for the supervising exercise professional. Exercising in the 2-hour period after injection of short-acting insulin may cause or increase the risk of exercise-related hypoglycemia. Injecting insulin into muscles that are actively utilized during exercise, such as injecting into the legs prior to a run or walk, may also cause or exacerbate hypoglycemia (4, 23). Generally, exercise should be planned to occur at times when blood glucose is at a peak. These periods can be elucidated by careful charting of daily blood glucose measurements and looking for patterns. The typical pattern of insulin

Table 10-8 Recommended Carbohydrates Proposed for Different Physical Activities Depending on Duration and Intensity (28)

Intensity/Duration	<20 Minutes	20–60 Minutes	>60 Minutes
<60% Max HR	NA	15 g	30 g/hr
60%–75% Max HR	15g	30 g	75 g/hr Insulin dose ↓ 20%
>75% Max HR	30g	75 g Insulin dose 0 to ↓ 20%	100 g/hr insulin dose ↓ 30%

Copyright © 2006 Diabetes & Metabolism. From Grimm JJ, Ybarra J, Berne C, Muchnick S, Golay A. A new table for prevention of hypoglycaemia during physical activity in type 1 diabetic patients. Diabetes Metabol. 2004;30:465-470. Reprinted with permission from Diabetes & Metabolism, Elsevier Masson, Masson Editeur.

use in T1D involves a bolus of long-acting insulin in the morning, followed by doses of short-acting insulin with each meal, and a long-acting dose before bedtime. This pattern provides 3 to 4 hour postprandial windows of time that are most acceptable for decreased risk of exercise-induced hypoglycemia.

Recently, a simple supplementation program to prevent exercise-related hypoglycemia was proposed. This program is aimed specifically at aerobic or cardiovascular endurance exercise, which includes circuit types of resistance training in individuals with T1D (28). A plan for supplementing carbohydrates and changing the insulin dose according to the intensity and duration of exercise is shown in Table 10-8.

Increased awareness and attention to foot care and wound care is extremely important in T1D. High-quality, exercise-specific footwear, including special attention to socks, is essential for those with T1D to help prevent blisters and other wounds that may prove difficult to heal in the presence of diabetic neuropathy and other microvascular complications. Socks specifically designed for diabetics are non-binding, minimize constriction around the ankles and feet, and are made from natural materials. Close attention must be paid to preventing injuries that may occur from the impact of weights or objects that could be dropped on the feet or otherwise cause injury.

SAMPLE 24-WEEK PROGRAM

The initial evaluation prior to resistance training should include all of the exercise testing data collected in the examinations recommended above, as well as risk factors for coronary artery disease, orthopedic risk factors, and exercise history. An initial strength evaluation that can be repeated for evidence of progress is essential. This test can use 1RM, or a submaximal test with ratings of perceived exertion (RPE) may be used, or testing may require the use of an arbitrary starting weight to assess muscular endurance (32, 33). All of these testing procedures can be used as the initial evaluation to formulate the exercise program.

In general, multiple-joint, large muscle group exercises should be prioritized. This program also assumes there are no musculoskeletal or other health concerns that might contraindicate these exercises. Thus this program utilizes exercises in each session that assumes barbells, dumbbells, and selectorized machines are available for the bench press, bent-over row, shoulder press, lat pulldown, dumbbell shoulder press, assisted chin-up, incline press, leg press or squat, lying leg curl or seated leg curl, leg extension, cable leg lift, cable hip adduction, deadlift, abdominal crunch, and back extension.

Weeks 1 through 8

The focus for the first 8 weeks is muscular endurance. Complete 2 to 3 sets of 12 to 15 repetitions for each exercise. Complete 2 sets of 25 to 50 repetitions for crunches and back extensions.

Weeks 9 through 16

Focus on strength and muscular hypertrophy. Complete 3 to 4 sets of 8 to 12 repetitions for each exercise. Complete 2 sets of 25 to 50 repetitions for crunches and back extensions.

Weeks 17 through 24

Focus is on strength and power. Complete 4 to 6 sets of 2 to 6 repetitions for each exercise. Complete 2 sets of 25 to 50 repetitions for crunches and back extensions.

CASE STUDY

Mr. B, a 40-year-old male, was transported by paramedics to the Emergency Room in a confused and semiconscious state after an episode of near syncope preceded by participation in a new exercise program at the local fitness center. Mr. B has a 23-year history of T1D with insulin use, and he reports a recent history of fatigue, blurred vision, polyuria, and polydipsia. He also states that his T1D had been well controlled until recently, when stresses at work and home, and some chronic bouts of upper-respiratory infections, made it difficult for him to control his diet and comply with his exercise program. He reports having discontinued his regular exercise program almost 6 months previously. Mr. B has mild, stable retinopathy and is being treated for hypertension that is well-controlled with medication. He also has mild albuminuria and a history of hypercholesterolemia that is controlled with exercise, diet, and medication. He has early signs of neuropathy, including numbness and discomfort in toes and feet, and no history of tobacco abuse or cardiovascular disease.

Mr. B's T1D is currently being treated with long-acting insulin in the mornings at breakfast, and he uses rapid-acting insulin three times per day with meals, using a sliding scale according to blood glucose. He had maintained good glycemic control, as determined by glycated hemoglobin levels averaging below 6.5 percent prior to this incident. His most recent glycated hemoglobin was 8.9 percent, and he has had several similar episodes in the previous 6 months that have resolved quickly with glucose supplementation without medical intervention. The previous episodes were not characterized by confusion or near-syncope. His BMI is 28.2, and his waist circumference is 38.25 inches.

The Emergency Room nurse arranged for a follow-up appointment with Mr. B's primary care physician the following week. His physician recommended no change in insulin dose, a dietary/nutritional consultation, and suggested that Mr. B begin a supervised cardiovascular rehabilitation fitness program.

Upon entry into the cardiac rehab program, Mr. B underwent cardiopulmonary exercise testing, and an exercise prescription was prepared based on heart rate at the ventilatory threshold. Recommendations were made regarding the time of exercise each day (3 to 4 hours after meals), maintenance of preexercise blood glucose levels between 120 and 250, and glucose supplementation should blood glucose drop below 120 before his exercise session. Because Mr. B has had a previous history of compliance to a resistance-training program, an exercise professional recommended that he integrate resistance training with cardiovascular endurance training. Mr. B was admitted to the program after orientation, and a combined exercise program was prescribed.

During the first 2 weeks of exercise, Mr. B had difficulties managing his blood glucose, with measurements both before and after exercise below 120 mg/dl. With input from his physician, Mr. B changed his insulin schedule. He decreased short-acting insulin in the early morning dose, because he had chosen mid-morning as his preferred exercise time. He also changed the content of his breakfast, adding protein and decreasing fat and simple carbohydrates, and he decreased the initial intensity of both cardiovascular endurance and resistance training. Mr. B's control of his blood glucose improved significantly, and he had no more incidents of low blood glucose postexercise after these adjustments. As a result, he was progressed over the next 8 weeks in both resistance training and cardiovascular endurance exercise. His program now consists of 60 minutes of cardio resistance training, warming up on a treadmill first then alternating resistance training with treadmill, bicycle, and elliptical exercise. The resistance portion of the program was similar to the 24-week sample program, with the above-mentioned addition of the circuit training for additional cardiovascular endurance training.

After 8 weeks, Mr. B was transitioned to the local fitness center and continues to comply with his exercise program. He has progressed further with respect to both cardiovascular endurance fitness and muscular strength and endurance. His glycated hemoglobin normalized at 6.2 percent since his Emergency Room visit, and his insulin routine has stabilized.

Mr. B has increased muscular endurance, strength, and cardiovascular endurance. His 1RM on the bench press increased 28 percent, and the leg press by 19 percent, after 10 weeks of training. These increases are consistent with expected levels of improvement in similar programs after 10 to 12 weeks of regular compliance and tight glycemic control.

Summary

Diabetes, particularly T2D, is a chronic disease that is epidemic in the United States. Although T2D represents the greatest proportion by far of diagnosed cases of diabetes, T1D represents between 5 to 10 percent of all cases. T1D is an autoimmune disease that impairs insulin production through destruction of insulin-producing beta cells in the pancreas. This process ultimately requires life-sustaining exogenous insulin supplementation for glycemic control. Maintaining tight control of blood glucose and healthy lifestyle behaviors that include appropriate diet and exercise reduces the risk of microvascular, macrovascular, and other complications of T1D.

The research on the optimal protocols for, and benefits of, resistance training for people with T1D is sparse and inconclusive. Since the pathophysiological correlates, complications, and comorbidities of T1D and T2D are similar, the literature on resistance training in T2D and its effects on vascular function, inflammation, blood pressure, lipids, and insulin-receptor sensitivity is pertinent. Resistance training produces changes in these physiological parameters and is beneficial for individuals with T1D. Resistance training is especially effective when coupled with cardiovascular endurance exercise. Lifestyle intervention, including attention to healthy exercise and diet is, in fact, a critical component of efficacious therapy for almost everyone with either type of diabetes mellitus.

Key Terms

Apoptosis
Autoimmune diabetes
Beta cells
C-peptide
Exogenous insulin
Glycemic control
Glycated hemoglobin
Hyperglycemia
Hyperinsulinemia
Hypoglycemia
Hypoinsulinemia
Insulin
Insulin-dependent diabetes mellitus
Insulin receptors
Ketoacidosis
Late-onset, postexercise hypoglycemia
Nephropathy
Neuropathy

Study Questions

1. What is the primary pathological process involved with T1D, and how is it manifested with respect to signs, symptoms, and physiology?

2. What is the primary treatment for T1D? What are the common comorbidities?

3. What are the specific effects of resistance training that may affect the pathophysiology of T1D?

4. What guidelines can assist in preventing an abnormal glycemic response to exercise in individuals with T1D?

5. Why is it important to include both cardiovascular endurance exercise and resistance training in exercise programs for individuals with diabetes?

References

1. Albright A, Franz M, Hornsby G, et al. American College of Sports Medicine position stand: Exercise and type 2 diabetes. *Med Sci Sports Exerc.* 2000;32:1345-1360.

2. Allen C, LeCaire T, Palta M, et al. Risk factors for frequent and severe hypoglycemia in type 1 diabetes. *Diabetes Care.* 2001;24:1878-1881.

3. American College of Sports Medicine position stand. Progression models in resistance training for healthy adults. *Med Sci Sports Exerc.* 2002;34(2):364-380.

4. American College of Sports Medicine. *ACSM's Guidelines for Exercise Testing and Prescription.* 7th ed. Philadelphia: Lippincott, Wilkins & Williams; 2005:207-212.

5. American College of Sports Medicine. *ACSM's Resource Manual for Guidelines for Exercise Testing and Prescription.* 5th ed. Philadelphia: Lippincott, Wilkins & Williams; 2005:470-479.

6. American Diabetes Association. 2004 clinical practice recommendations. *Diabetes Care* 2004;27:S1-142.

7. American Diabetes Association. Physical activity/exercise and diabetes. *Diabetes Care.* 2004;27:S58-62.

8. Atkinson MA, Eisenbarth GS. Type 1 diabetes: New perspectives on disease pathogenesis and treatment. *Lancet.* 2002;358:221-229.

9. Braith RW, Stewart KJ. Resistance exercise training: Its role in the prevention of cardiovascular disease. *Circulation.* 2006;113:2642-2650.

10. Brunner H, Cockcroft JR, Deanfield D, et al. Endothelial function and dysfunction. Part II: Association with cardiovascular risk factors and diseases. A statement by the Working Group on Endothelins and Endothelial Factors of the European Society of Hypertension. *J Hypertens.* 2005;23:233-246.

11. Bussau VA, Ferreira LD. The 10-s maximal spring: A novel approach to counter an exercise-mediated fall in glycemia in individuals with type 1 diabetes. *Diabetes Care.* 2006;29:601-606.

12. Camacho RC, Galassetti P, Davis SN, Wasserman DH. Glucoregulation during and after exercise in health and insulin-dependent diabetes. *Exer Sport Sci Rev.* 2005;33:17-23.

13. CDC Web site. 2007 National Diabetes Fact Sheet. Available at: http://www.cdc.gov/diabetes/pubs/estimates07.htm. Accessed 6-27-2008.

14. Chan NN, Vallance P, Colhoun HM. Endothelium-dependent and -independent vascular dysfunction in type 1 diabetes: Role of conventional risk factors, sex and glycemic control. *Arterioscler Thromb Vasc Biol.* 2003;23:1048-1054.

15. Conley MS, Rozenek R, and National Strength and Conditioning Association. National Strength and Conditioning Association Position Statement. Health aspects of resistance exercise and training. *Strength and Conditioning Journal.* 2001;23(6):9-23.

16. Daneman D. Type 1 diabetes. *Lancet.* 2006;367:847-858.

17. Devendra D, Liu E, Eisenbarth GS. Type 1 diabetes: recent developments. *BMJ.* 2004;328:750-754.

18. Diabetes Control and Complications Trial Research Group. The effect of intensive treatment of diabetes on the development and progression of long-term complications in insulin-dependent diabetes mellitus. *N Engl J Med*. 1993;329(14):977-986.

19. Diabetes Control and Complications Trial Research Group. Hypoglycemia in the Diabetes Control and Complications Trial. *Diabetes Care*. 1995;18:361-376.

20. Diabetes Control and Complications Trial Research Group. Epidemiology of diabetes interventions and complications research group: Effect of intensive therapy on the microvascular complications of type 1 diabetes mellitus. *JAMA*. 2002;287(19):2563-2569.

21. Diabetes Control and Complications Trial. Epidemiology of diabetes interventions and complications research group: Intensive diabetes treatment and cardiovascular disease in patients with type 1 diabetes. *N Engl J Med*. 2005;353:2643-2653.

22. Durak EP. Randomized crossover study of effect of resistance training on glycemic control, muscular strength and cholesterol in type 1 diabetic men. *Diabetes Care*. 1990;13:1039-1043.

23. Elder CL, Pujol TJ, Barnes JT. Exercise considerations for individuals with type 1 diabetes. *Strength and Conditioning Journal*. 2004;26(5):16-18.

24. Eves ND, Plotnikoff RC. Resistance training and type 2 diabetes: Consideration for implementation at the population level. *Diabetes Care*. 2006;29(8):1933-1941.

25. Ghosh J, Weiss MB, Kay RH, Frishman WH. Diabetes mellitus and coronary artery disease: therapeutic considerations. *Heart Dis*. 2003;5(2):119-128.

26. Gillespie KM. Type 1 diabetes: pathogenesis and prevention. *Can Med Assoc J*. 2006; 175(2):165-170.

27. Goldberg IJ, Dansky HM. Diabetic vascular disease. *Arterioscler Thromb Vasc Biol*. 2006;26:1693-1701.

28. Grimm JJ, Ybarra J, Berne C, Muchnick S, Golay A. A new table for prevention of hypoglycemia during physical activity in type 1 diabetic patients. *Diabetes Metab*. 2004;30:465-470.

29. Guelfi KJ, Jones TW, Fournier PA. Intermittent high-intensity exercise does not increase the risk of early postexercise hypoglycemia in individuals with type 1 diabetes. *Diabetes Care*. 2005;28:416-418.

30. Guelfi KJ, Jones TW, Fournier PA. The decline in blood glucose levels is less with intermittent high-intensity compared with moderate exercise in individuals with type 1 diabetes. *Diabetes Care*. 2005;28:1289-1294.

31. Huebschmann AG, Regensteiner JG, Vlassara H, Reusch JEB. Diabetes and advanced Glyco-oxidation end products. *Diabetes Care*. 2006;29(6):1420-1432.

32. Kraemer WJ, Adams K, Cafarelli E, et al. American College of Sports Medicine Position Stand. Progression models for resistance training for healthy adults.. *Med Sci Sports Exerc*. 2002;34(2):364-380.

33. Kraemer WJ, NA Ratamess. Fundamentals of resistance training: progression and exercise prescription. *Med Sci Sports Exerc*. 2004;364(4):674-688.

34. Knowler WC, Barrett-Connor E, Fowler SE, et al., and Diabetes Prevention Program Research Group. Reduction in the incidence of type 2 diabetes with lifestyle intervention or metformin. *N Engl J Med*. 2002;346(6):393-403.

35. Leslie DG, Castelli MD. Age-dependent influences on the origins of autoimmune diabetes. *Diabetes*. 2004;53:3033-3040.

36. Libby P., Nathan DM, Abraham K, et al. Report of the National Heart, Lung, and Blood Institute-National Institute of Diabetes and Digestive and

Kidney Diseases Working Group on Cardiovascular Complications of Type 1 Diabetes Mellitus. *Circulation.* 2005;111:3489-3493.

37. Lisle DK, Trojian TH. Managing the athlete with type 1 diabetes. *Curr Sports Med Rep.* 2006;5(2):93-98.

38. Macdonald MJ. Postexercise late-onset hypoglycemia in insulin-dependent diabetic patients. *Diabetes Care.* 1987;10(5):584-588.

39. Madamanchi NR, Vendrov A, Runge MS. Oxidative stress and vascular disease. *Arterioscler Thromb Vasc Biol.* 2005;25:29-38.

40. Mayo Clinic Web site. Diabetes symptoms: When to consult your doctor. Available at: http://www.mayoclinic.com/health/diabetes-symptoms/DA00125. Accessed July 11, 2008.

41. Centers for Disease Control and Prevention Web Site. National diabetes fact sheet, US, 2005. Available at: http://www.cdc.gov/diabetes/pubs/factsheet05.htm. Accessed Dec 12, 2008.

42. Olson TP, Dengel DR, Leon AS, Schmitz KH. Moderate resistance training and vascular health in overweight women. *Med Sci Sports Exerc.* 2006;38(9):1558-1564.

43. Ramalho AC, de Lourdes M, Nunes F, et al. The effect of resistance versus aerobic training on metabolic control in patients with type 1 diabetes mellitus. *Diabetes Res Clin Pract.* 2006;72:271-76.

44. Rewers M, Norris J, Dabelea D. Epidemiology of type 1 diabetes mellitus. In: Eisenbarth GS, ed. *Immunology of Type 1 Diabetes.* 2nd ed. Kluwer Academic/Plenum Publishers, New York, NY; 2004: 219-246

45. Schalkwijk CG, Stehouwer CDA. Vascular complications in diabetes mellitus: The role of endothelial dysfunction. *Clin Sci.* 2005;109:143-159.

46. Taskinen MR. Quantitative and qualitative lipoprotein abnormalities in diabetes mellitus. *Diabetes.* 1992;41(suppl 2):12-17.

47. Ter Braak EWMT, Appelman AMME, van de Laak MF, et al. Clinical characteristics of type 1 diabetic patients with and without severe hypoglycemia. *Diabetes Care.* 2000;23:1467-1471.

48. Zgibor JC, Piatt GA, Ruppert K, et al. Deficiencies of cardiovascular risk prediction models for type 1 diabetes. *Diabetes Care.* 2006;29:1860-1865.

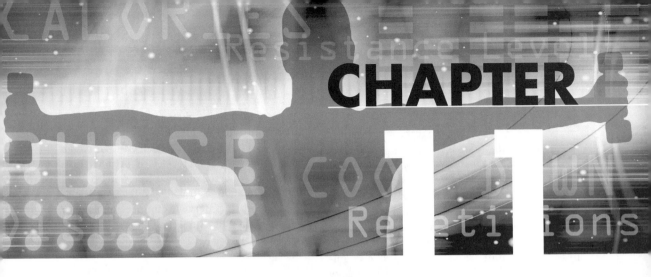

RESISTANCE-TRAINING STRATEGIES FOR INDIVIDUALS WITH TYPE 2 DIABETES

Objectives

Upon completion of this chapter, the reader will be able to:

○ Identify the prevalence and health impact of type 2 diabetes and the economic impact of this impending epidemic

○ Describe the current understanding of the health benefits and limitations of resistance training for individuals with type 2 diabetes based on the latest research

○ Describe the importance of resistance training in the control and prevention of type 2 diabetes, particularly with regard to changes in insulin action

○ Explain the specific factors to consider for preexercise screening, exercise testing, and exercise prescription when designing a resistance-training program for diabetic individuals

○ Be able to design a resistance-training program for type 2 diabetic individuals, taking into account health status and the presence of certain diabetes-related health complications, safety issues, and appropriate progression

INTRODUCTION

Regardless of the type of diabetes an individual has, the outcome is the same: abnormal elevations in blood glucose levels. There are two main types of diabetes. **Type 1 diabetes (T1D)** most often appears during childhood or adolescence and results from the autoimmune destruction of pancreatic beta cells, which leaves the pancreas unable to make insulin (3). **Insulin** is a hormone that allows glucose to enter cells and either be converted to energy or stored. **Type 2 diabetes (T2D)** is characterized by the development of insulin resistance—that is, a decreased ability to use the insulin the body produces—as well as lower insulin production over time. T2D comprises 90 to 95 percent of all cases and is more common in individuals over age 40, although younger individuals, including children and teens, are now manifesting the disease (3). Women may also experience a transient diabetic state known as **gestational diabetes** during the latter stages of pregnancy, and doing so puts them at much higher risk of developing permanent diabetes at some point after the pregnancy (3).

PREVALENCE AND ECONOMIC IMPACT OF TYPE 2 DIABETES

The current prevalence of diabetes in the United States is estimated to be 20.8 million individuals, or 7 percent of all Americans; close to a third of these are still undiagnosed, according to statistics from the Centers for Disease Control and Prevention (11). Over 1.5 million new cases of diabetes were diagnosed in adults in the United States in 2005 alone, most of them type 2 (11). Moreover, the lifetime risk for type-2 diabetes for individuals born in the United States in the year 2000 or later has risen to one in three; in certain minority groups, such as Hispanic females, the risk is closer to one in two (41). One in five adults over age 65 has diabetes, and African-American, Hispanic, American-Indian, and Alaska-Native adults are two to three times

more likely than white adults to have diabetes (41). In addition to the millions of Americans already diagnosed with the disease, an estimated 41 million American adults ages 40 to 74 have **prediabetes**, a condition in which blood sugar levels are elevated but not high enough to be classified as diabetes (10, 41). Without intervention, individuals with prediabetes have an extremely high lifetime risk of developing diabetes.

Diabetes is also a major precursor to other medical conditions, because when it is not well controlled, glucose and fats remain elevated in the blood and cause damage to vital organs over time. Consequently, diabetes can result in vascular damage throughout the body, leading to early heart disease, strokes, blindness, kidney failure, pregnancy complications, loss of central nerve function, loss of feeling in the feet or hands, lower-extremity amputations, premature death, and more (10, 11, 27, 49). Many undiagnosed individuals with type 2 diabetes first learn of their condition after their first heart attack (27). In fact, heart disease is the leading cause of diabetes-related deaths, and death rates among individuals with diabetes are about two to four times higher than for those without the disease who are the same age (27). The World Health Organization recently announced that diabetes kills more individuals worldwide than was ever suspected before: Currently 3.2 million deaths per year, or about six deaths every minute, result from diabetes—and that figure is likely an underestimate (56). Mortality attributable to diabetes is also likely to be three times higher than estimates based on death certificate data (48).

As of 2002, the total direct and indirect health care costs for treating diabetes in the United States amounted to an estimated $132 billion annually (11). Direct medical costs were $92 billion, and disability, lost time from work, and premature death accounted for another $40 billion per year (11). The estimated annual health care costs for an individual with diabetes amount to $13,243 compared with only $2,560 for someone without the chronic condition—a difference of more than $10,000 per person per year (11).

ETIOLOGY OF TYPE 2 DIABETES

Type 2 diabetes generally develops first as prediabetes, an insulin-resistant state that progresses over time to overt hyperglycemia at the point at which insulin production can no longer overcome the decrease in insulin action (3). Lifestyle and other environmental factors weigh heavily into the eventual loss of pancreatic beta-cell function and the resulting state of relative insulin deficiency. It is imperative that hyperglycemia be controlled with blood glucose levels kept in normal or near-normal ranges to prevent diabetes-related health complications from occurring (3, 27).

The problem with current diabetes care, however, is that most individuals never achieve or maintain optimal control over their blood glucose. "Optimal control" can be defined as average blood glucose in a normal or near-normal range, or a **glycated hemoglobin**—a measure of overall blood glucose levels over the previous 2 to 3 months—of no more than 7 percent. In fact, according to a recent report (49), only 37 percent of individuals in the United States with diagnosed diabetes ever achieve this level of control, and the many undiagnosed individuals are likely also unaware of the damage that diabetes is already causing to their bodies. Diabetes-related health problems are not inevitable, but they are a reality for many individuals living with diabetes, especially those unable or unwilling to control their blood glucose levels, or those unaware of the need for good control— and that is where resistance training is important.

BENEFITS OF RESISTANCE TRAINING FOR INDIVIDUALS WITH TYPE 2 DIABETES

Any type of exercise can potentially help improve insulin action in diabetic individuals, but resistance training can be particularly beneficial over the long run because of its ability to result in increased muscle mass (5, 7, 29). The main insulin-sensitive tissues in the body are muscle and adipose tissue, or fat cells. By increasing the quantity and sensitivity of skeletal muscle to available insulin through resistance training, an individual will likely experience better blood glucose control (30, 55), not to mention improvements in other coexisting conditions such as hypertension, elevated blood cholesterol, and excess body fat (40).

Literature Review of Research Supporting Resistance Training for Type 2 Diabetes

The most beneficial health effect of resistance training is, by far, its ability to enhance the action of insulin in individuals with T2D, thereby allowing them to maintain more normal blood glucose levels and avoid the majority of diabetic complications. Despite the fact that intense resistance training can acutely raise blood glucose levels due to its exaggerated counterregulatory hormonal response (32), resistance training improves overall glycemic control and insulin sensitivity through a number of training adaptations. Resistance training done by either healthy or diabetic subjects increases levels of GLUT4 in trained muscle, along with increasing insulin receptors, protein kinase B, glycogen synthase, and glycogen synthase total activity (12, 26). Resistance training also helps control systemic inflammation also associated with insulin resistance, and it increases adiponectin levels, which are directly associated with improved metabolic control (7). These adaptations allow for a greater insulin-stimulated uptake and utilization of blood glucose in resting skeletal muscle, which keeps blood glucose levels more normalized.

Because the hormone insulin stimulates most of the uptake of blood glucose into resting skeletal muscle, maintenance and enhancement of insulin action is critical to the control of blood glucose levels (7, 42, 50). Thus, an insulin-resistant state contributes to higher levels of insulin and blood glucose in individuals with T2D. Research has shown that resistance training has the capacity to improve the action of insulin and thereby lower insulin resistance and blood glucose levels (7, 9, 22, 28, 30). In non-obese subjects with T2D, an improvement in insulin sensitivity was documented following 4 to 6 weeks of moderate-intensity, high-volume resistance training 5 days per week despite minimal change in maximal aerobic capacity (30). In another study, 16 weeks of twice-weekly progressive resistance training done by older men newly diagnosed with T2D resulted in a 46 percent increase in insulin sensitivity, along with a 7 percent reduction in fasting glucose and significant loss of visceral fat, in spite of an average 15.5 percent higher calorie intake (28). Moreover, when 4 months of resistance exercise was added to an existing aerobic training program undertaken by overweight older men in a study by Ferrera and colleagues (22), insulin release in response to an oral glucose load decreased by 25 percent compared with no change in men who engaged in aerobic activities only, demonstrating that the resistance training exerted an even more significant total effect on the effectiveness of insulin. Likewise, Cauza and colleagues (9) found that resistance training resulted in greater improvements in overall glycemic control and insulin resistance than moderate aerobic training in T2D participants.

In examining glycemic control specifically, others have found that resistance training combined with weight loss is most effective, but physical activity appears to have a greater effect than weight loss (18, 19). Dunstan and associates studied sedentary, overweight men and women with T2D who underwent either high-intensity progressive resistance training plus moderate weight loss or weight loss without exercise (19). They found that when combined with moderate weight loss, resistance training was more effective for improving overall glycemic control—measured by glycated hemoglobin, or HbA_{1c}—than moderate weight loss without resistance training, an observation not explainable by differences in body weight, waist circumference, and fat mass changes during the study. Furthermore, the addition of resistance training contributed to the preservation of lean body mass during moderate weight loss. In fact, any type of regular exercise training in overweight, older, or diabetic individuals can improve insulin sensitivity even without significant weight loss (18, 47, 53). In individuals

with obesity and T2D, exercise combined with weight loss increases skeletal muscle mitochondrial capacity; and physical activity alone results in favorable alterations in lipid partitioning in skeletal muscle and enhanced oxidation of lipids within muscle via a greater oxidative capacity, giving muscle the ability to enhance insulin action without weight loss (18). Significant weight loss without increased physical activity improves insulin action as well, but it does not increase muscle mitochondrial capacity or fat oxidation (53).

In terms of maximizing gains in insulin action, the intensity of exercise does not appear to be as important as the total duration of, and caloric expenditure during, the activity (6, 22, 30, 42). Acute improvements in insulin sensitivity in women with T2D have been found whether they engaged in low-intensity or high-intensity aerobic exercise—such as walking versus running—as long as the total exercise energy expenditure was equal in both exercise conditions (6). Similar results were found after 24 weeks of moderate-intensity (60 percent of VO_2 max) or high-intensity (80 percent of VO_2 max) exercise with three 400-kilocalorie sessions per week (42). Moreover, in individuals with T2D, insulin sensitivity has been shown to improve 48 percent after 4 to 6 weeks of only low-intensity (40 to 50 percent of VO_2 max) resistance training with minimal change in body fat or muscle (30). In older women with T2D, the combination of aerobic and resistance training results in even greater improvements in insulin action and glucose use and a larger decrease in abdominal fat than aerobic training alone (15). Sigal and colleagues (50) also recently reported greater benefits to overall glycemic control from thrice-weekly combined aerobic and resistance training, although some improvement was seen in older adults with T2D who underwent a similar 6-month program of either supervised aerobic or resistance training only. In that study, though, the participants doing combined training had a greater total duration of exercise, which may explain some or all of their results.

Enhanced insulin action often occurs in conjunction with increases in muscle mass, which can result from varying intensities of resistance exercise. For older, unfit individuals, heavy weight training is especially beneficial to reversing or preventing further loss of skeletal muscle (55). For instance, after a 16-week resistance-exercise intervention in older Latinos, overall body strength increased by 33 percent, and an average of 1.2 kg of lean body mass was gained by participants doing thrice-weekly training that consisted of 3 sets of 8 repetitions done at 70 to 80 percent of the one-repetition maximum (1RM) (8). Both high-load (8 repetitions done at 80 percent of 1RM) and high-repetition (16 repetitions at 40 percent of 1RM) resistance-training protocols have been shown to be effective in improving muscular strength and size in postmenopausal women, indicating that low-intensity resistance training can be beneficial for the muscular fitness in women for whom high-intensity exercise is contraindicated (5). Similarly, in men and women aged 60 to 83 years, significant and similar improvements in strength, endurance, and stair-climbing time can also be attained by either high- or low-intensity resistance training (54). However, greater metabolic gains result from higher intensity work (20). In older adults with T2D, home-based, progressive resistance training was effective for maintaining the gymnasium-based improvements in muscle strength and mass but not glycemic control. Reductions in program adherence and exercise training volume and intensity may impede the effectiveness of home-based training for maintaining improved glycemic control (20). The results of this home-based study, and other similar resistance-training studies, are summarized in Table 11-1.

To fully understand the contribution of muscle-mass gains or muscle-mass retention to insulin action, the glycemic effects of resistance versus aerobic training can be examined. Poehlman and colleagues demonstrated that in nonobese young women, 6 months of either aerobic or resistance training improved muscular glucose disposal, or use, albeit by different mechanisms (45). An increase in fat-free mass from resistance training contributed to glucose uptake without altering the intrinsic capacity of muscle to respond to insulin. Conversely, aerobic training enhanced glucose disposal independently of changes in fat-free mass or maximal aerobic capacity, suggesting that such changes may result from an enhancement in insulin sensitivity. The study concluded that resistance training benefits

insulin action through increases in insulin-sensitive muscle mass. Other research has documented the ability of resistance training to enhance or retain muscle mass (5, 7, 29), which is particularly critical given that adults with long-standing diabetes may experience accelerated loss of muscle strength and muscle quality (43). Given that not all individuals experiencing improved insulin action as a result of resistance work have measureable gains in muscle mass (40), it appears that the advantages of resistance training for diabetic individuals may be realized in combination with other mechanisms beyond these anatomical adaptations.

In summary, regular physical activity, whether aerobic or resistance training, is imperative for individuals with T2D. Both types of training improve insulin sensitivity to some extent and may help maintain blood glucose levels in normal ranges, although intense resistance workouts can increase blood glucose levels, albeit temporarily. The effects of a single workout may last for an hour after short, mild exercise and up to a day or two for prolonged, intense activities. The effects of regular training, however, begin to reverse within just 2 to 3 days, even though muscle mass may have increased following training (31). Thus, maintaining a regular exercise program is critical to keep the benefits of increased muscle mass and insulin sensitivity that are so important to the individual with T2D.

DESIGNING RESISTANCE-TRAINING PROGRAMS FOR INDIVIDUALS WITH TYPE 2 DIABETES

The main factors to consider when designing resistance-training programs for individuals with T2D include 1) the current activity level of the individual; 2) the primary goals of the training program; 3) any medications that the individual may be taking that can affect, or be affected by,

Table 11-1 Resistance Training Studies for Individuals with Type 2 Diabetes

Authors	N	Gender & Mean Age	Frequency & Program Length	Repetitions & Sets	Strength Gains & Other Outcomes
Castaneda et al. (8)	62	22 M, 40 F; 66 years	3×/week × 16 weeks	70–80% of 1RM, 3 sets of 8 reps, 5 exercises	Whole-body muscle strength ↑ 33%; lean body mass ↑ 1.2 kg; HbA_{1c} ↓ by 12.6%
Cauza et al. (9)	22	11 M, 11 F; 56.2 years	2×/week × 4 months	10–15 reps, 6 sets/week	Upper-body strength ↑ 29%, lower-body strength ↑ 48%; 21.3% ↓ in insulin resistance
Cuff et al. (15)	28	28 F; 60.9 years	3×/week × 16 weeks	2 sets of 12 reps + aerobic training	Upper-body strength ↑ 49%, lower-body strength ↑ 42%; glucose disposal rate ↑ by 77%
Dunstan et al. (19)	16	10 M, 6 F; 67.6 years	3×/week × 6 months	75–85% of 1RM, 3 sets of 8–10 reps	Upper-body strength ↑ 41.7%, lower body ↑ 28%; 3x greater ↓ in HbA_{1c} than weight loss alone
Dunstan et al. (20)	36	21 M, 15 F; 60 to 80 years	3×/week, 6 months of gym-based, then 6 months of home training	60–80% of 1RM, 3 sets of 8–10 reps	Upper-body strength ↑ 30.7 kg, lower body ↑ 8.2 kg (maintained at home); no change in insulin sensitivity with training; included weight loss
Herriott et al. (25)	9	5 M, 4 F; 50.6 years	3×/week × 8 weeks	50–70% of 1RM, 3 sets of 8–12 reps	Upper-body strength ↑ 36%, lower body ↑ 41% no change in HbA_{1c}
Holten et al. (26)	10	10 unreported gender; 62 years	3×/week × 6 weeks, one-legged training	70–80% of 1RM, 4 sets of 8–12 reps	Knee extensions ↑ by 42%, leg press by 75%, insulin-stimulated leg glucose clearance ↑ by ~20% in trained leg

Table 11-1 Resistance Training Studies for Individuals with Type 2 Diabetes (continued)

Authors	N	Gender & Mean Age	Frequency & Program Length	Repetitions & Sets	Strength Gains & Other Outcomes
Ibañez et al. (28)	9	9 M; 66.6 years	2×/week × 16 wks	50–80% of 1RM; 3–4 sets of 10–15 reps	Upper-body strength ↑ 18.2%, lower-body strength ↑ 17.1%, insulin sensitivity ↑ by 46.3%
Ishii et al. (30)	9	9 M, 46.8 years	5×/week × 4 to 6 weeks	40–50% of 1RM, 2 sets of 10 reps (upper body) or 20 reps (lower body)	Quadriceps strength ↑ by 16%, insulin sensitivity ↑ by 48%
Maiorana et al. (37)	16	14 M, 2 F, 52 years	3×/week × 8 weeks	55–65% of 1RM, 15 reps, circuit (resistance + aerobic)	Sum strength on 7 resistance exercises ↑ by 13.2%, HbA_{1c} ↓ by 7%
Sigal et al. (50)	64	40 M, 24 F; 54.7 years	3×/week × 6 months	2–3 sets of 7–9 reps, 7 exercises	Strength improvements not reported, HbA_{1c} ↓ by 5%

physical activity; and 4) the existence of any related health comorbidities. Each of these factors should be assessed and considered prior to a diabetic individual beginning a resistance-training program.

The current activity level of an individual is important to consider, and it dictates the overall muscular fitness and strength gains that can be attained. A sedentary individual is likely to experience greater gains than a person who is already physically active. Individuals who are sedentary must be started on a low-intensity exercise program to protect them from exercise-related injuries. Although active individuals may not experience as much of an absolute change in muscle strength from a new resistance-training program, they are more likely to be able to perform moderate- to high-intensity work safely. Higher intensity training will result in even greater gains in

muscle strength compared to lower intensity training (20). Thus, the intensity of the exercise that can be undertaken will largely depend on an individual's previous activity level.

To achieve the most benefit, the main goals of the resistance training should be determined prior to the development of any specific program. Resistance-training benefits are specific to the types of exercises performed and the muscle groups that are exercised. Thus, if the goal of training is better glycemic control, then activities that utilize large muscle groups and result in increases in muscle mass would be ideal.

The medications an individual takes can potentially affect their risk for **hypoglycemia**, defined as a blood glucose level of 65 mg/dl or lower, and medications may also alter exercise performance. High-intensity exercises, such as repeated interval training, result in significant depletion of muscle glycogen and increase the risk for hypoglycemia (39), particularly if certain diabetic medications are taken, such as supplemental insulin or longer-lasting sulfonylureas (35). In addition, beta-blockers and other heart medications can artificially lower resting and exercise heart rates, making measurement of exercise intensity using heart rate problematic. The potential exercise-related side effects of any prescribed medications should be discussed with the client's physician or other health care professional prior to the initiation of any type of exercise training program. Finally, the presence of other chronic health concerns, such as hypertension and elevated blood cholesterol levels, is common in individuals with T2D. These comorbidities must also be considered when prescribing resistance training for such individuals.

Exercise Testing Considerations

In setting up a resistance-training program, testing is helpful to determine an individual's maximal strength (1RM) on each exercise so that an appropriate weight or resistance can be chosen for the desired number of repetitions. Maximal testing, however, can cause exaggerated rises in blood pressure, particularly in individuals who have preexisting hypertension, which is sometimes present in T2D; therefore repetition-maximum testing using 3RM or 10RM is better suited for this population. A maximal exercise stress test may also be helpful in determining if an upper limit to safe exercise exists, such as if there is a heart rate above which ischemia is present. Individuals with diabetes are more likely to experience a condition known as **silent ischemia,** which is a painless and symptom-free reduction in blood flow to the heart muscle through the coronary blood vessels. Thus, when prescribing exercise for diabetic individuals, an exercise stress test may be of particular importance to determine if any abnormalities occur during exercise. Furthermore, physician approval should be obtained before anyone with known cardiovascular

disease begins a new exercise program. For individuals who have been diagnosed with T2D for longer than 5 years, such exercise testing would be recommended for diagnostic purposes and to determine their functional capacity (2).

The American College of Sports Medicine (ACSM) recommends that individuals with T2D be screened for cardiovascular disease before beginning resistance training (2). In middle-aged and older diabetic individuals who have a high risk of cardiovascular disease, the safety of higher-intensity resistance exercise has been questioned by some medical practitioners, but research does not support this notion. For instance, even in men with known coronary ischemia and ECG changes inducible by moderate aerobic exercise, resistance training near maximal intensity does not induce the same negative ECG changes (21). In fact, between 1999 and 2001 in the United States, not a single one of the 20 deaths associated with resistance training were related to cardiac events (36).

Resistance Training Considerations

Individuals with T2D who are beginning a resistance-training program may have special concerns and may need to take certain precautions related to their diabetic state, particularly if any diabetes-related health complications are present. A summary of exercise precautions for individuals with T2D is presented in Table 11-2. In normal individuals or for those with T2D that is controlled with diet and exercise alone, the risk of developing hypoglycemia during exercise is minimal. Prolonged exercise, however, has a greater potential to cause significant lowering of blood glucose levels both during and after exercise, particularly in individuals who use insulin. When extraneous insulin is taken, extra care must be taken to prevent hypoglycemia, particularly during exercise. Since the absorption and release of injected insulin cannot always be effectively controlled or anticipated, the additional uptake of blood glucose by muscle contractions and excess insulin may result in hypoglycemia (12, 16). For regular, planned exercise, short-acting

Table 11-2 Exercise Precautions for Resistance Training with Type 2 Diabetes

- Consult with a physician prior to exercising if any of the following conditions are present:
  - Proliferative retinopathy or current retinal hemorrhage
  - Neuropathy (nerve damage), either peripheral or autonomic
  - Foot injuries, including ulcers
  - High blood pressure
  - Serious illness or infection
- Have a blood glucose meter accessible to monitor glycemia before, during, and after exercise or anytime symptoms of hypoglycemia occur.
- Immediately treat hypoglycemia with glucose tablets or soft drinks.
- Stay properly hydrated with frequent intake of small amounts of cool water.
- Seek immediate medical attention for chest pain or any pain that radiates down the arm, jaw, or neck that may indicate a heart attack.
- With hypertension or unstable proliferative retinopathy, avoid activities that cause excessive increases in blood pressure, such as heavy resistance work, head-down exercises, and breath holding.
- Never exercise with active retinal hemorrhages, and stop exercise if visual changes occur.
- Wear proper footwear, and check feet daily for signs of trauma such as blisters, redness, or other signs of irritation.

preexercise insulin doses will likely need to be lowered to prevent hypoglycemia. Newer, synthetic insulin analogs also induce more rapid and greater decreases in blood glucose concentrations than regular human insulin due to a faster absorption (57). Consequently, diabetic exercisers must check their blood glucose levels before, occasionally during, and after exercise to monitor the effects of exercise and compensate with appropriate dietary and/or medication regimen changes. If only longer-acting insulins are used, immediate declines in blood glucose during exercise are not as likely.

Hypoglycemia after exercise is a greater concern for diabetic individuals who participate in any type of exercise. High-intensity exercises such as repeated interval training result in significant depletion of muscle glycogen. After exercise, the use of blood glucose to restore muscle glycogen levels increases the risk for hypoglycemia. The effects of declining blood glucose after exercise may be compounded by supplemental insulin (35). Thus, diabetic individuals should regularly check

their blood glucose levels after exercise to protect against hypoglycemic situations. Furthermore, consuming moderate amounts of carbohydrates during and within 30 minutes after exhaustive, glycogen-depleting exercise will help lower hypoglycemia risk and will allow for more efficient restoration of muscle glycogen (24).

A recommendation from the American Diabetes Association (ADA) (3, 51), states that carbohydrate ingestion is needed when preexercise blood glucose levels are less than 100 mg/dl. However, this recommendation only applies to individuals with T1D or those with T2D using supplemental short- or rapid-acting insulin injections. For individuals whose blood glucose levels are controlled with diet or oral diabetic medications alone, hypoglycemia is not common, and extra carbohydrates are not generally required during exercise lasting less than an hour. However, it is recommended that insulin users ingest at least 15 grams of carbohydrates prior to exercise for a starting blood glucose level of 100 mg/dl or lower, but the exact quantity will depend on other variables, such as when the injected insulin peaks and the duration of the activity. In all cases, intense, short-term exercise requires less carbohydrate intake, if any, due to a greater release of counterregulatory hormones (23, 32). Alternately, insulin pump users simply may choose to reduce or eliminate their basal infusion of insulin during exercise rather than consume extra carbohydrates.

Another ADA recommendation addresses exercise undertaken during hyperglycemic conditions (3, 51). Any blood glucose value in excess of 125 mg/dl (6.9 mM) qualifies as hyperglycemia, however, abnormal responses to exercise are not usually experienced until levels exceed twice that value (250 mg/dl, or 13.9 mM). In such cases, exercise should be avoided, because any physical activity performed under such conditions would likely result in an exaggerated counterregulatory hormone response, causing blood glucose levels and ketones to rise excessively (4). Aerobic exercise has been shown to be beneficial in handling acute hyperglycemia that occurs following a meal by increasing muscle glucose uptake (34, 46).

Mounting evidence shows that older individuals with chronic health problems respond just as well to exercise training as their younger counterparts (2, 33, 58), yet many older individuals still choose not to be physically active (14). One reason may be their health, because 85 percent of individuals over the age of 65 have some health problem that they may view as a deterrent to exercise (14). However, recent literature has shown that exercise is beneficial for individuals with most diseases, including those with diabetes (37, 38, 58). In addition to improving diabetes-related health, regular exercise lessens the potential impact of most of the other cardiovascular risk factors, including elevated blood lipids (cholesterol and other blood fats), insulin resistance, obesity, and hypertension (44).

Many individuals who suffer from diabetes or prediabetes may also have cardiovascular disease (49). Resistance training was previously not prescribed to patients with cardiovascular disease because of fears of increasing blood pressure and placing the individual at greater risk for an adverse event. Resistance training, however, is now recommended for individuals with known cardiovascular disease and even for those who have suffered a heart attack or stroke (38). In individuals with T2D, resistance training increases blood pressure more than aerobic training, but it decreases submaximal heart rate, resulting in greater blood flow to the heart and less work performed by the heart (37). Thus for individuals diagnosed with coronary artery blockage from plaque buildup, moderate resistance training may actually be a safer activity than high-intensity aerobic training.

Diabetic individuals with cardiovascular disease should use the onset of angina as a guide in limiting exercise intensity or duration. In general, if reaching a certain heart rate measured in beats per minute (bpm) causes the development of chest pain, exercise should be limited to an intensity that keeps heart rate at least 10 bpm below the pain threshold.

Diabetes can also cause peripheral vascular disease (PVD), a cardiovascular condition that limits blood flow to the lower extremities. Individuals who have PVD often report leg pain while walking or standing that limits their exercise performance. Thus resistance exercises, such as seated exercises, may need to be chosen to decrease leg pain. If an individual experiences these symptoms during or after physical activity and has not been diagnosed with PVD, he or she should confer with a physician before proceeding with any exercise program (3, 51).

Hypertension is a problem that affects many individuals with T2D. Regular physical activity can result in lower blood pressure and reduced circulating levels of insulin. If a diabetic individual has preexisting hypertension, avoid high-intensity or heavy resistance exercises that may cause blood pressure to rise dangerously and precipitate a stroke or other cardiovascular event. Activities best avoided include heavy resistance training, near-maximal exercise of any type, or any resistance exercise that results in prolonged breath holding (1).

Loss of sensation in the feet or hands—known as **peripheral neuropathy,** or nerve damage—is common in individuals with diabetes. The loss of sensation increases an individual's risk of damage to the feet during exercise. Peripheral nerve damage blunts the usual symptoms of pain that would normally result from high impact on feet or friction and pressure from footwear, facilitating the development of a blister or sore. In some cases, a simple blister can progress to an infected abscess or ulcer and ultimately result in a lower-limb amputation if not properly cared for in time. Diabetic individuals should use a silica gel or air mid-soles in their shoes, along with polyester or polyester-blend (cotton-polyester) socks, to prevent the formation of blisters and to keep feet dry during physical activity (1). Feet should be checked daily for signs of trauma. Should any injury occur, it must be treated aggressively to prevent any worsening of the problem. If an individual suffers from severe neuropathy or unhealed foot ulcers, weight-bearing exercises performed while standing should be replaced by seated resistance or other non–weight-bearing exercises.

Diabetes-related damage to the central nervous system, called **autonomic neuropathy,** can result in silent ischemia, hyperthermia, or light-headedness during exercise. Severe autonomic neuropathy may cause difficulty in changing body position, such as going from sitting to standing or from lying to sitting, without experiencing **orthostatic hypotension,** which can result in light-headedness or fainting during activities. Hyperthermia during exercise, more common in autonomic neuropaths, can also lead to severe dehydration. Furthermore, this type of nerve damage may result in **gastroparesis,** a lessened ability to digest and absorb food, and an inability to absorb carbohydrates may increase the incidence and severity of hypoglycemia. Lastly, autonomic neuropathy may cause an elevated resting heart rate as well as a lesser rise in heart rate during physical exertion (13).

If autonomic nerve damage is present, a conservative approach to exercise is recommended. Individuals who suffer from this form of neuropathy should avoid rapid changes in movement that may result in fainting, and they must engage in longer warmups and cooldown periods, especially for more intense resistance training. Extra fluids may need to be consumed to protect against hyperthermia.

Eating large meals before exercise could result in delayed emptying of food and should be avoided; thus only small food portions before exercise are recommended. Individuals should use rapidly absorbed glucose tablets to treat hypoglycemia, and when blood glucose levels decrease to 100 mg/dl, to prevent severe hyperglycemia. Finally, exercise intensity should be monitored by means other than heart rate alone, such as subjective ratings of perceived exertion; because heart rate may no longer rise as much as expected, it may not be the best way to monitor intensity, unless maximal heart rate is determined (13).

Individuals with diabetes are prone to developing eye complications, including cataracts and proliferative retinopathy. While cataracts can obscure vision and make participation in certain activities more dangerous, such as cycling outdoors or using certain free weights, they are not a contraindication to participation in most types of resistance training. However, exercise may be contraindicated in individuals with more severe forms of eye disease, such as proliferative **diabetic retinopathy,** in which the eyes have weak, abnormal blood vessels in the retina that can break, tear, or bleed into the vitreous fluid in the center of the eye.

While exercise itself has not been shown to accelerate the proliferative process, certain exercise precautions may be needed to prevent intraocular hemorrhages or retinal tears. If eye disease is only mild or moderate, with no active bleeds, individuals should avoid activities that dramatically increase intraocular blood pressure, such as heavy resistance training or head-down activities in which the head is lower than the heart. Individuals with moderate to severe diabetic eye disease should avoid all jumping, jarring, or breath-holding activities that can cause more bleeding and increase the risk of retinal tears or retinal detachment, and this would include heavy resistance training and other aerobic activities (1, 51). If an individual experiences an active retinal hemorrhage or notices dramatic, sudden changes in sight, he or she should either forego exercise at that time or immediately stop the activity and consult an eye specialist for further guidance about safely resuming activity.

Many individuals who suffer from diabetes develop varying degrees of diabetic nephropathy, or kidney disease, from microalbuminuria to end-stage renal failure. Exercise, however, does not appear to worsen diabetic nephropathy in individuals with diabetes. If an individual is in the later stages of kidney disease, intense exercise is not usually recommended due to limited exercise capacity. Light to moderate exercise is recommended even for patients on dialysis. If an individual requires dialysis, exercise is contraindicated if the blood levels of hematocrit, calcium, or potassium become unbalanced as a result of the treatments (1). Individuals who have undergone kidney transplants can safely restart exercise training 6 to 8 weeks after surgery, once they are stable and free of signs of rejection of the new kidney.

Diabetes is also characterized by a higher risk of joint-related injuries, as well as overuse problems like tendonitis. Conditions such as frozen shoulder, trigger finger, and other acute joint problems can also come on with no warning, and for no readily apparent reason, in diabetic individuals. The best defense is to prevent all of these injuries with good glycemic control and flexibility exercises, along with resistance exercise that helps emphasize and maintain a full range of motion in all the joints (25).

Arthritis is also more common in individuals with T2D due in part to extra body weight (17). Lower extremity joints are most often affected, and when present, osteoarthritis can severely limit exercise. However, research has clearly shown that exercise is an effective way to manage all forms of arthritis (52, 59). Diabetic individuals are advised to start with range-of-motion exercises to increase joint mobility and light resistance work to increase the strength of the muscles surrounding the affected joints. After activities, ice may need to be applied to arthritic joints, particularly the knees, for 15 to 20 minutes to reduce swelling and help prevent soreness, or hydrotherapy may be used (52). Nonsteroidal anti-inflammatory medications, such as aspirin and ibuprofen, may also be beneficial to temporarily lessen any discomfort related to recent workouts.

Training Program Components

The ACSM has recommended the use of progressive resistance training at least two to three times per week as part of a well-rounded exercise program of endurance and resistance exercise for those with T2D without significant complications or limitations (1). Progressive resistance training involves training in which the resistance utilized is progressively increased over time. A resistance-training program will improve muscular strength and endurance and body composition by increasing or maintaining fat-free mass. It will also minimize cardiovascular risk factors by improving glucose tolerance and insulin sensitivity (26, 28, 30, 55).

A progressive resistance-training program for individuals with diabetes should incorporate a minimum of 8 to 10 exercises, involving all the major muscle groups in the upper and lower body, with a minimum of a single set of 10 to 15 repetitions to near fatigue, although the incorporation of 3 or more sets of 8 to 10 repetitions to near fatigue will likely be more effective (19, 28, 51). Frequency should begin at twice a week, with at least 1 day of rest between sessions, increasing to three times per week as tolerated. Increased intensity of exercise, additional sets, or combinations of volume and intensity may produce greater benefits, but training volume and intensity should be determined based on an individual's health and prior training status.

Adequate rest and recovery are critical to optimizing the benefits of resistance training (1, 2, 51). In addition, a conservative approach should be used with diabetic individuals who have been sedentary and with those who have significant health complications. Starting out slowly involves beginning with a single set of 10 to 15 repetitions two to three times per week at moderate intensity for several weeks, followed by 2 sets, and finally 3 sets, of 8 to 10 repetitions using weights that cannot be lifted more than 8 to 10 times before fatigue (51). In addition, each resistance-training session should be preceded and followed by a 5-minute period of light aerobic exercise to warm up and cool down. Initial supervision and periodic reassessment of strength by a qualified exercise professional are recommended to optimize health benefits while minimizing risk of injury.

Specific recommended exercises include upper-body, lower-body, and core work. For the upper body, exercises should include all of the major muscle groups—deltoids, trapezius, latissimus dorsi, biceps, and triceps—and should work groups of muscles before individual muscles. Examples of recommended exercises are the overhead press, lat pulldown, incline press, biceps curl, and triceps curl. For lower-body exercises, work the main muscles—quadriceps, hamstrings, gluteals, and calf muscles—with exercises like the leg press, squat, leg extension, leg curl, and calf raise. To increase core body strength and prevent low back pain, exercises to include are the abdominal crunch, twist, and back extension.

SAMPLE 24-WEEK PROGRAM

For this 24-week program, a minimum of 2 sets are recommended to be completed for each exercise, with the first set serving as a warm-up set at a lower intensity and the second set done at the recommended intensity, usually 50 to 80 percent of 1RM.

Weeks 1 through 4

Begin week 1 with baseline 1RM testing for all exercises included in the program. Training should take place 2 days per week separated by at least 48 hours. It should involve a single set of 12 to 15 repetitions at 40 to 45 percent of 1RM, followed by a second set of 12 to 15 repetitions at 50 percent of 1RM.

Weeks 5 through 8

Continue with two workouts per week with 48-hour rest intervals in between. Complete a single set of 12 to 15 repetitions at 50 percent of 1RM, followed by a second set of 12 to 15 repetitions at 60 percent of 1RM.

Weeks 9 through 12

Begin week 9 by reevaluating 1RM for each exercise and resetting the weight used on each exercise according to new 1RM levels. Continue with two workouts per week, and increase the number of sets to three. Complete a single set of 12 to 15 repetitions at 55 percent of 1RM, followed by 2 sets of 12 to 15 repetitions at 60 percent of 1RM.

Weeks 13 through 16

Continue with two workouts per week. Complete a single set of 12 to 15 repetitions at 60 percent of 1RM, followed by 2 sets of 12 to 15 repetitions at 70 percent of 1RM.

Weeks 17 through 20

Begin week 17 by reevaluating 1RM for each exercise and resetting the weight used on each exercise according to new 1RM levels. Continue with two workouts per week, but reduce repetitions to 8 to 12 to exhaustion. Complete a single set of 8 to 12 repetitions at 75 percent of 1RM, followed by 2 sets of 8 to 12 repetitions at 80 percent of 1RM.

Weeks 21 through 24

Continue with two workouts per week and consider increasing sets to 4 at least once per week. Complete a single set of 8 to 12 repetitions at 75 percent of 1RM, followed by 2 to 3 sets of 8 to 12 repetitions at 80 percent of 1RM.

CASE STUDY

A 72-year old sedentary woman, Mrs. W, who is moderately obese (BMI = 32) is interested in participating in a resistance-training program. Her medical history questionnaire indicates that she was diagnosed with T2D 10 years earlier, but no other comorbidities or diabetic complications are present. Due to Mrs. W's age and length of diagnosed disease, she needed to obtain her physician's approval, and needed to undergo an exercise stress test, prior to beginning an exercise program. During the stress test, she reportedly experienced mild chest pain at a heart rate of 120 bpm.

Research has suggested that resistance training can be performed safely and effectively for individuals with T2D and exercise-induced angina if proper precautions are taken. Mrs. W should monitor her blood glucose levels before, during, and after exercise. Close monitoring of blood glucose will reduce the likelihood of hypoglycemic or hyperglycemic conditions and will allow her to better understand the unique effect of resistance training on her glucose levels. Second, Mrs. W will need to monitor her heart rate during exercise to ensure that she does not perform any exercise that increases her heart rate above 110 bpm to protect against angina or ischemia caused by physical activity.

Mrs. W's recommended resistance workout will consist of a full-body progressive resistance-training program, along with aerobic training and flexibility exercises. The resistance-training portion will be particularly important for increasing fat-free mass and thereby improving her glucose uptake and overall glycemic control. Furthermore, her increased muscle mass will result in strength gains that will aid in maintaining her independence and function as she ages.

Mrs. W's recommended resistance-training program will begin twice a week with a single set of 12 to 15 repetitions at 40 to 50 percent of her estimated 1RM, including full-body exercises such as the seated leg press, chest press, and lat pulldown. Due to the fact that she is elderly and inactive, along with having exercise-induced angina, the recommendation will be for her to monitor her heart rate to make sure that this workload does not cause her heart rate to rise above 110 bpm. In addition, her resistance-training program will need close monitoring and frequent adjustments to ensure that she is performing the exercises correctly and increasing her intensity, repetitions, and sets in a correct manner. Mrs. W will increase her workload even more slowly than is usually recommended to monitor for and prevent the onset of exercise-induced angina.

Her ultimate goal, given her cardiovascular limitations, will be to work up to doing 3 sets of exercises twice a week, up to 15 repetitions per set, using the heaviest resistance that she can without increasing her heart rate above 110 bpm. Such a program will result in improvements in her muscular strength, insulin sensitivity, and overall glycemic control and will increase her ability to function and perform daily self-care activities without limitations.

Summary

Resistance training has been shown to be the best exercise to maintain muscle mass and to prevent losses of muscle mass and strength. Resistance training in individuals with diabetes is recommended due to the potential for increases in muscle mass and enhanced insulin sensitivity. Increased muscle mass generally results in increased resting blood glucose uptake and better glycemic control in individuals with both T2D and prediabetes. Full-body resistance training may actually be more beneficial than aerobic training due to the increased utilization of all muscle fibers. Individuals who suffer from T2D often have health comorbidities. Thus, when prescribing a resistance-training program, these other potential health concerns should likewise be considered to minimize risks and ensure safety.

Key Terms

Autonomic neuropathy
Diabetic retinopathy
Gastroparesis
Gestational diabetes
Glycated hemoglobin
Hypoglycemia
Insulin
Orthostatic hypotension
Peripheral neuropathy
Peripheral vascular disease (PVD)
Prediabetes
Silent ischemia
Type 1 diabetes (T1D)
Type 2 diabetes (T2D)

Study Questions

1. What are the benefits and drawbacks of resistance training as a treatment modality for T2D?

2. How does resistance training impact insulin action in people with T2D, and why are these changes important to the control of diabetes?

3. What elements are important to address prior to starting someone with T2D on a resistance-training program?

4. What components should be included in an effective resistance-training program for individuals with T2D?

References

1. Albright A, Franz M, Hornsby G, Kriska A, Marrero D, Ullrich I, Verity L. Exercise and type 2 diabetes. *Med Sci Sports Exerc.* 2000;32:1345-1360.

2. American College of Sports Medicine position stand. Exercise and physical activity for older adults. *Med Sci Sports Exerc.* 1998;30: 992-1008.

3. American Diabetes Association. Diagnosis and classification of diabetes mellitus. *Diabetes Care.* 2008;31:S55-S60.

4. Avogaro A, Gnudi L, Valerio A, et al. Effects of different plasma glucose concentrations on lipolytic and ketogenic responsiveness to epinephrine in type 1 (insulin-dependent) diabetic subjects. *J Clin Endocrinol Metab.* 1993;76:845-850.

5. Bemben DA, Fetters NL, Bemben MG, Nabavi N, Koh ET. Musculoskeletal responses to high- and low-intensity resistance training in early postmenopausal women. *Med Sci Sports Exerc.* 2000;32:1949-1957.

6. Braun B, Zimmerman BM, Kretchmer N. Effects of exercise intensity on insulin sensitivity in women with non–insulin-dependent diabetes mellitus. *J Appl Physiol.* 1995;78:300-306.

7. Brooks N, Layne JE, Gordon PL, Roubenoff R, Nelson ME, Castaneda-Sceppa C. Strength training improves muscle quality and insulin sensitivity in Hispanic older adults with type 2 diabetes. *Int J Med Sci.* 2006;4:19-27.

8. Castaneda C, Layne JE, Munoz-Orians L, et al. A randomized controlled trial of resistance exercise training to improve glycemic control in older adults with type 2 diabetes. *Diabetes Care.* 2002;25:2335-2341.

9. Cauza E, Hanusch-Enserer U, Strasser B, et al. The relative benefits of endurance and strength training on the metabolic factors and muscle function of people with type 2 diabetes mellitus. *Arch Phys Med Rehabil.* 2005;86:1527-1533.

10. Centers for Disease Control and Prevention. Diabetes 2008: Disabling disease to double by 2050. Available at: http://www.cdc.gov/nccdphp/publications/aag/ddt.htm. Accessed December 17, 2008

11. Centers for Disease Control and Prevention. National diabetes fact sheet: United States 2005. Available at: http://www.cdc.gov/diabetes/pubs/factsheet05.htm. Accessed December 17, 2008

12. Christ-Roberts CY, Pratipanawatr T, Pratipanawatr W, Berria R, Belfort R, Mandarino LJ. Increased insulin receptor signaling and glycogen synthase activity contribute to the synergistic effect of exercise on insulin action. *J Appl Physiol.* 2003;95:2519-2529.

13. Colberg SR, Swain DP, Vinik AI. Use of heart rate reserve and rating of perceived exertion to prescribe exercise intensity in diabetic autonomic neuropathy. *Diabetes Care.* 2003;264: 986-990.

14. Crombie IK, Irvine L, Williams B, et al. Why older people do not participate in leisure time physical activity: A survey of activity levels, beliefs and deterrents. *Aging.* 2004;33: 287-292.

15. Cuff DJ, Meneilly GS, Martin A, Ignaszewski A, Tildesley HD, Frohlich JJ. Effective exercise modality to reduce insulin resistance in women with type 2 diabetes. *Diabetes Care.* 2003;26:2977-2982.

16. Dela F, Mikines KJ, Larsen JJ, Galbo H. Glucose clearance in trained skeletal muscle during maximal insulin with superimposed exercise. *J Appl Physiol.* 1999;87:2059-2067.

17. Dillon CF, Rasch EK, Gu Q, Hirsch R. Prevalence of knee osteoarthritis in the United States: Arthritis data from the Third National Health and Nutrition Examination Survey 1991-1994. *J Rheumatol.* 2006;33:2271-2279.

18. Dubé JJ, Amati F, Stefanovic-Racic M, Toledo FG, Sauers SE, Goodpaster BH. Exercise-induced alterations in intramyocellular lipids and insulin resistance: The athlete's paradox revisited. *Am J Physiol Endocrinol Metab.* 2008;294:E882-E888.

19. Dunstan DW, Daly RM, Owen N, et al. High-intensity resistance training improves glycemic control in older patients with type 2 diabetes. *Diabetes Care.* 2002;25:1729-1736.

20. Dunstan DW, Daly RM, Owen N, et al. Home-based resistance training is not sufficient to maintain improved glycemic control following supervised training in older individuals with type 2 diabetes. *Diabetes Care.* 2005;28:3-9.

21. Featherstone JF, Holly RG, Amsterdam EA. Physiologic responses to weight lifting in coronary artery disease. *Am J Cardiol.* 1993;71:287-292.

22. Ferrara CM, McCrone SH, Brendle D, Ryan AS, Goldberg AP. Metabolic effects of the addition of resistive to aerobic exercise in older men. *Int J Sport Nutr Exerc Metab.* 2004;14:73-80.

23. Guelfi KJ, Jones TW, Fournier PA. Intermittent high-intensity exercise does not increase the risk of early postexercise hypoglycemia in individuals with type 1 diabetes. *Diabetes Care.* 2005;28:416-418.

24. Halse R, Bonavaud SM, Armstong JL, McCormack JG, Yeaman SJ. Control of glycogen synthesis by glucose, glycogen, and insulin in cultured human muscle cells. *Diabetes.* 2001;50:720-726.

25. Herriott MT, Colberg SR, Parson HK, Nunnold T, Vinik AI. Effects of 8 weeks of flexibility and resistance training in older adults with type 2 diabetes. *Diabetes Care.* 2004;27: 2988-2989.

26. Holten MK, Zacho M, Gaster M, Juel C, Wojtaszewshi JF, Dela F. Strength training increases insulin-mediated glucose uptake, GLUT4 content, and insulin signaling in skeletal muscle in patients with type 2 diabetes. *Diabetes.* 2004;53(2):294-305.

27. Hu G, Jousilahti P, Barengo NC, Qiao Q, Lakka TA, Tuomilehto J. Physical activity, cardiovascular risk factors, and mortality among Finnish adults with diabetes. *Diabetes Care.* 2005;28:799-805.

28. Ibañez J, Izquierdo M, Argüelles I, et al. Twice-weekly progressive resistance training decreases abdominal fat and improves insulin sensitivity in older men with type 2 diabetes. *Diabetes Care.* 2005;28:662-667.

29. Iglay HB, Thyfault JP, Apolzan JW, Campbell WW. Resistance training and dietary protein: Effects on glucose tolerance and contents of skeletal muscle insulin signaling proteins in older persons. *Am J Clin Nutr.* 2007;85: 1005-1013.

30. Ishii T, Yamakita T, Sato T, Tanaka S, Fujii S. Resistance training improves insulin sensitivity in NIDDM subjects without altering maximal oxygen uptake. *Diabetes Care.* 1998;21: 1351-1355.

31. King DS, Baldus PJ, Sharp RL, Kesl LD, Fleymeyer TL, Riddle MS. Time course for exercise-induced alterations in insulin action and glucose tolerance in middle-aged people. *J Appl Physiol.* 1995;78:17-22.

32. Kreisman SH, Halter JB, Vranic M, Marliss EB. Combined infusion of epinephrine and norepinephrine during moderate exercise reproduces the glucoregulatory response of intense exercise. *Diabetes*. 2003;52:1347-1354.

33. Kruk J. Physical activity in the prevention of the most frequent chronic diseases: An analysis of the recent evidence. *Asian Pac J Cancer Prev*. 2007;8:325-338.

34. Larsen JJ, Dela F, Madsbad S, Galbo H. The effect of intense exercise on postprandial glucose homeostasis in type 2 diabetic patients. *Diabetologia*. 1999;42:1282-1292.

35. Larsen JJ, Dela F, Madsbad S, Vibe-Petersen J, Galbo H. Interaction of sulfonylureas and exercise on glucose homeostasis in type 2 diabetic patients. *Diabetes Care*. 1999;22:1647-1654.

36. Lombardi VP, Troxel RA. US deaths and injuries associated with weight training. *Med Sci Sports Exerc*. 2003;35:S203.

37. Maiorana A, O'Driscoll G, Goodman C, Taylor R, Green D. Combined aerobic and resistance exercise improves glycemic control and fitness in type 2 diabetes. *Diab Res Clin Pract*. 2002;56:115-123.

38. McCartney N. Acute responses to resistance training and safety. *Med Sci Sports Exerc*. 1999;31:31-37.

39. McMahon SK, Ferreira LD, Ratnam N, et al. Glucose requirements to maintain euglycemia after moderate-intensity afternoon exercise in adolescents with type 1 diabetes are increased in a biphasic manner. *J Clin Endocrinol Metab*. 2007;92:963-968.

40. Misra A, Alappan NK, Vikram NK, et al. Effect of supervised progressive resistance exercise training protocol on insulin sensitivity, glycemia, lipids and body composition in Asian Indians with type 2 diabetes. *Diabetes Care*. May 5, 2008 [E-pub ahead of print].

41. Narayan K, Boyle J, Thompson T, Sorensen SW, Williamson DF. Lifetime risk for diabetes mellitus in the United States. *JAMA*. 2003;290:1884-1890.

42. O'Donovan G, Kearney EM, Nevill AM, Woolf-May K, Bird SR. The effects of 24 weeks of moderate- or high-intensity exercise on insulin resistance. *Eur J Appl Physiol*. 2005;95:522-528.

43. Park SW, Goodpaster BH, Strotmeyer ES, et al. Accelerated loss of skeletal muscle strength in older adults with type 2 diabetes: The health, aging, and body composition study. *Diabetes Care*. 2007;30:1507-1512.

44. Paterson DH, Jones GR, Rice CL. Aging and physical activity: Evidence to develop exercise recommendations for older adults. *Can J Public Health*. 2007;98:S69-S108.

45. Poehlman ET, Dvorak RV, DeNino WF, Brochu M, Ades PA. Effects of resistance training and endurance training on insulin sensitivity in nonobese, young women: A controlled randomized trial. *J Clin Endocrinol Metab*. 2000;85:2463-2468.

46. Poirier P, Mawhinney S, Grondin L, et al. Prior meal enhances the plasma glucose lowering effect of exercise in type 2 diabetes. *Med Sci Sports Exerc*. 2001;33:1259-1264.

47. Pruchnic R, Katsiaras A, He J, Kelley DE, Winters C, Goodpaster BH. Exercise training increases intramyocellular lipid and oxidative capacity in older adults. *Am J Physiol Endocrinol Metab*. 2004;287:E857-E862.

48. Roglic G, Unwin N, Bennett PH, et al. The burden of mortality attributable to diabetes: realistic estimates for the year 2000. *DiabetesCare*. 2005;28:2130-2135.

49. Saydah SH, Fradkin J, Cowie CC. Poor control of risk factors for vascular disease among adults with previously diagnosed diabetes. *JAMA*. 2004;291:335-342.

50. Sigal RJ, Kenny GP, Boulé NG, et al. Effects of aerobic training, resistance training, or both on glycemic control in type 2 diabetes: A randomized trial. *Ann Intern Med.* 2007;147:357-369.

51. Sigal RJ, Kenny GP, Wasserman DH, Castaneda-Sceppa C. Physical activity/exercise and type 2 diabetes. *Diabetes Care.* 2004;27:2518-2539.

52. Silva LE, Valim V, Pessanha AP, et al. Hydrotherapy versus conventional land-based exercise for the management of patients with osteoarthritis of the knee: A randomized clinical trial. Physical Therapy. 2008;88:12-21.

53. Toledo FG, Menshikova EV, Azuma K, et al. Mitochondrial capacity in skeletal muscle is not stimulated by weight loss despite increases in insulin action and decreases in intramyocellular lipid content. *Diabetes.* 2008;57:987-994.

54. Vincent KR, Braith RW, Feldman RA, et al. Resistance exercise and physical performance in adults aged 60 to 83. *J Am Geriatr Soc.* 2002;50:1100-1107.

55. Willey KA, Singh MA. Battling insulin resistance in elderly obese people with type 2 diabetes: Bring on the heavy weights. *Diabetes Care.* 2003;26:1580-1588.

56. World Health Organization. Global strategy on diet, physical activity, and health. Available at: http://www.who.int/dietphysicalactivity/publications/facts/diabetes/en/. Accessed December 17, 2008.

57. Yamakita T, Ishii T, Yamagami K, et al. Glycemic response during exercise after administration of insulin lispro compared with that after administration of regular human insulin. *Diab Res Clin Pract.* 2002;57:17-22.

58. Yau MK. Tai chi exercise and the improvement of health and well-being in older adults. *Med Sci Sport Exerc.*2008;52:155-165.

59. Zhang W, Moskowitz RW, Nuki G, et al. OARSI recommendations for the management of hip and knee osteoarthritis, part II: OARSI evidence-based, expert consensus guidelines. *Osteoarthritis Cartilage.* 2008;16:137-162.

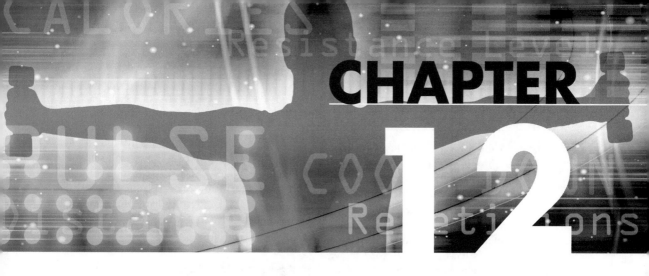

CHAPTER 12

RESISTANCE-TRAINING STRATEGIES FOR INDIVIDUALS WITH CORONARY HEART DISEASE

Objectives

Upon completion of this chapter, the reader should be able to:

- ○ Discuss the public health implications of coronary heart disease
- ○ Identify the etiology of coronary heart disease
- ○ Describe research supporting the safety and efficacy of resistance training for individuals with coronary heart disease
- ○ Describe different methods of resistance training and special considerations to enhance participant safety during exercise testing and training
- ○ Describe program variables used to design resistance training programs, as well as the relationship between the number of repetitions, number of sets, rest period between sets, and training intensity, velocity, and frequency
- ○ Explain the concept of periodization and its application to the design of resistance-training programs for individuals with coronary heart disease
- ○ Design safe, effective, and progressive resistance-training programs for individuals with coronary heart disease

INTRODUCTION

Coronary heart disease (CHD) is one of the most prevalent and chronic conditions in the United States. This condition is caused by **atherosclerosis,** a hardening of the arteries that reduces blood flow through coronary arteries to the heart muscle typically resulting in chest pain and/or heart damage. The growing number of individuals in the United States with CHD has led to the need for exercise programs that provide the most positive physiologic change, as efficiently as possible, with the lowest risk of adverse side effects. Numerous studies and clinical exercise authorities support the efficacy of aerobic and resistance training for individuals with CHD (3-6, 13, 16, 23, 26, 27, 32, 57). Due to the high prevalence of this disease in the United States, exercise professionals should develop resistance-training programs as one of the cornerstones of a program that also includes cardiovascular exercise, proper eating, and other lifestyle modifications that include stress management and smoking cessation to support health and fitness.

PREVALENCE OF CHD

CHD is the leading cause of death in the United States for both men and women (40). About every 29 seconds, someone in the United States suffers from a CHD-related event, and about every minute someone dies from such an event (40). The lifetime risk of having CHD after age 40 is 49 percent for men and 32 percent for women (40). As women get older, the risk increases to almost that of men (40).

ETIOLOGY OF CHD

CHD usually results from the buildup of fatty material and plaque in the coronary arteries, a process called *atherosclerosis,* in which deposits form in the inner layer of the arteries (40). As the coronary arteries narrow, the flow of blood to the heart can slow or stop, causing chest pain—known

as stable **angina**—shortness of breath, heart attack, or other symptoms (40). CHD derives from a myriad of factors ranging from family history to poor diet and lack of exercise. Excess cholesterol, smoking, and diabetes are established risk factors for CHD. Over time, these factors cause plaque buildup in a slow process that can lead to hardening, cracking, and complete blockage of arteries (40).

BENEFITS OF RESISTANCE TRAINING FOR INDIVIDUALS WITH CHD

Individuals with CHD are ideal candidates for **cardiac rehabilitation.** Cardiac rehabilitation consists of a comprehensive, long-term program involving medical evaluation, prescribed exercise, cardiac risk-factor modification, education, and counseling (19, 44). These programs are designed to limit the physiologic and psychological effects of cardiac illness, to reduce the risk for sudden death or a second infarction, to control cardiac symptoms, to stabilize or reverse the atherosclerotic process, and to enhance the psychosocial and vocational status of individuals. Cardiac rehabilitation programs have been developed to incorporate the latest research in exercise prescription for individuals with CHD using an environment staffed by exercise professionals and medical clinicians to insure the safety of the individual (44).

Literature Review of Research Supporting Resistance Training for CHD

Research supports the safety of resistance training from a cardiovascular standpoint even in individuals with advanced forms of heart disease (2, 9-12, 29, 41, 48, 49, 56). Studies show that resistance training significantly improves mood and muscular strength and limits the occurrence of angina, ST segment depression, and cardiovascular and pulmonary complications (12, 22, 24, 33, 49, 53). These research findings indicate that with proper drug therapy, and with effective management and monitoring from exercise professionals, individuals with a recent cardiac intervention can safely and effectively perform resistance-training activities without the fear of additional cardiac risk. The need for total-body strength to perform activities of daily living and job-related activities reinforces the need for a well-designed resistance-training program for individuals with CHD (11-14). Studies suggest that along with an improved mood, strength, and quality of life, individuals with CHD can increase strength, which will alleviate the stress of performing basic activities after a cardiac intervention or illness (22, 24).

Resistance training has the added benefits of increasing bone density (14, 38, 51, 52) and increasing lean body mass (17, 31, 36, 54). Braith and colleagues found that in heart transplant patients, a resistance-training protocol increased bone density, which is vital due to the patient's need for immunosuppressive therapy that leads to bone loss (14). The effects of resistance training occur in a timely manner in individuals with CHD, similar to individuals without the disease. As measured by muscular endurance and strength, recent bypass and myocardial infarction patients have been shown to benefit from resistance training initiated shortly after a cardiac event (2, 10, 11).

Finally, some research has shown that resistance training creates more favorable blood lipid levels (57), increases cardiovascular conditioning (1), lowers blood pressure (39, 41), enhances insulin uptake (21, 37, 42, 43, 51), and improves quality of life (12, 22, 24). Details of the studies on resistance training and CHD are listed in Table 12-1.

Table 12-1 Resistance-Training Studies in CHD Populations

Reference	Patient Subject Group or Risk Factor(s)	Program Length/ Weeks or Months	Intensity	Significant Research Findings
2	Cardiac Rehab Phase 2	8 weeks	High Intensity	No BP/ECG abnormalities, increase in strength, no muscle soreness/injury
10	Cardiac Rehab Phase 2	1RM Assessment	High Intensity	No BP/ECG abnormalities, no muscle soreness/injury
11	Cardiac Rehab Phase 2	8 weeks	High Intensity	No BP/ECG abnormalities, no muscle soreness/injury
12	Cardiac Rehab Phase 2	12 weeks	High Intensity	No BP/ECG abnormalities, increases in strength, muscular endurance, improvement in body composition
57	Cardiac Rehab Phase 2	6 months	Moderate Intensity	Increases in cardiovascular endurance in aerobic and strength training groups
41	CHF (Congestive Heart Failure)	Strength Assessment	Low and High Intensity	Increased stability of left ventricle of well compensated, optimally medicated patients during strength training

Low Intensity = Less than 60% 1RM, Moderate Intensity = 60-80% 1RM, High Intensity = 80% 1RM and above

DESIGNING RESISTANCE-TRAINING PROGRAMS FOR INDIVIDUALS WITH CHD

All individuals with CHD should have a physical that includes a cardiopulmonary exercise test before starting an exercise program (5). These tests will alert the exercise professional to any potential health issues that should be addressed, and they will serve as the basis for developing the exercise program. The American College of Sports Medicine (ACSM) outlines specifics for exercise testing and risk categorization (5).

Exercise Testing Considerations

Finding a one-repetition maximum (1RM) in each key exercise will give the exercise professional the most effective means of designing a resistance-training program, increasing resistance in regular intervals, and recording progress (1, 2, 8, 10, 11, 34). However, some exercise professionals may be reluctant to perform a 1RM assessment on individuals with CHD due to the fear of injury or adverse cardiovascular effects. Research shows that a 1RM assessment can be used for individuals with CHD without injury, muscle soreness, or cardiac abnormalities (2, 9, 10). Maximal strength testing is routinely performed on individuals with CHD 2 to 4 weeks after a cardiac event (2, 9, 10). The exercise professional may choose a reasonable repetition maximum (RM), but it should fall within the range of 8RM to 15RM to ensure assessment of strength rather than muscular endurance (8, 25, 45). The chances of injury or adverse effect due to the assessment process will be decreased if proper exercises are selected, proper coaching is offered, and the individual is allowed to become familiar with the exercise.

Following surgical procedures, individuals with CHD are susceptible to arrhythmia; thus it is important to monitor the cardiovascular response to the RM testing procedure. In the cardiac rehabilitation facility, monitoring the electrocardiograph (ECG) to evaluate

ST segment changes and other data is helpful to determine if the response to testing is within normal limits. If ECG monitoring is not available, monitoring heart rate (HR) and blood pressure (BP) will allow assessment of the response to the testing procedure. During the testing procedure, HR should not exceed 20 to 30 beats per minute (bpm) above resting values and should return to baseline or near baseline values during rest periods (2, 9, 10). For individuals who are also hypertensive, monitoring BP during assessment of 1RM is important and is strongly recommended as a safety precaution. During the testing procedure, increases in systolic BP should not exceed 30 mm Hg and should return to baseline or near baseline values during rest periods (1, 2, 9, 10, 34). Table 12-2 outlines an example of the adapted testing procedure to assess RM in individuals with CHD (2, 8, 10, 11).

The method in Table 12-2 may be performed on a regular basis to show progression and to change the workload to maintain overload as skill and strength increase. The 1RM assessment method has been performed many times and has been shown to be reliable and safe for use in individuals with CHD (2, 8-10). However, other methods of assessment are likely to be encountered and may be used to design resistance-training programs. Some programs will simply start at a light weight to familiarize the individual with the movement; then, when a goal number of repetitions are completed with this weight, the load is increased and the repetitions decreased (3). The individual will then strive to complete more repetitions with each training session and increase the weight when the goal is once again achieved. This method is not optimal for maximizing outcomes, because it can activate pulmonary fatigue before adequately training the muscles. However, if exercise professionals are not permitted to perform 1RM assessments due to facility policy, this method may be utilized to develop the resistance-training program. In this case, the number of repetitions performed or the weight used must be increased on a session-by-session basis. Detailed records must be kept of the weight used during each training session to increase the demands placed on the body and therefore realize the desired training effect.

Table 12-2 Assessing Repetition Maximum for Individuals with CHD

Verbally describe the process and the reason why the test is being performed. Inform the individual that ECG (if available), heart rate (HR) and blood pressure (BP) will be collected to ensure the safety of the assessment and to measure improvement. If no ECG monitoring is available, HR and BP will be checked immediately following exercise completion. Prior to testing, a baseline resting HR and BP should be obtained.

1. Demonstrate the exercise to the individual by performing the exercise or having a colleague perform the exercise while you describe correct form.

2. Allow the individual to perform the exercise with little or no weight to get familiar with the movement. Try to limit the number of repetitions at this time to approximately 8 to 10 to decrease the likelihood of fatigue. BP and HR should be checked after the completion of each attempt. BP should not increase more than 30 to 40 mm Hg. HR should not increase more than 20 to 30 beats per minute (bpm).

3. Allow approximately 2 to 4 minutes rest before attempting the next set. During each rest period, HR and BP should be assessed to make sure a return to baseline or near-baseline value is realized. If vital signs do not return to near baseline values, assess the individual and terminate the testing session if necessary.

4. Add a slight amount of weight to the exercise and have the individual perform 3 to 5 repetitions to further increase the familiarity of the exercise.

5. Rest 2 to 4 minutes before attempting the next set.

6. Add weight to the exercise in an effort to limit the performance of the exercise to the number of repetitions set as the goal, such as 8RM to 15RM.

7. If the target RM is achieved easily, add more weight to the exercise and allow the individual to rest 2 to 4 minutes before performing the exercise again.

8. Continue this process until target RM is achieved.

9. Try to limit the number of attempts at achieving the target RM to approximately 5 sets.

10. Assess the individual's HR and BP prior to discharge to be sure the individual has returned to baseline values.

11. All data from the testing session, including cardiovascular and strength measurements, should be recorded and used to assess progress.

Training Program Components

Exercise selection is of paramount importance in developing a resistance-training program. For individuals with CHD, exercise selection takes on more importance. Some exercises are not appropriate due to the anatomical structures stressed, the general age of this population, and the need to incorporate exercises that mimic activities of daily living. Exercises usually included in resistance-training programs for athletes and the general public may not be as

beneficial for individuals with CHD (1 ,2, 8-10, 34). Exercises chosen must increase the strength and lean body mass while minimizing adverse effects. The bench press or chest press is an excellent exercise for most populations, because it strengthens much of the upper-body musculature. However, for individuals with CHD, the bench press may cause soreness in the pectoral region along the sternum that may be mistaken for angina. Along these same lines, bypass-surgery patients who have had the sternum cut to gain access to the heart would not be candidates for using the chest press to strengthen the musculature of the upper body. In this case, the shoulder press would be an alternative exercise to increase shoulder and arm strength while minimizing stress on the sternum.

In addition to exercise selection, proper performance of the exercise must be continually emphasized. Individuals with CHD may be older and may have preexisting orthopedic problems. Also, due to advanced age, surgery, and medications, some individuals may have difficulty remembering how to perform the exercises properly. To stress the proper muscles and avoid stressing preexisting injuries, proper form must be used on each exercise. The exercise technique should be reinforced on a regular basis to maximize benefits and minimize the potential adverse effects of the program.

For resistance training to carry over into everyday life, exercises should mimic activities of daily living as much as possible. Many individuals who live in nursing homes and assisted living facilities do so because they simply do not have the strength to live on their own (24). For example, many individuals can walk for extended periods of time when they reach a standing position; however, attaining the standing position is difficult for them. This finding is a reflection of a decrease in strength that no longer allows them to overcome their own body weight when trying to perform an activity of daily living, such as standing up or climbing stairs (1). One effective exercise that will increase lean body mass, increase lower-body strength, and help participants perform activities of daily living is the step-up. This exercise works all major muscles of the lower body and mimics the action of walking up and down stairs. By adding a movement that mimics an activity routinely encountered to the resistance-training routine, the exercise becomes functional. Table 12-3 lists examples of exercises that mimic activities of daily living.

Table 12-3 Exercises that Simulate Activities of Daily Living

Exercise	Primary Movers	Activity of Daily Living Simulated
Leg press	Quadriceps, hamstrings, glutes	Pushing off to move from a seated to a standing position
Deadlift	Spinal erectors, quadriceps, hamstrings, glutes	Proper technique for picking up something from the floor or getting out of a chair
Step-up	Quadriceps, hamstrings, glutes	Walking up and down stairs
Squat	Quadriceps, hamstrings, glutes, spinal erectors	Getting out of a chair
Shoulder press	Deltoids, triceps	Putting something on a top shelf, such as dishes
Seated row	Latissimus dorsi, brachialis	Pulling something toward the body, such as opening a door
One arm row w/ dumbbell	Latissimus dorsi, brachialis, biceps	Pulling something toward the body, such as opening a door
Lat pulldown	Latissimus dorsi, brachialis, biceps	Pulling oneself to a seated position using shower safety bars in case of a fall
Chest press	Pectorals, deltoids, triceps	Pushing a lawnmower up hill or around obstacles
Biceps curl	Brachialis, biceps	Picking up a jug of milk and putting it in a cart

A major goal of resistance training for individuals with CHD should be to gain muscular strength. The benefits of a properly designed resistance-training program include an increase in lean body mass, increased coordination, and an increase in functional capacity. To maximize these benefits, loads assigned should be great enough to limit the number of repetitions to fall in the range of 8 to 15. A consensus among research studies agrees that a repetition range of 8 to 15 repetitions will produce gains in strength and muscle mass (4, 7, 25, 48, 49). If too many repetitions are performed, endurance is maximized but strength is not increased.

The research on resistance training has produced much debate over the number of sets required to produce gains in strength and muscle mass. Research indicates no significant difference between performing one set or multiple sets of resistance-training exercises in novice lifters and individuals with CHD in 8- to 12-week studies (3, 4, 7, 18, 23, 25, 48, 49, 55). Research also indicates that adherence may be increased due to less overall time required to perform resistance training when a one-set protocol is used (35). Due to time constraints encountered in many cardiac rehabilitation programs, one-set programs are most commonly used; however, research indicates multiple sets are required to increase strength and muscle mass in experienced lifters (7, 8, 25, 30), so additional sets may be used as the individual progresses and if time allows.

To improve strength and enhance lean body mass, a minimum amount of time must be spent resting between sets. In order for the anaerobic components of metabolism to be emphasized, the individual should rest a minimum of 2 minutes between sets (7, 8, 25). If less rest occurs between sets, cardiovascular limitations might decrease the benefit of resistance training. If longer rest periods are observed, the individual may cool down and any cardiovascular benefit will diminish.

Research supports 2 to 3 days per week of resistance training if full-body workouts are performed (3, 4, 7, 48, 49, 55). By working the entire body in each training session, the individual will have several days to recover, thus allowing adaptation.

Research indicates performing resistance training 2 nonconsecutive days per week is almost as effective as training 3 nonconsecutive days per week (15). This program frequency emphasizes getting the most gain for the amount of time invested, which will increase adherence.

Performing resistance training prior to cardiovascular exercise allows the individual to use the heaviest weights and produce the greatest gains in strength and muscle mass (7). On the other hand, for clinicians in the cardiac rehabilitation setting, insurance and the number of individuals in the program may dictate the placement of the resistance-training program (3). In this setting, resistance training may need to be performed after cardiovascular training or even in the middle of cardiovascular training. Such an example might include 15 minutes of cardiovascular exercise on a treadmill, performance of resistance training, and finally completing 15 additional minutes of cardiovascular exercise on a bike. If at all possible, keep the format the same each training session, as this will allow the body to adapt to the demand placed on it and will aid in completing the exercise program.

SAMPLE 24-WEEK PROGRAM

The overall program design for individuals with CHD is similar to any other balanced conditioning program. It should include cardiovascular conditioning and resistance training while being concise to increase adherence. Table 12-4 outlines a 24-week sample program. In the cardiac rehabilitation setting (traditional phase 2), ECG data should be monitored continuously to ensure safety and to help the individual exercise within an individualized training HR zone. BP should be checked before, during, and after exercise and should be checked at approximately the midpoint of each cardiovascular exercise, while the individual is in the training HR zone. After completing a resistance-training exercise, BP should be checked to make sure it is within limits established by the graded exercise test (2, 3, 5, 6, 9, 10).

Table 12-4 Sample 24-Week Resistance-Training Program

Week 1	Commence cardiovascular training three days per week at 60-80 percent of heart rate reserve, up to 30 minutes per day
Week 2	Continue cardiovascular training, maintaining frequency, intensity and duration for the remainder of the 24 week program
Week 3	Begin twice-weekly resistance training. Establish 1RM during first weekly session of week 1. Day 2, use 60% of 1RM for 1 set of 12 repetitions.
Week 4	Use 70% of 1RM for 1 set of 8 repetitions.
Week 5	Use 80% of 1RM for 1 set of 8 repetitions.
Week 6	Weight is selected to allow no more than 8 repetitions per exercise on each training day.
Week 7	Test for new 1RM on the first training day of week 7. Skip second training day.
Week 8	Use 60% of 1RM for 1 set of 12 repetitions.
Week 9	Use 70% of 1RM for 1 set of 8 repetitions.
Week 10	Use 80% of 1RM for 1 set of 8 repetitions.
Week 11	Weight is selected to allow no more than 8 repetitions for each exercise on each training day.
Week 12	Test for new 1RM first resistance training day of week 12. Skip second training day.
Week 13	Begin thrice-weekly schedule at 60% of 1RM for 1 set of 12 repetitions.
Week 14	Use 70% of 1RM for 1 set of 8 repetitions.
Week 15	Use 80% of 1RM for 1 set of 8 repetitions.
Week 16	Weight is selected to allow no more than one set of 8 repetitions for each exercise.
Week 17	Test for new 1RM on the first training day of week 17. Use 60% of 1RM for 1 set of 12 repetitions for the next two workouts.
Week 18	Use 70% of 1RM for 1 set of 8 repetitions.
Week 19	Use 80% of 1RM for 1 set of 8 repetitions.
Week 20	Weight is selected to allow no more than 1 set of 8 repetitions for each exercise.
Week 21	Test for new 1RM on the first training day of week 17. Use 60% of 1RM for 1 set of 12 repetitions for the next two workouts
Week 22	Use 70% of 1RM for 1 set of 8 repetitions.
Week 23	Use 80% of 1RM for 1 set of 8 repetitions.
Week 24	Weight is selected to allow no more than 1 set of 8 repetitions for each exercise.

In the fitness-center setting or maintenance cardiac rehabilitation setting, ECG monitoring might not be available or cost effective. Alternative monitoring includes a manual radial pulse check to help the individual exercise within a training HR zone. BP may be checked in this setting before, during, and after exercise, as it was in the monitored cardiac rehabilitation setting (2, 3, 5, 6, 9, 10).

Weeks 1 through 2

The goal of the first 2 weeks of the training program is to monitor the cardiovascular response to exercise. The use of cardiovascular training will also serve to limit the amount of muscle soreness when resistance training is added in week 3. The frequency will be three times per week at an intensity of 60 to

80 percent of the HR reserve (maximum heart rate minus resting heart rate) using the Karvonen method. The maximum HR achieved on the cardiopulmonary exercise test should serve as the basis for developing the training HR zone. Each exercise session will be increased up to 30 minutes in duration as tolerated. The cardiovascular component of the program will be maintained throughout the 24-week program.

Week 3

After 2 weeks of cardiovascular exercise without any complications, resistance training may begin on two nonconsecutive days. During the first session, a 1RM will be established on the exercises specific to the individual's condition. Exercise selection will be different for each individual to avoid soreness in any areas healing after surgery and to avoid causing pain in the sternal area that might be mistaken for angina. On the second training day of week 3, perform a single set of each exercise with 60 percent of the 1RM for 12 repetitions.

Weeks 4 through 6

Continue training on two nonconsecutive days, increasing workloads incrementally. Week 4 involves a single set of each exercise at 70 percent of the 1RM for 8 repetitions. For week 5, a single set of each exercise at 80 percent of 1RM for 8 repetitions should be done. Week 6 should comprise 1 set of each exercise with a weight that limits performance of the exercise to 8 repetitions.

Week 7

On the first training day of week 7, reassess 1RM for each exercise. This new 1RM will allow the workload to be adjusted for the next cycle of training. Only cardiovascular training will be completed on the second session of the week to allow for recovery before the start of a new cycle of training.

Weeks 8 through 11

Continue with 2 days per week. During week 8, perform 1 set of each exercise at 60 percent of 1RM

for 12 repetitions. During week 9, perform 1 set of each exercise at 70 percent of 1RM for 8 repetitions. Week 10 will include 1 set of each exercise at 80 percent of 1RM for 8 repetitions. Week 11 should include 1 set of each exercise with a weight that limits performance of the exercise to 8 repetitions.

Week 12

On the first training session of week 12, reassess 1RM for each exercise. This new 1RM will allow the workload to be adjusted for the next cycle of training. Only cardiovascular training will be completed on the second session of the week to allow for recovery before the start of a new cycle of training.

Weeks 13 through 16

After 12 weeks of cardiovascular and resistance training, individuals should have no restrictions in terms of resistance-training exercises that can be performed in their exercise program. Those previously told to avoid direct chest exercises can be allowed to utilize an exercise such as the chest press at this point. The remaining exercises could be supplemented by adding exercises that work on specific areas that need additional strengthening. As an example, someone requiring more leg strength to perform his or her job might have additional leg exercises added to the resistance-training program. The exercises selected should follow the rules outlined previously on exercise selection and should not require a great amount of additional time. In addition, a third nonconsecutive day of resistance training can be added at this time. However, continued success of any exercise program requires a high degree of adherence. Therefore, adding additional exercises and increasing the number of days per week should be approached judiciously so as not to make the program too demanding and therefore decrease adherence.

Begin 3 days per week frequency on nonconsecutive days if possible. Week 13, complete 1 set of 12 repetitions at 60 percent of 1RM. Week 14, complete 1 set of 8 repetitions at 70 percent of 1RM. Week 15, complete 1 set of 8 repetitions at 80 percent of 1RM. Week 16, complete 1 set with a weight that allows no more than 8 repetitions per exercise.

Weeks 17 through 20

Continue training 3 days per week. Reassess 1RM for each exercise on the first session of week 17. Complete 1 set of 12 repetitions at 60 percent of 1RM during remaining workouts for week 17. Week 18, complete 1 set of 8 repetitions at 70 percent of 1RM. Week 19, complete 1 set of 8 repetitions at 80 percent of 1RM. Week 20, complete a single set with a weight that allows no more than 8 repetitions per exercise.

Weeks 21 through 24

Continue training 3 days per week. Reassess 1RM for each exercise on the first session of week 21. Complete 1 set of 12 repetitions at 60 percent of 1RM during remaining workouts of week 21. Week 22, complete 1 set of 8 repetitions at 70 percent of 1RM. Week 23, complete 1 set of 8 repetitions at 80 percent of 1RM. Week 24, complete a single set with a weight that allows no more than 8 repetitions per exercise.

CASE STUDY

Mr. B is a 55-year-old male who had a myocardial infarction while shoveling snow but did not go to the hospital until the next day. His symptoms were shortness of breath, sweating, weakness, and fatigue, but he denies chest pain or pain radiating to the left arm. He was not a candidate for thrombolytic agents or angioplasty due to the amount of time that elapsed from the onset of symptoms until admission to the hospital. He was cleared to enter cardiac rehabilitation by his cardiologist 2 weeks after his cardiac event. His vital signs included a resting HR of 70 bpm, normal sinus rhythm with random PVCs, BP of 144/84, an oxygen saturation of 96 percent, and a weight of 185 pounds. Mr. B achieved 7 METs on a Bruce Protocol Stress Test. His maximum HR was 132 bpm, with a peak BP of 184/88. No chest pain or other symptoms were noted during the stress test. He was instructed that if

he did not exhibit any cardiovascular abnormalities during the initial 2 weeks of cardiac rehabilitation, he would have no restrictions in terms of exercise selection for resistance training. The first 12 weeks of his exercise prescription are presented below.

Cardiovascular: A thrice-weekly supervised and monitored exercise program was recommended with 2 to 4 days per week of home exercise. Intensity of cardiovascular training was set at 60 to 80 percent of HR reserve with a training HR zone of 107 to 120 bpm. Duration of training began at 10 minutes, to be increased up to 30 minutes maximum as tolerated.

Resistance Training: On the first day of resistance training, a 1RM was established. Because Mr. B did not have chest pain or a recent bypass, he did not have any exercise restrictions. A resistance-training program that worked all major muscle groups of the body was utilized in this order: deadlift or modified deadlift, leg press, lat pulldown, seated cable row, chest press, shoulder press, and biceps curl. This routine works the largest muscle groups of the body first before proceeding to the smallest muscle groups.

Summary

CHD is the leading cause of death in the United States for both males and females. Following revascularization and myocardial infarction, individuals enrolled in cardiac rehabilitation programs benefit with an increased quality of life and better cardiovascular functioning. In the past, cardiac rehabilitation focused mainly on cardiovascular exercise, and little attention was given to resistance training. However, cardiac rehabilitation programs now focus on a balanced program of cardiovascular and resistance training to help individuals with CHD return to an active lifestyle. To get the most out of the allotted time in cardiac rehabilitation, patients should have medical clearance before entering the program and should then begin a program of cardiovascular exercise supplemented with resistance training exercises that mimic activities of daily living. A one-set protocol two or three times per week utilizing a repetition range of 8 to 15 will increase strength and create muscular hypertrophy while encourage the highest adherence. Rest periods of 2 to 4 minutes between exercises will allow weights heavy enough to achieve the goals of strength and hypertrophy without being limited by cardiovascular capabilities. Regular testing of some kind should be utilized to document patient progress, program effectiveness, and weak muscle groups requiring additional attention.

Key Terms

Angina
Atherosclerosis
Cardiac Rehabilitation
Coronary heart disease

Study Questions

1. How can a resistance-training program help an individual with CHD? Is resistance training safe for individuals with CHD? If so, why?

2. What is atherosclerosis? How does it relate to and affect a person with CHD?

3. Why would the bench press be considered an inappropriate exercise for an individual with CHD? What alternative exercises can be used in place of the bench press?

4. What repetition range should be used to gain the most strength and lean muscle? Why would completing more repetitions not be as effective?

References

1. Adams KJ, Swank AM, Berning JM, Sevene-Adams PJ, Barnard KL, Shimp-Bowerman J. Progressive strength training in sedentary, older African-American women. *Med Sci Sports Exerc.* 2001;33(9):1567-1576.

2. Adams KJ, Barnard KL, Swank AM, Mann E, Kushnick MR, Denny DM. Combined high-intensity strength and aerobic training in diverse phase II cardiac rehabilitation patients. *J Cardiopulm Rehabil.* 1999;19(4):209-215.

3. American Association of Cardiovascular and Pulmonary Rehabilitation. *Guidelines for Cardiac Rehabilitation Programs.* 2nd ed. Champaign, IL: Human Kinetics; 1995.

4. American College of Sports Medicine. The recommended quantity and quality of exercise for developing and maintaining cardiorespiratory and muscular fitness in healthy adults. *Med Sci Sports Exerc.* 1990;22(2):265-274.

5. American College of Sports Medicine. *Guidelines for Exercise Testing and Prescription.* 5th ed. Baltimore, MD: Lippincott Williams & Wilkins; 1995.

6. American College of Sports Medicine position stand. Exercise for patients with coronary artery disease. *Med Sci Sports Exerc.* 1994;26(3):i-v.

7. American College of Sports Medicine position stand. Progression models in resistance training for healthy adults. *Med Sci Sports Exerc.* 2002;34(2):364-380.

8. Baechle T. *Essentials of Strength and Conditioning.* Champaign, IL: Human Kinetics; 1994.

9. Barnard KL, Adams KJ, Swank AM, Mann E, Denny DM. Injuries and muscle soreness during the one-repetition maximum assessment in a cardiac rehabilitation population. *J Cardiopulm Rehabil.* 1999;19:52-58.

10. Barnard KL, Adams KJ, Swank AM, Kaelin ME, Kushnik MR, Denny DM. Combined high-intensity strength and aerobic training in patients with congestive heart failure. *J Strength Cond Res.* 2000;14:383-388.

11. Beniamini Y, Rubenstein JJ, Faigenbaum AD, Lichtenstein AH, Crim MC. High-intensity strength training of patients enrolled in an outpatient cardiac rehabilitation program. *J Cardiopulm Rehabil.* 1999;19(1):8-17.

12. Beniamini Y, Rubenstein JJ, Zaichkowsky LD, Crim MC. Effects of high-intensity strength training on quality-of-life parameters in cardiac rehabilitation patients. *Am J Cardiol.* 1997;80:841-846.

13. Braith RW, Limacher MC, Leggett SH, Pollock ML. Skeletal muscle strength in heart transplant recipients. *J Heart Lung Transplant.* 1993;12:1018-1023.

14. Braith RW, Mills RM, Welsch MA, Keller JW, Pollock ML. Resistance exercise training restores bone mineral density in heart transplant recipients. *J Am Coll Cardiol.* 1996;28:1471-1477.

15. Braith RW, Graves JE, Pollock ML, et al. Comparison of 2 vs. 3 days/week of variable resistance training during 10- and 18-week programs. *Int J Sports Med.* 1989;10:450-454.

16. Butler RM, Palmer G, Rogers FJ. Circuit weight training in early cardiac rehabilitation. *J Am Osteopath Assoc.* 1992;92:77-89.

17. Byrne HK, Wilmore JH. The effects of a 20-week exercise training program on resting metabolic rate in previously sedentary, moderately obese women. *Int J Sport Nutr Exerc Metab.* 2001;11:15-31.

18. Carpinelli RN, Otto RM. Strength training: Single versus multiple sets. *Sports Med.* 1998;26(12):73-84.

19. Certo CM. History of cardiac rehabilitation. *Phys Ther.* 1985;65:1793-1795.

20. Daub WD, Knapik GP, Black WR. Strength training early after myocardial infarction. *J Cardiopulm Rehabil.* 1996;16:100-108.

21. Eriksson J, Tuominen J, Valle T, et al. Aerobic endurance exercise or circuit-type resistance training for individuals with impaired glucose tolerance? *Horm Metab Res.* 1998;30:37–41.

22. Ewart CK. Psychological effects of resistive weight training: implications for cardiac patients. *Med Sci Sports Exerc.* 1989;21:683-688.

23. Feigenbaum MS, Pollock ML. Prescription of resistance training for health and disease. *Med Sci Sports Exerc.* 1999;31:38-45.

24. Fiatarone MA, Marks EC, Ryan ND, Meredith CN, Lipsitz LA, Evans WJ. High-intensity strength training in nonagenarians. *JAMA.* 1990;263:3029-3034.

25. Fleck SJ, Kraemer WJ. *Designing Resistance Training Programs.* Champaign, IL: Human Kinetics; 1987.

26. Fletcher GF, Balady G, Froelicher VF, Hartley LH, Haskell WL, Pollock ML. Exercise standards. A statement for healthcare professionals from the American Heart Association. Writing Group. *Circulation.* 1995;91:580-615.

27. Goldberg AP. Aerobic and resistive exercise modify risk factors for coronary heart disease. *Med Sci Sports Exerc.* 1989;21:669-674.

28. Greer M, Dimick S, Burns S. Heart rate and blood pressure response to several methods of strength training. *Phys Ther.* 1984;64:179-183.

29. Harris KA, Holly RG. Physiological response to circuit weight training in borderline hypertensive subjects. *Med Sci Sports Exerc.* 1987;19:246-252.

30. Hass CJ, Garzarella L, de Hoyos D, Pollock ML. Single versus multiple sets in long-term recreational weight lifters. *Med Sci Sports Exerc.* 2000;32:235-242.

31. Hunter GR. Changes in body composition, body build and performance associated with different weight-training frequencies in males and females. *National Strength and Conditioning Association Journal.* 1985;7:26-28.

32. Hurley B. Aerobic or strength training for coronary risk factor intervention? *Ann Med.* 1994;26:153-155.

33. Izawa K, Hirano Y, Yamada S, Oka K, Omiya K, Iijima S. Improvement in physiological outcomes and health-related quality of life following cardiac rehabilitation in patients with acute myocardial infarction. *Circ J.* 2004;68:315-320.

34. Kaelin ME, Swank AM, Adams KJ, Barnard KL, Berning JM, Green A. Cardiopulmonary responses, muscle soreness, and injury during the one-repetition maximum assessment

in pulmonary rehabilitation patients. *J Cardiopulm Rehabil.* 1999;19:366-372.

35. King AC, Haskell WL, Young DR, Oka RK, Stefanick ML. Long-term effects of varying intensities and formats of physical activity on participation rates, fitness, and lipoproteins in men and women aged 50 to 65 years. *Circulation.* 1995;91:2596-2604.

36. McBride JM, Blaak JB, Triplett-McBride T. Effect of resistance exercise volume and complexity on EMG, strength, and regional body composition. *Eur J Appl Physiol.* 2003;90:626-632.

37. Maiorana A, O'Driscoll G, Goodman C, Taylor R, Green D. Combined aerobic and resistance exercise improves glycemic control and fitness in type 2 diabetes. *Diabetes Res Clin Pract.* 2002;56:115-123.

38. Marconi C, Marzorati M. Exercise after heart transplantation. *Eur J Appl Physiol.* 2003;90:250-259. [Epub 2003 Sep 6]

39. Martel GF, Hurlbut DE, Lott ME, et al. Strength training normalizes resting blood pressure in 65- to 73-year-old men and women with high normal blood pressure. *J Am Geriatr Soc.* 1999;47:1215-1221.

40. Medline Plus Medical Encyclopedia. Coronary heart disease. http://www.nlm.nih.gov/medlineplus/ency/article/007115.htm#Definition. Accessed December 17, 2008.

41. Meyer K, Hajric R, Westbrook S, et al. Hemodynamic responses during leg press exercise in patients with chronic congestive heart failure. *Am J Cardiol.* 1999;83:1537-1543.

42. Miller WJ, Sherman WM, Ivy JL. Effect of strength training on glucose tolerance and post-glucose insulin response. *Med Sci Sports Exerc.* 1984;16:539-543.

43. Miller JP, Pratley RE, Goldberg AP, et al. Strength training increases insulin action in healthy 50- to 65-yr-old men. *J Appl Physiol.* 1994;77:1122–1127.

44. Mutual of Omaha Insurance Company. Local Medical Review Policy. August 1999.

45. Nieman DC. *Exercise Testing and Prescription: A Health Related Approach.* 4th ed. Mountain View, CA: Mayfield Publishing Company; 1999.

46. Oliver D, Pflugfelder PW, McCartney N, McKelvie RS, Suskin N, Kostuk WJ. Acute cardiovascular responses to leg-press resistance exercise in heart transplant recipients. *Int J Cardiol.* 2001;81:61-74.

47. Parker ND, Hunter GR, Treuth MS, et al. Effects of strength training on cardiovascular responses during a submaximal walk and a weight-loaded walking test in older females. *J Cardiopulm Rehabil.* 1996;16:56-62.

48. Pollock ML, Franklin BA, Balady GJ, et al. AHA Science Advisory. Resistance exercise in individuals with and without cardiovascular disease: Benefits, rationale, safety, and prescription: An advisory from the Committee on Exercise, Rehabilitation, and Prevention, Council on Clinical Cardiology, American Heart Association; Position paper endorsed by the American College of Sports Medicine. *Circulation.* 2000;101:828-833.

49. Pollock ML, Evans WJ. Resistance training for health and disease: Introduction. *Med Sci Sports Exerc.* 1999;31:10-11.

50. Reynolds 4th, TH, Supiano MA, Dengel DR. Resistance training enhances insulin-mediated glucose disposal with minimal effect on the tumor necrosis factor-alpha system in older hypertensives. *Metabolism.* 2004;53:397-402.

51. Starkey DB, Pollock ML, Ishida Y, et al. Effect of resistance training volume on strength and muscle thickness. *Med Sci Sports Exerc.* 1996;28:1311-1320.

52. Stone MH. Implications for connective tissue and bone alterations resulting from resistance exercise training. *Med Sci Sports Exerc.* 1988;20:S162-S168.

53. Swank AM, Funk DC, Manire JT, DeGruccio LA, Dimitriadis CK, Denny DM. Echocardiographic evaluation of stress test for determining safety of participation in strength training. *J Strength Cond Res.* 2005;19:389-393.

54. Treuth MS, Ryan AS, Pratley RE, et al. Effects of strength training on total and regional body composition in older men. *J Appl Physiol.* 1994;77:614–620.

55. *Physical Activity and Health: A Report of the Surgeon General.* Atlanta, GA: Centers for Disease Control and Prevention, National Center for Chronic Disease Prevention and Health Promotion. US Dept of Health and Human Services; 1996. Publication S/N 017-023-00196-5

56. Werber-Zion G, Goldhammer E, Shaar A, Pollock ML. Left ventricular function during strength testing and resistance exercise in patients with left ventricular dysfunction. *J Cardiopulm Rehabil.* 2004;24:100-109.

57. Wosornu D, Bedford D, Ballantyne D. A comparison of the effects of strength and aerobic exercise training on exercise capacity and lipids after coronary artery bypass surgery. *Eur Heart J.* 1996;17:854-863.

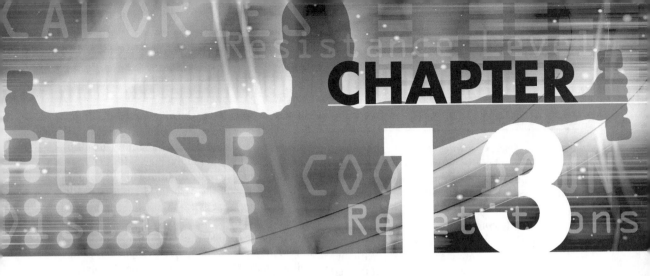

CHAPTER 13

RESISTANCE-TRAINING STRATEGIES FOR INDIVIDUALS WITH CHRONIC OBSTRUCTIVE PULMONARY DISEASE

Objectives

Upon completion of this chapter, the reader should be able to:

○ Define chronic obstructive pulmonary disease (COPD)
○ Identify the prevalence and costs associated with treating COPD
○ Describe the benefits of resistance training in individuals with COPD
○ Design a safe and effective resistance-training program for an individual with COPD that addresses the individual's goals and functional deficits

INTRODUCTION

Respiratory diseases such as **asthma, emphysema,** and **chronic bronchitis** are classified together under the name **chronic obstructive pulmonary disease (COPD).** They are progressive diseases characterized by gradual loss of lung function, airflow obstruction, dyspnea with exertion, weight loss associated with muscle wasting, recurrent bronchial infections, and chronic disability (10). Although all three conditions are classified as COPD, there is a difference between asthma and the others: Individuals with asthma can significantly reverse their airway obstruction utilizing bronchodilators, but only modest improvements at best are observed in individuals with emphysema and chronic bronchitis (6, 7, 28). Severity of impairment is generally quantified by measuring the **forced expiratory volume in one second (FEV$_1$),** defined as the volume of air expired during the first second of expiration, as seen in Table 13-1. In addition to respiratory dysfunction, individuals diagnosed with COPD are at higher risk of developing comorbidities such as congestive heart failure, osteoporosis, diabetes, depression, and anxiety due to medications utilized to control the symptoms and progression of their disease.

Individuals with COPD consistently report that the shortness of breath air is appropriate term here and fatigue associated with their disease interferes with performing daily tasks and participating in everyday events. As a result, their **quality of life,** defined as the gap between that which is desired in life and that which is achieved, is diminished (30, 32, 34). In comparison with other community-dwelling adults of similar age, individuals with COPD are less active and more deconditioned (17). Dyspnea with activity, and the associated anxiety, results in a curtailing of activities. Consequently, routine community activities and activities of daily living become more taxing, leading to greater decreases in aerobic capacity and muscular strength that fuel a downward spiral of inactivity, social isolation, and disability (32, 34).

In the past, endurance training was the primary exercise component of most pulmonary rehabilitation programs (34). However, the degree of exercise intolerance and functional limitations seen in individuals with COPD is not completely explained by cardiovascular factors (7). Skeletal muscle dysfunction and weakness play an integral role in the symptoms and functional impairments found in individuals with COPD (20, 25). The performance of activities of daily living requires both muscular strength and cardiovascular endurance. This chapter discusses resistance-training strategies for individuals with COPD. To maximize functional gains, the American College of Chest Physicians, the American Association of Cardiovascular and Pulmonary Rehabilitation, the American Thoracic Society, and the British Thoracic Society include resistance training as an important component of any pulmonary rehabilitation program (29, 30).

Table 13-1 Disease Severity Expressed as FEV$_1$ and VO$_2$ Max

Disease Severity	FEV$_1$	VO$_{2max}$: ml/kg/min	VO$_{2max}$: METs
Mild	≤60–79% predicted	between 20–25	5.7–7.14
Moderate	≤41–59% predicted	between 15–20	4.2–5.7
Severe	≤40% of predicted	<15 ml/kg/min	<4.2

(Adapted from reference 19); FEV$_1$ = Forced expiratory volume in one second

VO$_{2max}$ = Maximal oxygen uptake; METS = Metabolic equivalents of task

PREVALENCE AND ECONOMIC IMPACT OF COPD

Recent reports from the Centers for Disease Control and the *New England Journal of Medicine* illustrate the prevalence and economic impact of COPD in the United States (4, 8). Ten million adults report having a diagnosis of emphysema and/or chronic bronchitis; over 3 million are men and 6 million are women. Generally, people over the age of 50 are more likely to be considered disabled, however, the damage starts at an early age. Younger individuals with mild and moderate COPD, although not disabled, significantly contribute to the economic impact of these diseases (47). Furthermore, 11 million adults and 9 million children report having a diagnosis of asthma. Of these over 8 million are male and 11 million are female (4, 8, 45).

The economic impact of these diagnoses cannot be understated. Respiratory diseases are the third major cause of lost workdays and the fourth most common noncommunicable cause of disability (4, 38). Furthermore, the associated medical costs of treating these diseases—such as outpatient visits, emergency department visits, hospitalizations, physician fees, pharmacological management, nursing home care, and home health care—are well over $32 billion (8, 9, 18, 38). While these numbers are staggering, the actual number of individuals struggling with COPD is undoubtedly much higher due to underdiagnosis (24).

ETIOLOGY OF DISEASE

The three most prominent disease states associated with COPD are asthma, emphysema, and chronic bronchitis. While all three diseases are categorized by progressive expiratory flow obstruction, dyspnea with exertion, and some degree of airway hyperactivity, causation is specific to the disease state (1).

Asthma is characterized by airways that are hypersensitive to allergens, triggers such as air pollutants, pollen, tobacco smoke, chemical fumes, and exercise. Triggers act as antigens, resulting in airway inflammation, bronchospasm, and mucosal edema (1). Air pollutants, mold, pollens, tobacco smoke, dust mites, animal dander, chemical fumes, exercise, or exposure to cold air can all provoke an asthmatic episode or bronchospasm. The end result is a decrease in ventilation, a decrease in lung perfusion, and in severe cases, respiratory failure. The four hallmark signs of asthma are 1) coughing that includes frequent clearing of the throat; 2) wheezing, or a hoarse whistling sound heard during exhalation; 3) shortness of air; and 4) chest tightness. Guidelines for the care of asthma state that adherence to medical therapy is important for good clinical outcomes (35). Generally, with good pharmacological management, lung obstruction can be significantly reduced, resulting in near-normal or normal pulmonary function (13, 14, 35). More importantly, adherence to pharmacological therapy enables many asthmatics to gain control of their asthma, defined as minimal or no chronic asthma symptoms and no limitation of activities in patients (13, 14, 17, 35). However, some patients with long-standing asthma may possess a component of irreversible airflow obstruction due to airway remodeling despite optimal therapy (17).

Emphysema is characterized by the destruction of alveolar walls and the permanent enlargement of the airspaces distal to the terminal bronchioles (27). This process results in airflow limitations, impaired gas-exchange efficiency, loss of lung elasticity, increased intralumenal pressure, and loss of small-airway patency (1, 12, 27). The hereditary deficiency of $alpha_1$-antitrypsin accounts for only 1 percent of emphysema diagnoses. The rest are due to smoking, occupational exposures, and air pollution (12, 42). Clinical signs include progressive dyspnea, or shortness of air. In the early stages of emphysema, dyspnea only occurs during activity. However, as the disease progresses and lung function is further reduced, dyspnea is present at rest as well (27, 28). To overcome the loss of diffusion capacity, patients must maintain increased minute ventilation (1), the volume of air inhaled and exhaled in 60 seconds. In mild and moderate emphysema, arterial oxygen and carbon dioxide are generally well maintained (1). In severe cases, hypoxia—that is, oxygen deficiency—is a significant contributor to loss of function that eventually results in respiratory failure.

Chronic bronchitis is a hypersecretion of mucus characterized by a chronic, productive cough that continues for at least 3 months of the year for at least 2 consecutive years (28). Exposure to cigarette smoke and air pollution initiates a process of local inflammation and mucus production. This exposure results in an increase in the size and number of mucus glands and goblet cells and a thickening of the airway wall caused by edema, along with the accumulation of inflamed cells; decreased mucus clearance due to the loss of mucociliary escalator function; and an increase in respiratory infections as the sticky, mucous coating found in the airways serves as a good site for inhaled bacteria to become embedded (1, 28, 40). Clinically, patients will present with complaints of decreased exercise tolerance, wheezing, shortness of air, and a frequent productive cough. Disease progression can generally be stopped if exposure to the irritants—such as cigarette smoke and air pollution—can be eliminated. If these are not eliminated, the patient will run a long course of illness characterized by frequent respiratory infections, hypoventilation, dyspnea, and eventual right-sided heart failure.

BENEFITS OF RESISTANCE TRAINING FOR INDIVIDUALS WITH COPD

Individuals with COPD can expect the same benefits from resistance training as other populations. These benefits include but are not limited to increases in muscular strength, trabecular bone content, glucose tolerance, and lean body mass. Individuals with COPD who engage in resistance training can also expect to experience a decreased number of falls, enhanced ability to handle orthostatic challenges, and decreased effort performing activities of daily living (16, 21). The current literature on resistance training in pulmonary rehabilitation provides reviews of programs that utilize one-repetition maximum (1RM)

testing and periodization of exercise programming (32, 34, 39). The current literature reinforces one major theme: resistance training is a safe and effective modality to increase strength and improve quality of life for individuals with COPD. Although various studies have measured different outcomes and have shown varied degrees of improvement in outcomes, the ability of individuals with COPD to tolerate maximal testing and high-intensity resistance training is clearly illustrated. Safety is dependent upon clinicians selecting the appropriate exercises, training volumes, and intensities. Activities of daily living require both muscular strength and cardiovascular endurance; thus, exercise programming for individuals with COPD should include both types of training. Specific exercises and training tools utilized should reflect individual goals and deficits rather than offering a cookbook approach of applying the same lifts and endurance techniques to everyone.

Literature Review of Research Supporting Resistance Training for COPD

Current literature provides evidence that resistance training can benefit individuals with COPD. Table 13-2 lists the characteristics, methods, and outcomes documented in the current literature. The following studies highlight the findings of research to date.

Simpson and colleagues (36) randomized 34 individuals with severe COPD into either a control group or resistance-training group to determine the impact of resistance training on muscle fatigue, weakness, dyspnea, and performance of activities of daily living. Training subjects performed 3 sets of 10 repetitions of single-arm curls, single-leg extensions, and single-leg presses 3 times a week for 8 weeks. Initial training loads were 50 percent of 1RM and were increased to 85 percent of 1RM by the end of the study. The researchers found significant improvements in the training groups cycling power and ability to perform activities of daily living. They also found reduced dyspnea in the training group, but the control group had no change in any of these variables (36).

Table 13-2 Review of Studies of Resistance Training for Individuals with COPD

Author	n	Age in Years/ $FEV_1\%$ Predicted	Training Intensity	Strength Gains	Outcomes
Simpson (36)	34	71.5/38%	50–80% 1RM	73% max cycle ergometer test	Decrease in shortness of breath with activities of daily living
Bernard (5)	45	65.5/42.2%	60–80% 1RM	8–20%	No difference between groups
Clark (11)	43	49/77%	70% 1RM	increase in maximal lifts	Increased quality of life
Wright (43)	28	55.7/42%	Maximal	18.7%	Increased quality of life
Kaelin (21)	50	68/39%	RPE = 4–7	n/a	Increased physical function
Panton (33)	17	62/40%	32–64% 1RM	36%	Decreased effort with three of eight activities of daily living
Kongsgaard (23)	18	65–80/46%	Heavy RT	14–18%	Increased health
Ortega (31)	72	64/41%	70–85% 1RM	significant increases in all lifts	Fatigue and emotion
Mador (26)	32	74/44%	60% 1RM	17.5–26%	Increased health-related quality of life
Spruit (37)	48	64/40%	70% 1RM	20–40%	Increased health-related quality of life

Clark and colleagues (11) evaluated the efficacy of resistance training on performance of activities of daily living and 12-minute–walk results in a COPD population already performing aerobic exercise to determine if adding resistance training would result in greater improvements in function. Subjects were randomized into either a control group that performed aerobic exercise only twice a week or an experimental group that performed aerobic exercise with two additional resistance-training sessions a week. Experimental subjects' training sessions consisted of 3 sets of 10 to 12 repetitions at 32 to 64 percent of their 1RM on 12 exercises. The exercises employed were seated leg presses, calf presses, seated leg curls, leg extensions, chest presses, lat pulldowns, shoulder presses, seated rows, abdominal curls, back extensions, bicep curls, and tricep extensions. Functional outcomes were measured before and after training in both groups and consisted of the time required to complete eight standardized tests: buttoning and unbuttoning a shirt, folding 10 T-shirts into a pile, lifting 10 books from a table to a high shelf, arm raises performed in 1 minute, standing up and sitting down in 1 minute, a get-up-and-go test, a clothespin task, climbing stairs, and distance covered in a 12-minute walk. The number of arm raises performed in 1 minute, the number of times the individual could stand and sit down in 1 minute, the number of stairs climbed in 1 minute, and the distance covered in a 12-minute walk were significantly greater in the experimental group compared to the results achieved by the control group (11).

Kongsgaard and colleagues (23) randomized 18 elderly male COPD patients into either a control group or resistance-training group to examine the efficacy of resistance training on muscle size, strength, physical performance of activities of daily living, and health perception. The training group performed 60-minute training sessions twice a week for 12 weeks. Sessions consisted of 4 sets of 8 repetitions at 80 percent of 1RM of leg press, leg extension, and leg flexion exercises. The researchers found significant improvements in muscle size, muscle strength, power, physical performance of activities of daily living, and perceived health (23).

DESIGNING A RESISTANCE-TRAINING PROGRAM FOR INDIVIDUALS WITH COPD

Opportunities to train individuals with COPD occur in a variety of settings, including hospital-based rehabilitation programs, community health and wellness settings, and home-based personal training environments. Institutions and businesses should initiate policies and procedures that reflect current exercise guidelines to ensure safety. Additionally, policies and procedures should be consistently reviewed with staff members to ensure compliance to safety guidelines.

Before exercise training begins, physician clearance should be obtained. A thorough physical assessment should be performed, and baseline physiological measures should be recorded. These measures include but are not limited to heart rate, blood pressure, body composition, and **oxygen saturation,** also referred to as *oxygenation* or *aeration* of blood. Depending on the severity of the diagnosis, supplemental oxygen, oxygen delivery devices, and a pulse oximeter may be needed at the time of evaluation and during exercise. A **pulse oximeter** is a noninvasive electronic device that selectively measures oxygen saturation of blood. Heart rate, blood pressure, and oxygen saturation readings should be recorded at rest and during exercise for individuals with moderate to severe COPD. Having two types of oximetry measuring devices available ensures the most accurate results. Due to vasoconstriction and poor circulation, many individuals with COPD will register oxygen saturation well below normal limits in the extremities.

Evaluations of individuals with COPD prior to resistance training generally consist of reviewing a medical history that includes a list of current medications and dosages, a physical exam, assessment of cardiovascular endurance using a 6- or 12-minute walk, a maximal or submaximal cardiopulmonary exercise test, and evaluations of muscular strength, flexibility, and quality of life. Exercise professionals should spend a significant amount of evaluation time documenting and reviewing goals for rehabilitation and exercise participation. Individuals should be medically stable and willing to adhere to all facility rules and must becompliant with all prescribed medications, such as long-term oxygen therapy (2).

Exercise Testing Considerations

The safety and efficacy of 1RM assessments in individuals with COPD has been examined (20).

When proper testing and screening procedures are employed, even severely deconditioned individuals with COPD can be safely assessed using 1RM without incurring any abnormal cardiopulmonary responses, muscle injury, or significant muscle soreness (20). In studies, cardiopulmonary responses observed during 1RM testing were significantly lower than when the same individuals performed aerobic exercise at a submaximal level (20).

Training Program Components

Information collected during the evaluation and testing will be used to design an individualized exercise program. Training programs, in general, should attempt to achieve maximal physiologic training effects, but this approach may have to be modified because of disease severity, symptom-related limitations, comorbidities, and level of motivation (30). Based on the available research (see Table 13-2), resistance training for individuals with COPD should generally include 2 to 4 sets of 6 to 12 repetitions at intensities ranging from 50 to 85 percent of 1RM. Exercise professionals should be sure to employ exercises that have a mechanical similarity to functional deficits. The more similar training activities are to actual movements involved in daily living, the greater the likelihood of positive carryover to performance (3). Arranging exercise programs in the form of interval training is an appropriate exercise modality for individuals with COPD (21, 30, 44).

Psychological Issues with COPD

Individuals with COPD are at increased risk for developing anxiety and depression (30). They often experience fear and anxiety in anticipation of, and in association with, episodes of dyspnea. The anxiety can precipitate or exacerbate dyspnea, significantly increasing overall disability (30). The American Thoracic Society and European Respiratory Society recommend the following practice guidelines for

addressing anxiety and depression for individuals with COPD:

○ Individuals should be screened for anxiety and depression as part of an initial assessment.

○ Although mild or moderate levels of anxiety or depression related to the disease process may improve with pulmonary rehabilitation, individuals with significant psychiatric disease should be referred for appropriate professional care.

Given the natural progression of COPD and subjective reports of dyspnea with activity, the increased risk of depression and anxiety is easy to understand. The presence of anxiety and depression impact exercise program design in that exercise professionals must ease individuals into exercise at a lower intensity and duration than they can tolerate. Intensity and duration of training can be increased once the individual with COPD has become comfortable with the level of exertion (21, 30).

SAMPLE 24-WEEK PROGRAM

Resistance training should be performed on three nonconsecutive days per week. Aerobic exercise and flexibility training should also be included as appropriate.

Week 1

For the first training session, 1RM testing should be done. During the other two sessions, have the client perform a single set of 10 to 15 repetitions at 60 percent of 1RM for the following exercises: sit-to-stands, seated rows on an exercise machine, military presses, and step-ups.

Week 2

Week 2 should begin with 2 sets of 12 repetitions at 60 percent of 1RM for each exercise. Continue with the same exercises used in week 1, but add 1 to 2 sets of 15 repetitions of supine back extensions for core work.

Week 3

Continue with the same exercises, but increase exercise intensity to a single set of 8 to 12 repetitions at 80 percent of 1RM for each exercise.

Week 4

Continue with the same exercises, but increase exercise volume to 2 sets of 8 to 12 repetitions at 80 percent of 1RM for each exercise.

Week 5

Reassess 1RM for the first training session. During the remaining two sessions, perform 1 set of 15 repetitions at 60 percent of 1RM for each exercise. Continue with the same exercises, but substitute dumbbell deadlifts for sit-to-stand exercises. The addition of dumbbell exercises will increase the intensity and support efforts to enhance function.

Week 6

Begin with 2 sets of 12 repetitions at 60 percent of 1RM for each exercise.

Week 7

Begin with a single set of 8 to 12 repetitions at 80 percent of 1RM for each exercise.

Week 8

Begin with 2 sets of 8 to 12 repetitions at 80 percent of 1RM for each exercise.

Week 9

Reassess 1RM for the first training session. During the other two sessions, perform a single set of 15 repetitions at 60 percent of 1RM for the following exercises: dumbell deadlifts, bent-over rows with dumbbells, incline bench presses

with dumbbells, squats, bridging with 2 sets of 15 repetitions.

Week 10

Begin with 2 sets of 12 repetitions at 60 percent of 1RM.

Week 11

Begin with 1 set of 8 to 12 repetitions at 80 percent of 1RM.

Week 12

Begin with 2 sets of 8 to 12 repetitions at 80 percent of 1RM.

Week 13

Reassess 1RM for the first training session. During the other two sessions, perform 1 set of 15 repetitions at 60 percent of 1RM.

Week 14

Begin with 2 sets of 12 repetitions at 60 percent of 1RM.

Week 15

Begin with 1 set of 8 to 12 repetitions at 80 percent of 1RM.

Week 16

Begin with 2 sets of 8 to 12 repetitions at 80 percent of 1RM.

Week 17

Reassess 1RM for the first training session. During the other two sessions, begin with 1 set of 15 repetitions at 60 percent of 1RM.

Week 18

Begin with 2 sets of 12 repetitions at 60 percent of 1RM.

Week 19

Begin with 1 set of 8 to 12 repetitions at 80 percent of 1RM.

Week 20

Begin with 2 sets of 8 to 12 repetitions at 80 percent of 1RM.

Week 21

Reassess 1RM before the first session. During the other two sessions, perform 1 set of 15 repetitions at 60 percent of 1RM on the following exercises: push press with dumbbells, seated rows on an exercise machine, deadlifts with dumbbells, bridging with 2 to 3 sets of 15 repetitions.

Week 22

Begin with 2 sets of 12 repetitions at 60 percent of 1RM.

Week 23

Begin with 1 set of 8 to 12 repetitions at 80 percent of 1RM.

Week 24

Reassess 1RM, review the home exercise program, and perform 1 set of 15 repetitions at 60 percent of 1RM.

CASE STUDY

Mr. H is a 52-year-old male admitted to inpatient rehabilitation with a primary diagnosis of severe emphysema with an asthmatic component. He was transferred from an acute facility after a 12-day stay due to respiratory failure caused by a bout of pneumonia. Hospital notes report 10 days of mechanical ventilation with difficult extubation and a prolonged weaning period. Mr. H has a prior smoking history, but he has not smoked for the last 5 years. Pulmonary function tests performed prior to hospital admission show a predicted FEV_1 of 39 percent, with an increase up to 42 percent with administration of a bronchodilator. In addition to emphysema, Mr. H has hypertension that is controlled with medication. He has no other cardiac risk factors or history of diabetes.

Pulmonary rehabilitation reports that Mr. H covered 140 feet during a 6-minute walking test with oxygen saturations of 86 to 94 percent while on 2 liters per minute of supplemental oxygen. Heart rate and blood pressure were within normal limits, and Mr. H reported a rating of perceived exertion of 7 out of 10 on the dyspnea scale. He required moderate assistance to perform a sit-to-stand transfer from a chair and had several episodes of lost balance. During muscular strength assessment, heart rate, blood pressure, and oxygen saturations were within normal ranges. His 1RM measurements included a 5-pound military press, 20-pound seated rows, and one sit-to-stand. Mr. H indicated that his goals were to take care of himself, get off the supplemental oxygen, and return home.

The treatment team agreed to a 3-week stay for Mr. H and set the following training goals: 1) to be independent with self-care tasks and to be able to ambulate household distances with oxygen saturation within normal limits; 2) a demonstrated tolerance of 10 to 20 minutes of continuous aerobic exercise at 1 to 3 METs; 3) to be independent with purse-lip breathing and diaphragmatic breathing. In an attempt to wean Mr. H from supplemental oxygen, his physician ordered supplemental oxygen to be titrated to keep saturation above 90 percent.

Mr. H met with the inpatient pulmonary rehabilitation team daily. On Monday, Wednesday, and Friday, he performed the aerobic, resistance training, and flexibility components of his exercise program. Tuesday and Thursday sessions were devoted to aerobic conditioning and education on disease management. The resistance-training program was consistent with the first 3 weeks of the program presented in the 24-week sample discussed previously.

Mr. H was discharged from inpatient care on day 21 and continued with rehabilitation on an outpatient basis. He reported to the center three times per week for exercise conditioning and education. To aid in outpatient exercise prescription, 6-minute walk and 1RM testing were readministered. He ambulated 800 feet in 6 minutes with one rest break, had a rating of perceived exertion of 4 out of 10 on the dyspnea scale, and required 2 liters per minute of supplemental oxygen to keep saturation above 90 percent. 1RM exercises were performed with 20-pound chest presses, 50-pound seated rows, and step-ups with 3-pound dumbbells in each hand.

At the end of 12 weeks, Mr. H was discharged from the monitored outpatient program and agreed to continue coming to the rehabilitation center two times per week for independent, unmonitored sessions. He would perform his third exercise session at home. After 24 weeks, he reported increased activity around his house and community and demonstrated both an increase in 1RM testing and functional evaluations.

Summary

COPD is a chronic disease with no known cure. However, limitations in exercise capacity, quality of life, and participation in activities of daily living are many times lower than would be expected from changes in lung function. While optimal bronchodilation is the first step in the treatment of patients with COPD, greater treatment effects—that is, improvements in exercise performance, symptoms, and health-related quality of life—are often achieved only after the addition of pulmonary rehabilitation that addresses all facets of the disease. Exercise programs for individuals with COPD should contain an endurance, strength, and flexibility component. Recent reports in the literature provide many treatment modalities to improve functional mobility. However, the key to positive outcomes requires a thorough interview and physical exam. Individuals with COPD can only be helped if they actively participate in rehabilitation and exercise sessions. Therefore, treatment plans should enable individuals to reach their goals. Training programs, in general, should attempt to achieve maximal physiologic training effects, but

this approach may have to be modified because of disease severity, symptom limitation, comorbidities, and level of motivation. Furthermore, even though high-intensity targets are advantageous for inducing physiologic changes in patients who can reach these levels, low-intensity targets may be more important for long-term adherence and health benefits for a wider population.

Key Terms

Asthma
Chronic bronchitis
Chronic obstructive pulmonary disease (COPD)
Emphysema
Forced expiratory volume in one second (FEV_1)
Oxygen saturation
Pulse oximeter
Quality of life

Study Questions

1. Define COPD and the different conditions included in such a diagnosis.

2. How do clinicians quantify the severity of COPD?

3. What role does periodization play in the development of a resistance-training program for individuals with COPD?

4. What evidence is present to support 1RM testing for individuals with COPD?

5. Why is it important that resistance-training activities mimic functional deficits?

References

1. American College of Sports Medicine. *Guidelines for Exercise Testing and Prescription*. 3rd ed. Baltimore MD: Williams & Wilkins; 1998.

2. Atis S, Tutluoglu B, Bugdayci R. Characteristics and compliance of patients receiving long-term oxygen therapy (LTOT) in Turkey. *Monaldi Arch Chest Dis*. 2001;56(2):105–109.

3. Bachele TR, and Earle RW *Essentials of Strength Training and Conditioning.* Champaign, IL: Human Kinetics;1994.

4. Barnes P. Medical progress: chronic obstructive pulmonary disease. *N Engl J Med.* 2000; 343:269–280.

5. Bernard S, Whittom F, LeBlanc P, et al. Aerobic and strength training in patients with chronic obstructive disease. *Am J Resp Crit Care Med.* 1999;159:896–901.

6. Casaburi R. *Principles and Practice of Pulmonary Rehabilitation.* Philadelphia, PA: W. B. Saunders;1993.

7. Casaburi R. Skeletal muscle dysfunction in chronic obstructive pulmonary disease. *Med Sci Sports Exerc.* 2001;33(suppl7):S662–S670.

8. Centers for Disease Control and Prevention. *Surveillance for Asthma: United States, 1980–1999.* Atlanta, GA: *Morbidity and Mortality Weekly Report.* 2002.

9. *Chronic Obstructive Pulmonary Disease Surveillance: United States, 1971–2000. Morbidity and Mortality Weekly Report.* 8/2/200. 51(SS-6):1–16.

10. *Chronic Obstructive Pulmonary Disease: Fact Sheet.* Bethesda, MD: National Institutes of Health. Heart, Lung, and Blood Institute; 2003. NIH Publication No. 03-5229.

11. Clark CJ, Cochrane LM, Mackay E, Payton B. Skeletal muscle strength and endurance in patients with mild COPD and effects of weight training. *Eur Respir J.* 2000;15(1):92–97.

12. DeMeo DL, Mariani TJ, Lange C, et al. The serpine2 gene is associated with chronic obstructive pulmonary disease. *Am J Hum Genet.* 2006;78:253–264.

13. National Asthma Education and Prevention Program. Expert Panel Report: Guidelines for the diagnosis and management of asthma. Bethesda, Md.: National Institutes of Health,

National Heart, Lung, and Blood Institute. NIH Publication 91-3042,1991.

14. National Asthma Education and Prevention Program. Expert Panel Report 2: Guidelines for the diagnosis and management of asthma. Bethesda, Md.: National Institutes of Health, National Heart, Lung, and Blood Institute. NIH Publication 97-4051,1997.

15. Faryniarz K, Mahler DA. Writing an exercise prescription for patients with COPD. *J Respir Dis.* 1990;11(7):644–648.

16. Fiatarone MA. High-intensity strength training in nonagenarians: effects on skeletal muscle. *JAMA.* 1999;263(22):3029–3034.

17. Fish JE, Peters SP. Airway remodeling and persistent airway obstruction in asthma. *Allergy Clin Immunol.* 1999;104(suppl 3 pt 1): 509–516.

18. Friedman M, Hilleman DE. Economic burden of chronic obstructive pulmonary disease: impact of new treatment options. *Pharmacoeconomics.* 200119(3):245–254.

19. Hodgkin JE, Connors GL, Bell CW, eds. *Pulmonary Rehabilitation: Guidelines to Success.* 2nd ed. Philadelphia, PA: Lippincott, Williams & Wilkins; 1993.

20. Kaelin ME, Swank AM, Adams KJ, Barnard KL, Berning JM, Green A. Cardiopulmonary responses, muscle soreness, and injury during the one-repetition maximum assessment in pulmonary rehabilitation patients. *J Cardiopulm Rehabil.* 1999;19:366–372.

21. Kaelin ME, Swank AM, Barnard KL, Adams KJ, Beach P, Newman J. Physical fitness and quality of life outcomes in a pulmonary rehabilitation program utilizing symptom-limited interval training and resistance training. *JEP online.* 2001;4(3)30–37.

22. Kaelin ME. Case study: early intervention for COPD patients is essential. *JEP online.* 2000;3(1).

23. Kongsgaard M, Backer V, Jorgensen K, Kjaer M, Beyer N. Heavy resistance training increases muscle size, strength and physical function in elderly male COPD patients: a pilot study. *Respir Med.* 1998;98(10):1000–1007.

24. Lindberg A, Jonsson AC, Ronmark E, Lundgren R, Larsson LG, Lundback B. Prevalence of chronic obstructive pulmonary disease according to BTS, ERS, GOLD and ATS criteria in relation to doctor's diagnosis, symptoms, age, gender, and smoking habits. *Respiration.* 2005;72(5):471–479.

25. Marin JT, Ortega F, Cejudo P, Elias T, Sanchez H, Montemayor T. Peripheral muscular strength in stable COPD patients: correlation with respiratory function variables and quality of life. *Arch Bronconeumol.* 1999;35(3):117–121.

26. Mador J, Bozkanat E, Aggarwal A, Shaffer M, Kufel TJ. Endurance and strength training in patients with COPD. *Chest.* 2004;125: 2036–2045.

27. Mannino DM. COPD: Epidemiology, prevalence, morbidity and mortality, and disease heterogeneity. *Chest.* 2002;121:121–126.

28. McCance KL, Huether SE. *Pathophysiology: The Biological Basis for Disease in Adults and Children.* 5th ed. St. Louis, MO: Elsevier; 2006.

29. Morgan MDL, Calverley PMA, Clark CJ, Davidson AC, Garrod R, Goldman JM, Roberts E, Sawicka E, Singh SJ, Wallace L, and White R. British Thoracic Society Statement: Pulmonary Rehabilitation. Thorax;56:827–834,2001

30. Nici L, Donner C, Wouters E, Zuwallack R, Ambrosino N, Bourbeau J, Carone M, Celli B, Engelen M, Fahy B, Garvey C, Goldstein R, Gosselink R, Lareau S, MacIntyre N, Maltais F, Morgan M, O'Donnell D, Prefault C, Reardon J, Rochester C, Schols A, Singh S, and Troosters T. American Thoracic Society/ European Respiratory Society Statement on Pulmonary Rehabilitation. Am J Respir Crit Care Med. 2006;173:390–1413,2006.

31. Ortega F, Toral J, Cejudo P, et al. Comparison of effects of strength and endurance training in patients with chronic obstructive pulmonary disease. *Am J Respir Crit Care Med.* 2002;166:669–674.

32. O'Shea SD, Taylor NF, Paratz J. Peripheral muscle strength training in COPD. *Chest.* 2004;126(3):903–914.

33. Panton LB, Golden J, Broeder CE, Browder KD, Cestaro-Seifer DJ, Seifer FD. The effects of resistance training on functional outcomes in patients with chronic obstructive pulmonary disease. *Eur J Appl Physiol.* 2004;91:443–449.

34. Rochester CL. Exercise training in chronic obstructive pulmonary disease. *J Rehabil Res Dev.* 2003;40(5):59–80.

35. Rubin BK. What does it mean when a patient says, "My asthma medication is not working?" *Chest.* 2004;126:972–981.

36. Simpson K, Killian K, McCartney N, Stubbing DG, Jones NL. Randomized controlled trial of weight-lifting exercise in patients with chronic airflow limitation. *Thorax.* 1992;47(2):70–75.

37. Spruitt MA, Gosselink R, Troosters T, De Paepe K, Decramer M. Resistance versus endurance training in patients with COPD and peripheral muscle weakness. *Eur Respir J.* 2002;19:1072–1078.

38. Strassels SA, Smith DH, Sullivan SD, Mahajan PS. The costs of treating COPD in the United States. *Chest.* 2001;119:344–352.

39. Taylor NF, Dodd KJ, Damiano DL. Progressive resistance exercise in physical therapy: a summary of systematic reviews. *Phys Ther.* 2005;85:1208–1223.

40. Tetley TD. Macrophages and the pathogenesis of COPD. *Chest.* 2002;121:156S–159S.

41. Troosters T, Casaburi R, Gosselink R, Decramer, M. Pulmonary rehabilitation in chronic obstructive pulmonary disease. *Am J Respir Crit Care Med.* 2005;172:19–38.

42. Tobin MJ, Cook PJ, Hutchison DC. Alpha$_1$-antitrypsin deficiency: the clinical and physiological features of pulmonary emphysema in subjects homozygous for Pi type. *Br J Dis Chest.* 1983;77(1):14–27.

43. Wright PR, Heck H, Langenkamp H, Franz KH, Weber U. Influence of a resistance training program on pulmonary function and performance measures of patients with COPD. *Pneumologie.* 2002;56(7):413–417.

44. Wilson M, Swank AM, Felker J. Exercise strategies for the individual with chronic obstructive pulmonary disease. *Strength and Conditioning Journal.* 2004;26(3):58–63.

45. Summary Health Statistics for U.S. children: National Health Interview Survey, 2002. Series 10, Number 221:2004 page 1549. Available at http://www.aaaai.org/media/statistics/asthma-statistics.asp

46. Centers for Disease Control and Prevention. National Center for Health Statistics. Asthma prevalence, health care use and mortality 2002. Available at: http://www.cdc.gov/nchs/products/pubs/pubd/hestats/asthma/asthma.htm. Accessed June 11, 2008.

47. COPD International. COPD statistical information. Available at: http://www.copd-international.com/library/statistics.htm. Accessed June 11, 2008.

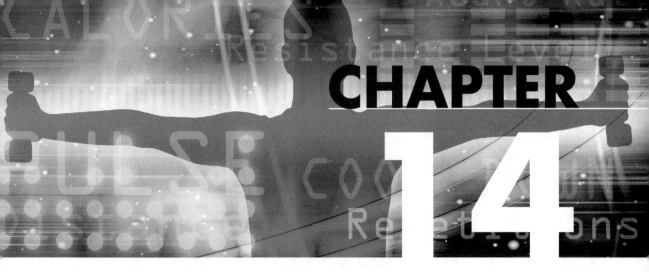

CHAPTER 14

RESISTANCE-TRAINING STRATEGIES FOR INDIVIDUALS WITH MENTAL RETARDATION

Objectives

Upon completion of this chapter, the reader should be able to:

○ Discuss the prevalence of mental retardation (MR) in its many forms
○ Describe how MR develops and is treated
○ Identify research evaluating the impact of resistance training for individuals with MR
○ Design a resistance-training program for individuals with MR, taking into account health status, readiness, safety issues, progression, and outcome assessment measures

INTRODUCTION

Developmental disabilities that develop before or after birth affect physical or mental development, and this term may refer to one or more of several potential disabilities that affect the normal development of a child. Some of the more common types of developmental disabilities include mental retardation, cerebral palsy, autism, spina bifida, and vision or hearing impairment. Of these conditions, **mental retardation (MR),** an intellectual and developmental disorder characterized by substandard IQ and need of support, is the most common developmental disorder in industrialized society (4, 12). In the past, diagnosis of MR was made according to an IQ score, using one of the standardized intelligence tests such as the Wechsler Adult Intelligence Scale or the Stanford-Binet Scale. Based on IQ scores, individuals were classified into four categories: mild MR, with IQ scores between 50 and 70; moderate MR, with IQ scores between 35 and 40; severe MR, with IQ scores between 25 and 40; and profound MR, with IQ scores below 25 (4, 12, 38). Although these classifications are still widely used and referred to, a new classification system has been adopted by the American Association on Mental Retardation. They define MR as being manifested by significantly subaverage intellectual functioning evident before age 18, existing concurrently with related limitations in two or more of the following adaptive skills areas: communication, self-care, home living, social skills, community use, self-direction, health and safety, functional academics, and leisure and work (1).

The Individuals with Disabilities Education Act (IDEA) adds schooling as a criteria and defines MR as significantly subaverage general intellectual functioning, existing concurrently with deficits in adaptive behavior manifested during the developmental period that adversely affect a child's educational performance. Significant subaverage general intellectual function is typically defined as an IQ of two standard deviations below the expected mean. Consequently, individuals with MR usually have an IQ below 70 and several deficits in adaptive skills. MR is developmental in nature but is no longer considered a static, unchangeable condition.

Although MR cannot be "cured" per se but is now recognized as a fluid condition, some individuals may, with early intervention, progress to the point where they would no longer be diagnosed with MR (4).

Under the current definition of MR, there are only two levels, mild and severe, instead of the traditional four levels. Classification is based primarily on how well the individual functions in the adaptive skill areas and the level of support the individual needs due to their deficit in adaptive skills (13). There are four designated levels of support: intermittent, requiring support on an as-needed basis, either high or low intensity; limited, in which support is needed consistently over time but of lesser intensity; extensive, requiring regular involvement in at least some environments; and pervasive, requiring constant high-intensity support across environments, or constant care. The more support a person requires, the less functional they are. Typically, those with mild MR have IQs between 35 and 70, need adaptive schooling, and have some minimal but not extensive reading, writing, and math capabilities. Most can be productive in unskilled or semiskilled jobs, and they may manage independent living but often live in group homes in the community.

PREVALENCE AND ECONOMIC IMPACT OF MR

The estimated prevalence of mental retardation in industrialized society is 3 percent of the total population (4, 12). If this estimate is correct, approximately 9 million individuals with MR live in the United States. Estimates classify over 90 percent of all people with MR as having mild MR (4, 13). Many of these individuals exhibit only marginal developmental disabilities, and other people may not consider them as having MR. Individuals with severe MR almost always have IQs below 50 and often have IQs below 35, and they are usually dependent on others for care. This group of individuals with MR will often exhibit gross motor deficits, anatomical deformities, and sensory deficits. Most individuals with severe MR will have substantial problems with simple self-care skills (4) and will need to live in a supported living environment. However, only 10 percent or less of the population with MR would be considered to have severe MR.

Most people with MR live in the community either independently, with family, in group homes, or in assisted-living facilities. This finding is a result of a movement for deinstitutionalization that has occurred over the past 30 to 40 years, and most large, institutional facilities have now been closed. As a result, most individuals with MR are fully or partially integrated in society, a process that has been aided by mainstreaming children with MR in public schools. Consequently, a high likelihood exists that exercise professionals will encounter individuals with MR either in school- or community-based programs (37).

Mortality rates are higher in populations with MR compared to populations without MR, and estimates vary between 1.5 to 4 times higher than expected (22, 41). Mortality is typically linked to low IQ and poor self-care skills. However, low levels of physical activity may also contribute to the higher mortality and morbidity of individuals with MR (17, 22). This finding is consistent with the fact that cardiovascular and pulmonary disorders are the most common medical problems in people with MR, except for those with **Down Syndrome (DS)**, a kind of MR characterized by an extra chromosome and specific physical characteristics (22, 32). For individuals with DS, infections, leukemia, and early development of Alzheimer's disease are the most frequent causes of both mortality and morbidity (10).

ETIOLOGY OF MR

Although many potential causes of MR are known, the specific cause is usually unknown. The most common cause of MR is **fetal alcohol syndrome,** a permanent birth defect resulting from prenatal maternal alcohol consumption, with an estimated incidence rate of 1 in 100 births—roughly one third

of all cases of MR (4, 27). Maternal drug abuse is the second leading cause of MR, followed by other causes that include birth trauma, as in cerebral palsy; infectious diseases, such as toxoplasmosis, rubella and herpes, which may occur in the mother during pregnancy or may affect the child after birth; maternal disorders; genetic disorders; chromosomal abnormalities, such as Down syndrome; poverty that results in malnutrition; severe stimulus deprivation; perinatal factors, such as prematurity or low birth weight; and postnatal factors, such as lead poisoning (4, 13, 27).

DOWN SYNDROME

Down syndrome (DS) is the most common manifestation of MR, with an incidence rate of approximately 1 in 800 to 1 in 1000 births (41). The risk of having a child with DS increases with maternal age, with an incidence rate of 1 in 400 for women over 35 years of age (4). This incidence rate increases to 1 in 45 in mothers aged 45 years (4). Individuals with DS present a special challenge to exercise professionals because of physical and physiological characteristics often associated with this condition that include short stature, short arms and legs, poor muscle tone, malformations of the feet and toes, and visual impairments. Most individuals with DS also exhibit joint laxity, which is especially important because of the common occurrence of **atlantoaxial instability,** an excessive mobility at the junction between the first and second cervical vertebrae due to either a bony or ligamentous abnormality, which can be a life-threatening condition. Most children with DS also have **skeletal muscle hypotonia,** a diminution of muscle tone marked by a diminished resistance to passive stretching. There have also been reports of **pulmonary hypoplasia,** an incomplete development of lung tissue resulting in reduced lung weight and volume, reduced alveolar count, and so on (41). More importantly, as many as half of all individuals born with DS have congenital heart disease (4, 41). Finally, reduced immune function, a much higher risk than normal of developing leukemia, and a higher risk of developing early Alzheimer's disease provide substantial challenges for exercise participation for people with DS (10, 27, 41).

BENEFITS OF RESISTANCE TRAINING FOR INDIVIDUALS WITH MR

The importance of physical activity for individuals with MR should not be underestimated. Although little research shows a direct relationship between physical activity and mortality in people with MR, physical activity likely plays an important role in developing and maintaining independent living in this population (11, 17, 37). Since muscle strength is very low in people with MR, resistance training can play an important role in not just increasing strength but also in increasing quality of life, independence, and vocational productivity (11).

Comparative Levels of Muscle Strength

Muscle strength has been extensively evaluated in people with MR of all ages using a variety of measurement tools including field tests, free weights, exercise machines, hand-grip dynamometry, hand-held dynamometry, leg and back dynamometry, and isokinetic dynamometry (9, 16, 21, 24, 25, 33, 35, 36, 44). Regardless of the type of measurement, the results are very uniform for all ages and genders. Individuals with MR have very low levels of strength, usually 30 to 50 percent of that of nondisabled individuals (24, 25, 35, 36). Individuals with DS exhibit even lower levels of muscle strength, typically 30 to 40 percent lower than their peers with MR and less than 50 percent of the expected strength levels of their nondisabled peers (3, 9, 36). These low levels of muscle strength are present in childhood (16, 24, 33) and persist into adulthood (9, 25, 36, 43). Interestingly, in individuals with MR who were extremely active and exhibited very high aerobic capacity, muscle strength was still

below expected levels—about 25 percent below the strength values of age- and activity-matched subjects without MR (20). This finding suggests that regardless of physical activity levels, people with MR have altered muscle function.

Only a few studies have evaluated muscle strength in children and adolescents with MR, and most of these have used isokinetic dynamometry to measure muscle strength (16, 24, 33), although one study used hand-held dynamometry (34). These studies consistently show reduced strength of the lower body in individuals with MR; upper-body strength was not measured. These findings may be especially important, because lower-body muscle strength is particularly important for efficient movement and independence (7, 37). Considering that lower-body muscle strength is a prerequisite for adequate performance and participation in recreational activities (23), physical activity levels appear to be associated with lower-body muscle strength (29).

Interestingly, the developmental trajectory of muscle strength in children with MR does not appear to be altered (34). This finding suggests that most children with MR increase muscle strength in an expected manner from childhood through late adolescence; however, the absolute level of muscle strength is still approximately 30 to 50 percent below the muscle strength of their nondisabled peers. This relationship is illustrated in Figure 14-1.

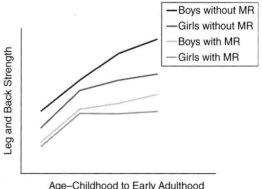

Figure 14-1

© Delmar/Cengage Learning

The low levels of muscle strength in adults with MR may have serious implications. Not only is muscle strength important for recreational activities, it may also be important for vocational productivity (8, 13, 30). Furthermore, muscle strength is related to aerobic capacity and endurance run performance in people with MR (16, 33, 35). This finding illustrates that typical endurance-type activities are probably also limited by poor muscle strength in this population. This relationship is not demonstrated in children and young adults without MR, because endurance performance and muscle strength are unrelated in nondisabled populations. However, this relationship has been shown in the frail elderly (17), suggesting that the low levels of muscle strength in populations with MR may contribute to early or accelerated aging. Thus, resistance-exercise programs may have very important implications for people with MR beyond simply increasing muscle strength.

Literature Review of Research Supporting Resistance Training for Individuals with MR

Early studies on individuals with MR used field tests including sit-ups, push-ups, and pull-ups to measure muscle function responses to exercise training programs. However, these tests are now recognized as primarily tests of muscle endurance and muscle strength. Nevertheless, Solomon and Pangle (42) showed substantial improvements in both sit-ups and chin-ups following an 8-week training program for boys with mild MR. These improvements were observed despite devoting only 15 minutes of physical education class activities, suggesting very low initial fitness levels or a substantial learning effect not related to actual improvements in muscle strength or endurance. Hussey and colleagues (26) showed similar improvements in sit-up performance in young adults (mean age 31 years). They conducted an intense 3-week program in a sheltered workshop setting, exercising the participants 1 hour per day, 5 days per week. Those individuals who participated in the program increased their performance by 58 percent, but controls from the same workshop did not change.

Montgomery and colleagues (28) also conducted an exercise program in a sheltered workshop setting in two phases. The first phase consisted of a 6-month program, and the second phase employed a 4-month program (with different participants). The program consisted of 40 minutes of overall fitness activities 3 days per week. Although sit-up and push-up performance increased substantially, no changes in hand-grip strength were observed, suggesting that muscle strength did not improve. However, hand-grip strength was not specifically addressed in the exercise program, thus improvements should not have been expected. In fact, the hand-grip test is probably not an appropriate test for measuring muscle strength improvements, because improved hand-grip strength is not normally targeted as an exercise goal during these types of programs. However, even non–strength-specific exercise programs clearly improve muscle endurance in people with MR. A more recent study (8) showed that using surgical tubing during the exercise sessions improved muscle strength. Thus, nontraditional muscle strength and endurance programs will have beneficial effects, but the effects will reflect the type of training conducted.

Using a more traditional resistance-training regimen, Rimmer and Kelly (40) conducted a 9-week circuit-resistance program consisting of two sessions per week using variable resistance machines. The exercise group improved muscle strength on all eight exercises used. The resistance-training group scored significantly higher than a control group on five of the eight exercises after the training program, showing the efficacy of more traditional resistance training for individuals with MR. However, this was not a randomized controlled study, thus self-selection may have played a role in the findings.

Suomi and colleagues (44) conducted the first randomized controlled trial on the effects of resistance training in men with mild MR (age ~30 years). The subjects exercised 3 days per week for 12 weeks using hydraulic exercise machines. The program utilized one set of 10 repetitions at the start, gradually increasing to 5 sets of 10 repetitions, an intensity equivalent to 70 to 80 percent of one-repetition maximum (1RM).

Peak muscle strength increased between 8 to 82 percent depending on the measurement used, whereas the control group showed strength changes from -5.6 to 15 percent.

In a follow-up study, Suomi (43) continued to train six of the men and also followed six controls for an additional period of 12 weeks of supervised training, followed by a period of 9 months of self-directed, unsupervised training. The exercise program was the same as described above. The exercise group showed improvements in muscle strength between 19 to 36 percent, whereas the control group *decreased* their mean strength after the initial 12 weeks. Following the 9-month, self-directed training program, neither group altered their strength levels, showing muscle strength was maintained during the self-directed portion of the program. These findings have important implications, because they show that self-motivated individuals with mild MR can successfully maintain strength gains on their own without supervised programming after a period of supervised exercise training in which they learned how to conduct the exercises.

Although traditional resistance-training programs have not been conducted with individuals with DS, several studies have shown changes in strength with a variety of training approaches. Peran and colleagues (31) found that a high-intensity sports-training program, consisting primarily of running activities and circuit-track training, had a beneficial impact on strength in individuals 17 to 21 years of age. After a year of training two to three times per week, an increase in strength of approximately 10 percent was observed. This increase was small compared with the 75 percent improvement in endurance, probably reflecting the nature of the program. Carmeli and colleagues (6) evaluated the effect of a walking program in institutionalized older individuals with DS (age ~63 years) using a randomized controlled design. Subjects in the walking group participated in a treadmill-walking program three times per week for 25 weeks. Muscle strength improved significantly more than for control subjects, ranging from 6.9 to 18 percent. The study also showed that participants in the

walking program improved balance and walking function. These fairly large changes resulting from a nonspecific endurance program were probably a reflection of severe initial deconditioning of the participants. Tsimaras and colleagues (45) recently conducted a 12-week training study in individuals with DS using jumping and balance activities. Participants in the training group improved muscle strength between 12 and 25 percent, whereas the control group did not change. Unfortunately, the groups were not randomly assigned, which detracted from the findings. However, the study also showed that dynamic balance was substantially improved with training, further substantiating the beneficial effects of the program. This type of jumping, high-intensity program might be difficult for many individuals with DS.

The best evidence for the effect of resistance training in individuals with DS was provided by Rimmer and colleagues (39). They conducted a randomized controlled study with 52 participants using a combination of endurance and resistance training. The participants exercised using endurance exercise—such as cycle ergometry, treadmill walking, or elliptical trainers—for 30 minutes each session, followed by one set of resistance training consisting of 10 to 20 repetitions at 70 percent of 1RM using a circuit-type program design three times per week. Following the 12-week program, the exercise group increased their bench press and leg press strength by 39 to 43 percent, whereas the control group did not change. Interestingly, neither group changed hand-grip strength, indicating this mode of strength testing is inappropriate to evaluate the effects of resistance training. However, this study, with supporting evidence from other studies presented above, clearly shows that individuals with DS can increase muscle strength with a variety of exercise training protocols. This finding may be partially attributed to the very low initial levels of strength in this population, because people with poor initial levels would be expected to improve more than someone with higher levels of strength at the start. Table 14-1 provides details of several related resistance-training studies involving subjects with MR.

Table 14-1 Review of Studies on Resistance Training in Individuals with Intellectual Disabilities

Study	Subjects	Program Design	Results
Croce et al. (8)	3 men (age 25 yrs) with MR	60 min/day; 3–4 days/wk, 24 wks 10 min warm up (stretching) 20 min resistance training (upper body using surgical tubing; 3 sets of 8–12 reps) 20 min aerobic exercise (65–85% HR_{max}) 10 min cool down	Exercise increased measures of muscular strength, aerobic capacity, and work productivity.
Rimmer et al. (39)	52 adults (age 39 yrs) with DS Exercise group (n = 30) Control (n = 22)	45 min/day, 3 days/wk, 12 wks 30–45 min aerobic exercise (50–70% VO_{2peak}) 15–20 min resistance training (70% 1RM, 10–20 reps)	The exercise group experienced increases in aerobic capacity, muscular strength, and muscular endurance.
Rimmer & Kelly (40)	24 adults (age 34 yrs) with MR Exercise group (n = 12) Control (n = 12)	60 min day, 2 days/wk, 9 wks Resistance training (machine based, 70% 1RM, 3 sets, 8–10 reps)	The exercise group experienced increases in muscular strength.
Suomi (43)	12 adults (age 27 yrs) with MR Exercise group (n = 6) Control (n = 6)	12 wks trainer-directed hydraulic resistance training, 1 yr self-directed hydraulic resistance training	The exercise group increased strength following supervised training and maintained the gain in strength following self-directed training.
Suomi et al. (44)	22 men (age 30 yrs) with MR Exercise group (n = 11) Control (n = 11)	12 wks hydraulic resistance training	The exercise group experienced increases in strength and total work.
Tsimaras et al. (45)	25 men (age 25 yrs) with DS Exercise group (n = 15) Control (n = 10)	30–35 min/day; 3 days/wk 12 wks of exercise training consisting of plyometric and balance tasks	The exercise group experienced increases in muscular strength, muscular endurance, and dynamic balance.

DESIGNING RESISTANCE-TRAINING PROGRAMS FOR INDIVIDUALS WITH MR

The most important factors to consider for program design in individuals with MR are 1) the level of understanding of the individual, 2) the individual's attention span, 3) the level of fitness or prior exercise experience, 4) the age of the individual, 5) any potential physical impairments or significant problems with coordination, 6) individualization of the program, 7) the reason for the program or the goals of the individual, and 8) medications.

The level of understanding of the individual is very important. This factor will influence the entire program process, because some individuals with MR may not understand why resistance training is important or why they should do it, or they may not understand instructions on how to conduct the program or how to perform individual exercises. The level of understanding is also influenced by the person's attention span and their socialization skills. Many individuals with MR have limited understanding and limited attention spans; but there is a wide range, and some will be completely able to understand and will have very good attention spans. Inappropriate social behavior is also common. These difficulties may include oppositional disorders, depression, phobias, sensitivity to noise, withdrawal behavior or shyness, dementia, hallucinations and altered psychotic perceptions, and self-talk. This factor must be taken into account, because of the potential impact not only on the individual but on others if the program is conducted in a public facility or as a group program.

Individuals with MR tend to be frail and have an earlier onset of aging than the general population (37). As a result, the age of the person will impact both the type of program used and the implementation of the program. Most people with MR will require a more prolonged initial phase of resistance training than the general population of a similar age, and they will require a slower progression thereafter.

This finding is directly tied to their prior exercise experience and level of muscular fitness. However, most individuals with MR are very sedentary, are more likely to be overweight or obese, and have very low levels of muscular strength (11, 13, 15, 17, 37, 38). Consequently, for most people with MR, the initial program needs to be low level with slow progression.

Exercise progression will also be influenced by the level of coordination of the individual and whether they have any physical impairment. Individuals with MR commonly have multiple disabling conditions, including serious motor dysfunction and/or metabolic problems such as diabetes. The disabling conditions will impact the type of program used, equipment choices, and the selection of specific exercises. Since motor problems are commonly manifested unilaterally, motor impairments in particular can be a challenge in appropriate program design. Consequently, individualization of the program is of primary importance, because most individuals will exhibit combinations of different levels of the conditions mentioned above.

Depending on the level of understanding of the individual, he or she may not be able to understand the importance of participating in resistance exercise and thus may exhibit limited motivation. Parents or caretakers commonly choose to have the person participate, thus participation may not be a personal choice, creating a substantial challenge for motivation and enjoyment of the program (11, 13, 37). This challenge includes motivation to perform the exercises correctly in the program, as well as motivation to stay with the program and prevent dropout. Programs should be supervised by qualified personnel for the first 6 months, not just to provide feedback and motivation during the sessions, but also to ensure proper exercise technique and breathing (14). Motivational techniques need to be individualized. Most people with MR enjoy music during their training, thus playing their favorite music can be a powerful motivational tool (14). For some individuals with MR, exercising in a group setting is a powerful motivator, whereas others do not have the attention capabilities to conduct group exercise successfully. An individual with MR rarely begins a program with personal goals of achievement, although this does occur, especially for those who participate in athletic competitions. Consequently, an exercise professional needs to invest substantial effort in individuals with MR to help them understand and enjoy the program, as well to set appropriate goals. Goal setting is an effective and essential part of a successful program, but it requires careful thought and planning.

Although most individuals with MR are not taking any medications, some may take various psychotropic medications, and antidepressants are fairly common. Some of these medications can be very strong, especially those used to control psychotic behavior. Standard cardiovascular medications are also used, as are diabetic medications. For instance, the use of beta blockers is common, especially in older individuals with MR; but interestingly, these may also be used in individuals who are still adolescents. A common complication in people with DS is hypothyroidism, thus these individuals will be on a thyroxine replacement therapy. Furthermore, since the prevalence of congenital heart problems may be as high as 50 percent in people with DS, this population will probably take a variety of cardiovascular medications. Most of the medications discussed above do not affect the response to resistance training per se, but heart rate and blood pressure responses may be slightly altered. These medications can also make the individual tired and may cause a loss of concentration, thus increasing the difficulty in motivating the individual during the exercise program.

Exercise Testing Considerations

Before participation in any exercise program, a thorough health history screening should be conducted. Screening questionnaires will usually need to be used in an interview format if the questions are asked directly of the individuals with MR. However, also interview the parent or guardian in addition to the participant to ensure that accurate information is provided. During this process, screen for any form of cardiovascular disease, diabetes,

cancer, lung disease, infectious diseases, some individuals with MR have reduced immune function and are prone to infections, neurological conditions, orthopedic conditions, medications, exercise history, and lifestyle history. Most standard health history questionnaires will cover this information (2). Because individuals with DS have an increased incidence of congenital heart disease, questions must be asked correctly to ensure that screening for these conditions, and not just atherosclerotic heart disease, is appropriately conducted. Congenital heart conditions encountered may include septal or valvular defects, aortic arch defects, and tetralogy of Fallot. Today, these conditions are surgically corrected in infancy, thus most of the individuals with DS who have these conditions may not know about it but should present with a visible scar.

Atlantoaxial instability makes individuals with DS susceptible to serious spinal cord injury, so screening for atlantoaxial instability is essential and may be a contraindication to resistance training. People with DS also have lax ligaments in general and are prone to joint hyperflexion and hyperextension, so this condition needs to be screened for and considered when designing the training program. For individuals with congenital heart disease, atlantoaxial instability, or any other medical condition that may jeopardize their safety during exercise, a physician's clearance should be obtained prior to commencing the exercise program. In some instances, exercise participation may be contraindicated.

Conditions such as difficulty with task understanding, short attention span, difficulty understanding directions, poor motivation to perform, and other behavioral problems make an appropriate familiarization process essential when working with individuals with MR (17). The familiarization process should focus on making the individual comfortable with the program setting, providing them with an opportunity to learn how to use the equipment appropriately, practicing the test protocols, and getting to know program and testing personnel. The familiarization process is highly individual and may require minimal time or several sessions before the testing is actually conducted. Without appropriate familiarization, testing will probably not yield any usable information. Suggestions for sequencing the familiarization process have been made (18, 37), however these recommendations have not been systematically investigated.

It is generally agreed that testing muscle strength should be conducted using weight machines or isokinetic equipment (14, 42, 43). However, isokinetic equipment is typically not available for training. Free weights may not be safe for use with many individuals with MR and are usually avoided. Thus, the most appropriate tests should be conducted on the same machines used for training. Although standard 1RM testing protocols have been used, using submaximal loads and estimating the 1RM is also appropriate. Considering potential problems with task understanding, motivation to perform, and lack of experience with maximal efforts, a 10- to 12-repetition set to fatigue can be successfully used, and 1RM can be estimated using standard formulas (5). Even with this approach, a true set to fatigue may be difficult to elicit in individuals with MR, especially for those with little prior exercise experience. Therefore, testing should be repeated on a consistent basis during the first 2 weeks of the training program. This procedure can easily be built into the training program, because 10 to 12 repetitions are commonly used for training. Eight to twelve exercises using major muscle groups should be tested and then used in the program. Depending on the capabilities of the person, this recommendation may be adjusted up or down as appropriate. American College of Sports Medicine (ACSM) or National Strength and Conditioning Association guidelines for resistance training should be followed with the above modifications (2, 5).

Training Program Components

To minimize the chance of injury and muscle soreness, the first step in any resistance-training program for individuals with MR must be to ensure that they can perform each exercise with appropriate form. Furthermore, proper breathing technique needs to be taught, because most individuals with MR will automatically perform the Valsalva maneuver when lifting a heavy weight. This training becomes part of the familiarization process and may take several weeks to accomplish. Intermittent reinforcement will probably be needed on a biweekly basis thereafter.

Considering that most individuals with MR are fairly deconditioned, the program should start with a 2- to 3-week period during which lighter weights are used to teach participants proper technique and get them used to conducting the exercises (39). Although no specific guidelines exist, an intensity of 40 to 50 percent of 1RM is an appropriate starting load. This intensity can easily be handled for 10 to 12 repetitions, and most participants will avoid undue muscle soreness using this load. During this time, proper breathing technique should also be continuously emphasized—inhale on the eccentric, and exhale on the concentric—possibly with the use of verbal cues, such as "breathe in" and "breathe out." Ensure that participants control both concentric and eccentric portions of the contraction, and instruct them not to simply drop the weight during the eccentric portion. The ACSM recommends a 3-second concentric contraction and a 3-second eccentric contraction (2). The initial period may need to be longer for those with poorer cognitive ability, and the length of the initial period must vary with the skill level of the individual and will be up to the discretion of the exercise professional.

In addition, a prolonged warm-up, both muscle specific and general, is also indicated and can easily be accomplished by having participants ride a cycle ergometer or walk on a treadmill for 5 to 7 minutes before starting their resistance training (5, 39). Warm-up should then be followed by an easy set for each resistance exercise (40 to 50 percent of 1RM), conducted before the normal sets. Include a flexibility program prior to and following the program, focusing on the muscle groups used during the resistance training. The exercise program after the first few weeks would then follow ACSM guidelines (2) for resistance programs for healthy adults, which includes training 2 to 3 days per week using 8RM to 12 RM (approximately 70 to 85 percent of 1RM) for 1 to 3 sets with 1 to 2 minutes rest between sets.

Frequent retesting to demonstrate strength improvements is also important. Retesting should not be difficult, because the program will normally employ an 8RM to 12RM approach, which means improvements can be easily documented. Increasing the resistance when appropriate during the program is necessary, otherwise improvements will be minimized. Most populations can easily be taught to monitor themselves, but this will probably not work for most people with MR. Gauging intensity can be difficult in this population, because participants may grimace and grunt excessively even during submaximal loads. Therefore, instead of assessing exercise intensity by attaining a rating of perceived exertion from the participant, the exercise professional can subjectively gauge signs of participant muscular fatigue—such as excessive slowing of the concentric–eccentric duty cycle, loss of proper form, "cheating" to complete repetitions, or failure to complete target repetitions—and adjust the load accordingly.

Consistent with published guidelines, exercises should be selected that stress all major muscle groups (2, 5). Due to the smaller stature of individuals with DS, ensure that all machines are adjusted properly prior to exercise initiation. Due to their smaller stature, the feet of participants with DS may not reach the floor during the performance of certain exercises, such as a machine chest press. This reduces overall stability. Given the possibility of poor balance in this population, additional raised platforms may be needed upon which participants may rest their feet to stabilize the torso. The platform may also serve as a step to help participants comfortably get into the machine. Sample exercises are listed in Table 14-2.

Spotting is particularly important in this population. Do not assume that machines are safer and require less supervision. Although not common, individuals with MR may lose interest halfway through a set, or even a repetition, and simply stop. For most machines, this does not pose a problem. However, for a select few exercises, stopping in the middle could result in injury, such as letting go of the bar during a lat pulldown. The supervising exercise professional should be thoroughly familiar with correct spotting

techniques for all exercises. The National Strength and Conditioning Associations' *Essentials of Strength and Conditioning* text includes a detailed description of spotting techniques (5).

SAMPLE 24-WEEK PROGRAM

Weeks 1 through 2

The initial 2 weeks will be used to familiarize the individual with the selected exercises, teach proper breathing techniques, and evaluate 1RM on each exercise. Training should take place on 3 nonconsecutive days each week with at least 1 day of rest between sessions. Individuals will complete 1 set of 12 to 15 repetitions at 40 to 50 percent of 1RM on each exercise.

Week 3

This week is a transitional period in which load is increased to 50 to 60 percent of 1RM. Continue with the same exercises completed three times a week, but increase to 3 sets of 12 to 15 repetitions, allowing 1 to 2 minutes rest between each set.

Weeks 4 through 12

During this period, the load is increased to 60 to 75 percent of 1RM. Continue with 3 sets, but widen the range of repetitions to 10 to 15 to allow for the heavier load. Remain on the same thrice-weekly schedule.

Week 13

Use this week to reassess 1RM on each exercise, and add new exercises as appropriate.

Weeks 14 through 24

Return to the thrice-weekly schedule. Complete 3 sets of 8 to 12 repetitions at 75 to 85 percent of the new 1RM measured during week 13.

Table 14-2 Sample Resistance Exercises and Suggestions for Optimal Performance

Muscle Group	Exercises	Tips
Chest Pectoralis major	Seated chest press*	If participant's feet do not reach the floor, place platforms on the ground as footrests to increase stability.
Back Latissimi dorsi	Lat pulldown (to the chest)	Due to possible shoulder joint laxity, it is advised to have participants perform this exercise to the front rather than behind the head.
Shoulders deltoids	Shoulder/military press*	If participant's feet do not reach the floor, place platforms on the ground as footrests to increase stability.
Arms Biceps brachii	Cable biceps curl*	
Arms Triceps brachii	Cable triceps extension*	
Legs Quadriceps, gluteals	Squat (warm up)	Start with a chair sit-to-stand; progress to a body-weight squat. Increase body-weight resistance using dumbbells or other handheld weights.
Legs Quadriceps, gluteals	Leg press machine*	Care should be taken when helping obese individuals into the machine. Due to possible joint laxity, verbally cue participants to terminate the eccentric contraction and initiate the concentric contraction (i.e., lower the weight until the knee forms a 45-degree angle).
Legs Quadriceps	Seated leg extension*	
Legs Hamstrings, quadriceps, gluteals	Seated leg curl*	Due to smaller limbs, participants with DS may not properly fit in a supine leg curl machine.
Abdominals Rectus abdominus	Crunch	Use of an abdominal frame may help ensure proper form.

*If gross muscular imbalances occur, exercises may be performed unilaterally.

CASE STUDY

Mr. J is a 24-year-old male with Down Syndrome. Following physician clearance, he is set to begin a resistance-training program for general health promotion. Mr. J lives at home and has a part time job at a local shopping center. His parents are very excited about the exercise program, however Mr. J is not motivated to participate in resistance training. After work, he takes part in several recreational and competitive activities at a local disability center, including softball and swimming. His functional capacity is exceptional.

Although Mr. J masters correct form and breathing technique for all exercises within the first week, a 3-week run-in period, as outlined above, is still carried out to reduce the risk of injury to joint connective tissue. Given his short stature, a platform is needed to increase his stability during such exercises as the seated chest press and shoulder press. An adjustable

aerobics step is used and adequately provides a stable surface on which he may plant his feet during exercise. Sessions are conducted three times per week, consisting of 3 sets of 10 to 12 reps at 75 to 85 percent of 1RM with 1 to 2 minutes rest in between each set. Each session lasts approximately 45 minutes.

To increase motivation, Mr. J is allowed to listen to his favorite music during the exercise session. The exercise professional also highlights how several exercises will help him become a better softball player and swimmer. They show how a squat may help him scoop up a ground ball faster and how a lat pulldown will help him with his freestyle stroke. The trainer also locates several pictures of his favorite athletes performing similar exercises. During the first 3 weeks, increases in strength that Mr. J experiences are presented to him in graphical form and increase his motivation substantially. As can be seen from Table 14-3, he experienced substantial strength gains from this exercise program.

Table 14-3 Strength Gains for Several Exercises from a 12-week Resistance Training Intervention in a Young Man with DS

Exercise	Baseline 1-RM	Post 1-RM	% Change
Squat (warm up)	-	-	-
Seated Chest Press - flat	70 lbs	120 lbs	71
Leg Press Machine	140 lbs	200 lbs	43
Lat Pull-Down - to the chest	70 lbs	90 lbs	29
Seated Leg Extension	50 lbs	70 lbs	40
Shoulder/Military Press	40 lbs	60 lbs	50
Supine Leg Curl	50 lbs	80 lbs	60
Cable Biceps Curl	30 lbs	40 lbs	33
Cable Triceps Extension	30 lbs	40 lbs	33

Summary

MR is the most common developmental disability in the industrialized world with a prevalence rate of approximately 3 percent. There are many causes of MR, but often the cause is not known, although one third of cases are caused by fetal alcohol syndrome. Individuals with MR tend to be sedentary, more obese, and exhibit low levels of physical fitness and low levels of muscle strength compared to individuals without disabilities. Individuals with Down syndrome have exceptionally low levels of muscle strength and also have a higher incidence of obesity. Low levels of muscle strength impact independent living in this population, thus increasing muscle strength is an important goal. It is clear that individuals with MR exhibit comparable responses to individuals without disabilities following resistance training, thus resistance training may be an important tool for increasing quality of life, independence, and vocational productivity in this population. A standard, progressive resistance-exercise program can be used; however, a lower starting exercise intensity may be indicated, and resistance-exercise machines are preferred over the use of free weights. It is essential that individuals with MR are familiarized with the exercise setting, personnel, and equipment to be used before testing or training begins. This process may require repeated familiarization sessions. Since task understanding and attention span are also reduced in this population, careful supervision is indicated during the first 6 months of the program.

Key Terms

Atlantoaxial instability
Development disabilities
Down syndrome (DS)
Fetal alcohol syndrome
Mental retardation (MR)
Pulmonary hypoplasia
Skeletal muscle hypotonia

Study Questions

1. What is the most common cause of mental retardation?

2. What pathologies commonly associated with Down syndrome should be considered when designing an exercise program?

3. If one does not have access to an isokinetic dynamometer, how can muscle strength be assessed in individuals with mental retardation?

4. What are the consequences of low muscular strength in individuals with mental retardation?

5. How should exercise intensity be gauged in individuals with mental retardation?

References

1. American Association on Mental Retardation. Classification in Mental Retardation. Washington, DC: American Association on Mental Retardation; 2002.

2. American College of Sports Medicine. *Guidelines for Exercise Testing and Exercise Prescription.* 6th ed. Philadelphia, PA: Lippincott, Williams & Wilkins; 2000.

3. Angelopoulou N, Matziari C, Tsimaras V, Sakadamis A, Souftas V, Mandroukas K. Bone mineral density and muscle strength in young men with mental retardation (with and without Down syndrome). *Calcif Tissue Int.* 2000;66:176–180.

4. Auxter D, Pfyfer J, Huettig C. *Principles and Methods of Adapted Physical Education and Recreation.* New York, NY: McGraw-Hill; 2001.

5. Baechle TR, Earle RW, Wathan W. Resistance training. In: *Essentials of Strength Training and Conditioning.* Baechle TR, Earle RW, eds. Champaign, IL: Human Kinetics; 2000.

6. Carmeli E, Kessel S, Coleman R, Ayalon M. Effects of a treadmill walking program on muscle strength and balance in elderly people with Down syndrome. *J Gerontol.* 2002;57A:M106–M110.

7. Clark H. Muscular power of the legs. *Phys Fitness Res Digest.* 1978;8:1–24.

8. Croce R, Horvat M. Effects of reinforcement-based exercise on fitness and work productivity in adults with mental retardation. *Adapt Phys Activ Q.* 1992;9:148–178.

9. Croce RV, Pitetti KH, Horvat M, et al. Peak torque, average power, and hamstring/quadriceps ratios in nondisabled adults and adults with mental retardation. *Arch Phys Med Rehabil.* 1996;77:369–372.

10. Eyman R, Call T. Life expectancy of persons with Down syndrome. *Am J Ment Retard.* 1991;95:603–612.

11. Fernhall B. Physical fitness and exercise training of individuals with mental retardation. *Med Sci Sports Exerc.* 1993;25:442–450.

12. Fernhall B. *Mental Retardation: ACSM's Exercise Management for Persons with Chronic Disease and Disability.* Champaign, IL: Human Kinetics; 1997.

13. Fernhall B. Mental retardation. In: Durstine J, Moore G, eds. *ACSM's Exercise Management for Persons with Chronic Diseases and Disabilities.* 2nd ed. Champaign, IL: Human Kinetics; 2003.

14. Fernhall B. Mental retardation. In: LeMura L, von Duvillard S, eds. *Clinical Exercise Physiology: Application and Physiological Principles.* Philadelphia, PA: Lippincott Williams & Williams; 2004.

15. Fernhall B, Figuerao A, Giannopoulou I, et al. Chronotropic incompetence and autonomic dysfunction in individuals with Down syndrome. *Med Sci Sports Exerc.* 2002;34(5):S47.

16. Fernhall B, Pitetti K. Leg strength is related to endurance run performance in children and adolescents with mental retardation. *Pediatr Exerc Sci.* 2000;12:324–333.

17. Fernhall B, Pitetti K. Limitations to work capacity in individuals with intellectual disabilities. *Clin Exerc Phys.* 2001;3:176–185.

18. Fernhall B, Tymeson G. Graded exercise testing of mentally retarded adults; a study of feasibility. *Arch Phys Med Rehabil.* 1987;63:363–365.

19. Fernhall B, Tymeson G, Millar AL, et al. Cardiovascular fitness testing and fitness levels of adolescents and adults with mental retardation including Down syndrome. *Education and Training in Ment Retard.* 1989;68:363–365.

20. Frey G, McCubbin JA, Hannigan-Downs S, et al. Physical fitness of trained runners with and without mild mental retardation. *Adapt Phys Activ Q.* 1999;16:126–137.

21. Guerra M, Roman B, Geronimo C, et al. Physical fitness levels of sedentary and active individuals with Down syndrome. *Adapted Physical Activity Quarterly.* 2000;17:310–321.

22. Hayden M. Mortality among people with mental retardation living in the United States: research review and policy application. *Ment Retard.* 1998;36:345–359.

23. Horvat M, Croce R. Physical rehabilitation of individuals with mental retardation: physical fitness and information processing. *Crit Rev Phys Rehabil Med.* 1995;7:233–252.

24. Horvat M, Croce R, Pitetti KH, et al. Comparison of isokinetic peak force and work parameters in youth with and without mental retardation. *Med Sci Sports Exerc.* 1999;31:1190–1195.

25. Horvat M, Pitetti KH, Croce R. Isokinetic torque, average power, and flexion/extension ratios in nondisabled adults and adults with mental retardation. *J Orthop Sports Phys Ther.* 1997;6:395–399.

26. Hussey C, Maurer JF, Schofield LJ. Physical education training for adult retardates in a sheltered workshop setting. *J Clin Psych.* 1976;32:701–705.

27. Krebs P. Mental retardation. In: Winnick J, ed. *Adapted Physical Education and Sport.* Champaign, IL: Human Kinetics; 1990:153–176.

28. Montgomery DL, Reid G, Seidl C. The effects of two physical fitness programs designed for mentally retarded adults. *Can J Sport Sci.* 1998;13:73–78.

29. Newcomer K, Sinaki M, Wollan PC. Physical activity and four-year development in back strength in children. *Am J Phys Med Rehabil.* 1997;76:52–58.

30. Nordgren B, Backstrom L. Correlations between muscular strength and industrial work performance in mentally retarded persons. *Acta Paediatr Suppl.* 1971;217:122–126.

31. Peran S, Gil JL, Ruiz F, Fernadez-Pastor V. Development of physical response after athletic training in adolescents with Down syndrome. *Scand J Med Sci Sports.* 1997;7:283–288.

32. Pitetti K, Campbell K. Mentally retarded individuals: a population at risk? *Med Sci Sports Exerc.* 1991;23:586–593.

33. Pitetti K, Fernhall B. Aerobic capacity as related to leg strength in youths with mental retardation. *Pediatr Exerc Sci.* 1997;9:223–236.

34. Pitetti K, Yarmer D. Lower-body strength of children and adolescents with and without mild mental retardation: a comparison. *Adapt Phys Activ Q.* 2002;19(1):68–81.

35. Pitetti KH, Boneh S. Cardiovascular fitness as related to leg strength in adults with mental retardation. *Med Sci Sports Exerc.* 1995;27:423–428.

36. Pitetti KH, Climstein M, Mays MJ, et al. Isoki netic arm and leg strength of adults with Down syndrome: a comparative study. *Arch Phys Med Rehabil.* 1992;73:847–850.

37. Pitetti KH, Rimmer JH, Fernhall B. Physical fitness and adults with mental retardation: an overview of current research and future directions. *Sports Med.* 1993;16:23–56.

38. Rimmer J. Fitness and rehabilitation programs for special populations. Dubuque, IA: Brown and Benchmark; 1994.

39. Rimmer JH, Heller T, Wang E, Valerio I. Improvements in physical fitness in adults with Down syndrome. *Am J Ment Retard.* 2004;109:165–174.

40. Rimmer J, Kelly L. Effects of a resistance training program on adults with mental retardation. *Adapted Physical Activity Quarterly.* 1991;8:146–153.

41. Roizen NJ, Patterson D. Down syndrome. *Lancet.* 2003;361(9365):1281–1289.

42. Solomon A, Pangle R. Demonstrating physical fitness improvement in the EMR. *Exceptional Children.* 1967;34:177–181.

43. Suomi R. Self-directed strength training: its effect on leg strength in men with mental retardation. *Arch Phys Med Rehabil.* 1998;79:323–328.

44. Suomi R, Surburg P, Lecius P. Effects of hydraulic resistance strength training on isokinetic measures of leg strength in men with mental retardation. *Adapted Physical Activity Quarterly.* 1995;12:377–387.

45. Tsimaras V, Fotiadou EG. Effect of training on the muscle strength and dynamic balance ability of adults with Down syndrome. *J Strength Cond Res.* 2004;18:343–347.

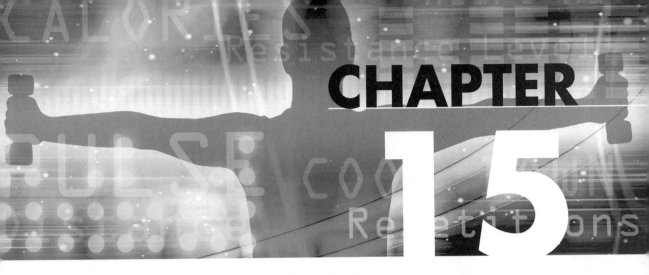

CHAPTER 15

RESISTANCE-TRAINING STRATEGIES FOR INDIVIDUALS WITH CANCER

Objectives

Upon completion of this chapter, the reader should be able to:

- ○ Explain the widespread prevalence of cancer in its many forms
- ○ Describe how cancers develop and are treated
- ○ Identify research evaluating the impact of resistance training on cancer symptoms or treatment side effects both during and following treatment
- ○ Design a resistance-training program for individuals with cancer, taking into account health status, readiness, safety issues, progression, and outcome assessment measures

INTRODUCTION

Cancer is a term that refers to a family of diseases marked by unregulated cell growth and proliferation that can affect virtually any bodily organ or system. With an aging population, the incidence of cancers may increase in coming years, but early detection, promising new treatments, and rehabilitation appear to be converting at least some cancers from fatal diseases to curable ones, or at least chronically manageable conditions. Cancer rehabilitation must contend not only with adverse effects of the disease but with the toxic effects of radiation and chemotherapy, including fatigue, impaired immune system function, and potential side effects of surgery that include disfigurement and functional loss (63). Recent descriptions of resistance-training prescriptions and the appropriate progression for both clinical and nonclinical populations underscore the significance of this intervention (47). This finding is indicated by the fact that with increasing age, physical strength is an important determinant of functional capabilities (29). With appropriate adaptations for specific medical conditions, resistance-training programs are efficient and can make a significant contribution to muscle mass, endurance, and strength. This chapter presents evidence-based strategies for using resistance training to benefit individuals with cancer.

PREVALENCE AND ECONOMIC IMPACT OF CANCER

Cancers are currently the second leading cause of death in the United States, exceeded only by heart disease (49). Recent statistics indicate that lifetime risk probabilities are approximately 50 percent for males and 33 percent for females (6), a significant proportion of the population. The most common cancer forms, and their incidence rates per 100,000 population, are prostate (72), breast (68.5), lung (63.9), and colorectal (50.6) cancers (61). According to recent statistics provided by the American Cancer

Society, nearly 1.4 million new cases of cancer were anticipated in 2005, excluding noninvasive and squamous-cell skin cancers (5). Although cancer accounted for nearly one quarter (22.8 percent) of all deaths in 2005 (49), overall death rates have declined in recent years, including those for the most common types of cancer—an encouraging development attributed to both early detection and improved treatment (55). Cancer is increasingly conceptualized as a chronic illness, and the focus of systematic rehabilitation programs is intended to maximize functional capabilities and quality of life. With few exceptions, cancer risk increases with age. For example, the overall median age at diagnosis is 68 for prostate cancer, 61 for breast cancer, 71 for lung cancer, and 71 for colorectal cancer, averaging several years less for African Americans (61).

The economic impact of cancers has steadily grown. An analysis published in 2001 reported that the total direct cost of cancer treatments increased from $1.28 billion in 1963 to $42.39 billion in 1996, consistently accounting for approximately 5 percent of total health expenditures over time (12). Person-years of life and corresponding income potential lost to cancer are substantial, although this is mitigated somewhat by the relatively late onset of most cancers.

ETIOLOGY OF CANCER

Currently, more than 100 forms of cancer have been identified (33), and the term actually refers to a collection of diseases rather than a single condition (30). Cancer genesis involves a multistep process resulting in an aggregate proliferation of abnormal cells triggered by exposure to either intrinsic or environmental **carcinogens**, cancer-causing agents that initially damage cellular DNA and culminate in tissue invasion virtually anywhere in the body. The process is under genetic control, a factor common to all cancers (14, 58). Early cancer research was stimulated by the Knudson hypothesis, which states that cancer results from accumulated cellular DNA mutations (44). Manifestations of unregulated growth may be site-specific, as with breast or prostate cancers, or systemic, as with leukemia and lymphoma. Treatment is specific with respect to the site and type of cancer and may involve surgery, radiation, and/or chemotherapy.

Because of the possibility of **metastasis,** or cancer cell migration, multiple sites may become involved. For example, individuals with breast cancer whose symptoms include limited muscle strength and fatigue could develop other impairments in the event of metastasis, especially if the central nervous system is affected. Further complicating rehabilitation are factors related to the stage at which intervention is initiated, whether prior to, during, or following treatment; treatment-related side effects, many of which are quite toxic; and individual variations in physical and psychological stamina affecting both motivation and compliance (64).

Staging is a method used to assess the range and severity of cancer progression. The TNM **staging system** for tumor, lymph node, and metastasis is among the most widely used and is endorsed by the National Cancer Institute and other regulatory groups (32). This system grades cancer according to 1) the size and scope of the primary tumor on a scale ranging from T1, the least extensive, to T4, which is highly extensive; 2) lymph node involvement, ranging from N0, or no involvement, to N3, or extensive involvement; and 3) presence (M1) or absence (M0) of metastasis. For example, a grading of T1N0M0 indicates a relatively circumscribed tumor without lymph node involvement or metastasis, whereas T3N2M1 would refer to a more advanced case with both lymph node involvement and metastatic distribution.

BENEFITS OF RESISTANCE TRAINING FOR INDIVIDUALS WITH CANCER

Increasingly early detection and treatment for cancer are cause for greater optimism concerning recovery and restoration of function, and the American Cancer Society (6) recently reported that not only are rates of prostate, breast, lung, and colorectal cancer declining but that preventive behaviors are on the rise. Significantly, this report targeted physical activity as an area in need of greater emphasis. In fact, research has demonstrated that physical activity aids the recovery process and is likely to be of benefit to nearly all individuals with cancer (15, 16, 18, 65, 66).

Resistance-training guidelines published by Feigenbaum and Pollock (26) recommend single-set programs of 8 to 10 exercises for the major muscle groups performed at least twice per week for healthy individuals of all ages and for many with chronic illnesses. With older individuals, emphasizing strength maintainance or even slowing the rate of decline that appears to be inevitable with age, as opposed to establishing goals based on progressively increasing strength, may be appropriate. This principle is relevant both in terms of age-related developmental effects and in the context of cancer treatment and recovery.

Literature Review of Research Supporting Resistance Training for Individuals with Cancer

Although research is sparse, resistance training may help alleviate both physical and psychological symptoms of cancer (38), especially with respect to breast cancer (53). An early study by Doyne and colleagues (22) demonstrated that both resistance training and running can help manage depression when practiced regularly, and research continues to demonstrate the positive effects of physical activity on psychological health in a wide range of medical patients. Most of the cancer rehabilitation literature to date (72) has focused on aerobic fitness programs for breast cancer (16) due to advances in early detection, treatment, and survivability. However, a recent review by Knols and colleagues (43), and evidence from comprehensive cancer rehabilitation programs (64), documents increasing attention to other exercise modalities and other cancer types, including prostate cancer, leukemia, and colorectal cancer.

Recent reviews (16, 17, 31, 43, 71) document the current status of research and exercise for cancer patients. Despite methodological limitations, variability in the types and stages of cancer studied, phase of treatment, and varying outcome measures, these reviews tend to suggest that physical activity is of benefit to cancer patients undergoing and following treatment in terms of physical status and quality of life. Research on cancer recurrence and mortality is limited (18). Table 15-1 lists representative studies evaluating the impact of resistance training, either alone or in combination with aerobic training, on various parameters associated with cancer treatment and rehabilitation. The table is divided into two sections: A) resistance training alone or combined with aerobics during treatment, and B) resistance training alone or combined with aerobics following treatment.

Collectively, these studies suggest placing increased emphasis on resistance training in cancer rehabilitation, either alone or in combination with aerobic training. Provided that exercise programs are individualized and supervised, studies reviewed by Knols and colleagues (43) suggest that both resistance and aerobic training are safe and well tolerated by males and females both during and following treatment.

DESIGNING RESISTANCE-TRAINING PROGRAMS FOR INDIVIDUALS WITH CANCER

The most important factor to consider in designing resistance training programs for individuals with cancer is that of individualization due in part to

Table 15-1 Resistance Training Studies with Cancer Patients A) During or B) Following Treatment

Author(s)	Cancer Type	N (Comp/ Enrolled)	Gender & Age	Program Length	Intensity	Strength Gains & Other Outcomes
A. During Treatment						
A.1. RT¹ Only						
Cunningham et al. (20)	Leukemia	30/40	F/M	3×/week × 5 wks		Sig. ↓ creatinine excretion (protein sparing)
McNeely et al. (52)	Head & Neck	17/20	F/M	3×/week × 12 wks	≤13 Borg Scale	↑ Ext. shoulder rotation;10% disability ↓
Segal et al. (67)	Prostate	135/ 155 R³	M; m = 68	3×/week × 12 wks	60–70% 1RM	↑ upper/lower body strength
A.2. Combined RT & AT²						
Adamsen et al. (2, 3)	Mixed		F/M	3×/week x 6 wks	85–95% 1RM	↑ 32% WBS

Table 15-1 Resistance Training Studies with Cancer Patients A) During or B) Following Treatment (continued)

Author(s)	Cancer Type	N (Comp/ Enrolled)	Gender & Age	Program Length	Intensity	Strength Gains & Other Outcomes
A.2. Combined RT & AT^2 (continued)						
Coleman et al. (13)	Multiple Myeloma	11/24 R	F/M; m=55	24 weeks (max.)	Borg Scale; intensity not specified	↑2.4% S (vs ↓12.6% Control)
Hayes et al. (35, 36)	Mixed		F/M;	3×/week × 12 wks	15RM–20RM wks 1–6; 8–12RM wks 8–12	↑FFM, no immune system impact
Kolden et al. (46)	Breast	/40	F; all >45	3×/week × 16 wks	Not specified	↑Fitness/vigor; ↑QOL
B. Post-Treatment						
B.1. RT Only						
Schmitz et al. (65)	Breast	69/85	m=53	2×/wk × 6 (delayed treat.) or 12 (imm. treat.) months	Upper body: light weights, progressing as tolerated; lower body: 8RM–10RM	Sig. ↑ in lean body mass; sig. ↓ body fat; sig. ↓ insulin-like growth factor (IGF) protein (a cancer risk factor)
B.2. Combined RT & AT						
Berglund et al. (8)	Breast	/30	F	2×/week × 10 wks	Light	Improved health status
Berglund et al. (9, 10)	Mixed	/188			Not specified	Improved health status
Durak & Lilly (23, 24)	Mixed	/20	F/M; m=50	2×/week × 20 wks	Progressive	↑43–73%; ↑WBS
Harris & Niesen-Vertommen (34)	Breast	/20	F	3×/week × 32 wks	Vigorous training	No lymphedema exacerbation

(continued)

Table 15-1 Resistance Training Studies with Cancer Patients A) During or B) Following Treatment (continued)

Author(s)	Cancer Type	N (Comp/ Enrolled)	Gender & Age	Program Length	Intensity	Strength Gains & Other Outcomes
B.2. Combined RT & AT (continued)						
McKenzie & Kalda (51)	Breast	14/14 R	F; m=56.6	3×/week x 8 wks	Light weights, progressing as tolerated	No change in arm circumference; Sig. ↑, SF-36 physical functioning, general health, vitality
Nieman et al. (56)	Breast	12/16 R	F; 35–72	3×/week x 8 wks	Moderate AT; progressive RT	No differences: natural killer cell cytotoxic activity; T and NK cell concentration
Turner et al. (70)	Breast	10/11	F; m=47	1×/week x 8 wks	Low to moderate	No change in lymphedema status; trend toward ↑ QOL and ↓ fatigue

[1]RT = Resistance Training; [2]AT = Aerobic Training; [3]R = randomized to intervention/control groups; m = mean age in years; QOL = quality of life; FFM = fat-free mass; Sig. = significant; WBS = whole body strength

the many potential forms of cancer and variations in treatment (64). The following is a list of factors to consider in program design: stage of illness; whether training is to occur before, during, or after treatment; prior exercise experience; age and general physical status; physical conditioning level; and goals, aspirations, and motivation.

Training during treatment must take into account the nature and side effects of primary and associated interventions, which may include surgery, radiation, bone marrow transplantation, and systemic interventions (64) that may include chemotherapy, hormone therapy, and immunotherapy (15). Both the American Cancer Society and the National Cancer Institute maintain frequently updated Web sites

(http://www.cancer.org and http:www.cancer.gov) containing useful information concerning treatment agents and side effects.

The experience of a critical illness such as cancer can engender mistrust or even fear of the body and body functions. Living through the experience of having previously normal functions go awry can promote anxiety when even minor physical or physiological aberrations are subsequently detected. Reactions can range from denial or avoidance to anxious consultation with health care providers. Such apprehension is understandable, the natural by-product of encountering a life-threatening illness. However, this response can pose a significant obstacle to exercise training.

Possible concerns expressed by cancer patients include fears that:

○ Exercise may somehow promote or hasten the spread of cancer

○ Exercise may further weaken an already compromised immune system

○ Exercise may increase the fatigue that most individuals experience

○ Physical impairments due to cancer and its treatment may be made worse by exercise

○ Exercise may cause additional impairment or injury

The exercise professional must be prepared to address such concerns as part of the process of designing and implementing a resistance-training program. This recommendation is important given that cancer can promote feelings of helplessness and psychological trauma. Moreover, long-term medical regimens required to treat cancer may engender a passive, stoic attitude in individuals who can take relatively little direct action other than to follow prescriptive medical advice. Thus, it is important to encourage the individual to actively participate in the process of designing and implementing a training program.

Individuals with cancer are often severely deconditioned as a result in part of the toxicity associated with chemotherapy and radiation. Surgery imposes its own constraints, and depending on the site, it can potentially affect strength and range of movement in any limb. These limitations underscore the importance of an individualized approach to exercise testing. Determining the individual's goals and needs is important to defining appropriate benchmark assessment criteria. Finally, do not assume that a baseline assessment will necessarily be followed by steady, regular progress, especially when implemented during treatment. Individuals with cancer routinely experience significant fluctuations in physical energy, mood, and treatment-related side effects that can markedly impact performance. Marked variations in energy, fatigue, and motivation on a session-by-session basis are common, and these may be intensified in comparison to such fluctuations in the general population that frequently result from daily stress (1).

Assessment measures should be selected with a measure of flexibility and must be consistent with individual capabilities. An alternative to a single, comprehensive baseline assessment might be to use multiple assessments for measuring improvement or decrements in performance.

Cancer staging carries important implications for both treatment and rehabilitation. The earlier cancer is detected, the less likely it is to have spread to the lymph nodes or other organ systems, a fact that simplifies treatment and recovery management. Conversely, lymph node involvement and metastasis necessitate more comprehensive management strategies. For example, breast cancer is often associated with lymph node involvement, and many who undergo either lumpectomies or mastectomies also have lymph nodes removed. The former may impair muscular strength, flexibility, and range of motion, depending on the amount of muscle and connective tissue removed to excise the tumor. The latter heightens the risk of **lymphedema**, a condition involving swelling of the arm due to inadequate draining of lymphatic fluid, which can be triggered by heavy upper-body exertion or even partial occlusion of the arm due to tight-fitting jewelry or clothing. Both of these factors need to be taken into account in planning resistance training, along with other possible behavioral or physiological symptoms in the event of any metastatic involvement. A study by McKenzie and Kalda (51) reported that an 8-week program of combined aerobic and resistance training for breast cancer patients with lymphedema resulted in significantly increased physical functioning without any increase in arm circumference, the hallmark of lymphedema.

Exercise Testing Considerations

Exercise testing of individuals with cancer should start with a health and medical history evaluation, a physical fitness assessment, and evaluations of lifestyle and activity to measure baseline performance and monitor exercise training progress.

For most individuals with cancer, assessing one-repetition maximum (1RM), although ultimately desirable, may not be necessary or appropriate during the initial phases of a resistance-training program. Several factors contribute to the inadvisability of performing 1RM testing early in the resistance-training program. First of all, fatigue, which is almost always present both during and following treatment, can significantly limit performance. Second, lack of familiarity with resistance-training equipment limits performance capabilities. Third, stressful exercise, whether in the context of an assessment or day-to-day training, can easily overtax musculoskeletal and immune systems already weakened by disease and treatment. Finally, individuals with cancer experience varying restrictions on range of motion. This can limit performance during concentric and eccentric movement as a result of any combination of disease site, chemotherapy, radiation, and surgery.

One alternative to consider is to refer to norms for body-weight percentage that can be used in various resistance-training exercises (64). As an additional alternative, the American College of Sports Medicine (ACSM) (7) describes procedures for exercise prescription without exercise testing, primarily via the use of ratings of perceived exertion (RPE) ratings. From a functional standpoint, exertion in areas rated light to somewhat hard on the Borg scale (11), ratings between 10 and 13, correspond to a level of moderate intensity; this may provide a useful baseline focal point, as well as a reference for periodic assessment of progress throughout the program.

ACSM guidelines for exercise testing of individuals with cancer advocate 1RM to 3RM measures to assess muscular strength prior to exercise prescription (66). Prior to assessing muscular strength, the range of motion required for any proposed exercises should be performed as a means of determining the feasibility of conducting a baseline strength assessment. Table 15-2 provides a template for assessing the range of motion for the major muscle groups (42). Following weight-free range-of-motion assessment, the next step in exercise testing is to assess baseline strength for major muscle groups.

Special Considerations for Exercise Training

The most prevalent forms of cancer affecting older adults include lung, colorectal, prostate, and breast cancers. In addition to risk of cancer, older adults are prone to other age-related comorbidities that may negatively affect muscle strength, power, and endurance. Among the most prominent of these conditions are sarcopenia, decreased metabolic rate, reduced bone density, insulin sensitivity, and aerobic capacity. Sarcopenia, a widely cited correlate of aging involving loss of muscle mass, becomes increasingly pronounced after age 50 and may have a significant impact on strength and ambulatory capabilities (62). Long-term resistance training has been found to have a positive impact on these factors (60) since the pioneering study by Fiatarone and colleagues (28) with elderly adults.

Along with progressively declining physical attributes, both cancer-specific and treatment-specific factors warrant consideration during exercise training. Cancer treatments, particularly radiation and chemotherapy, are notable for their toxic impact on many organ and physiological systems. Among the most significant physical side effects of cancer treatments are pain, fatigue, sleep problems, and lymphedema; these are frequently accompanied by anxiety, depression, and body-image issues (64).

Cancer survivors are not immune to other chronic conditions that become prevalent with advancing age including obesity, diabetes, high cholesterol, hypertension, and heart disease. The latter is of particular significance, owing to the cardiotoxic effects of both radiation and chemotherapy, which are known to include anemia, pericarditis, reduced ventricular function, tachycardia, and arrhythmias that can act in combination to further reduce the efficiency of an already overtaxed cardiovascular system (64).

Changes in strength for the individual with cancer need to be interpreted in light of both baseline levels and developmental trends. For example, resistance training for an individual with cancer

Table 15-2 Range-of-Motion Assessment for Establishing Feasibility of Resistance Training

Name: _____   Date: _____

Evaluate range of motion and teach correct form for each exercise <u>without</u> using weights. Assess bilateral symmetry as appropriate. Encourage slow and deliberate movements to become familiar with movement patterns and to develop sensitivity to proprioceptive feedback. Integrate limb movement and breathing: Exhale with exertion/contraction, inhale on release.

	LIMITED	MODERATE	FULL
CHEST/INCLINE PRESS			
SEATED ROW			
LAT PULLDOWN			
SQUAT (OVER CHAIR/BENCH)			
LOWER-LEG EXTENSION (SEATED)			
BICEPS CURL			
BENT-OVER ROW			
TRICEPS KICKBACK			
LATERAL RAISE			
FRONT RAISE			
POSTERIOR PRESS BACK			

just completing chemotherapy or radiation may involve little or no evident progress. In contrast, individuals with cancer who become involved in resistance training during or shortly after treatment may show little apparent improvement during a comparable time period. However, training may in fact be slowing or even reversing atrophic strength declines that would otherwise occur as a result of disuse or treatment side effects.

Fatigue is a key factor in cancer and its treatment and must be taken into account in planning resistance training. A recent review (19) concluded that diverse exercise programs, including resistance training, may help counteract cancer-related fatigue. Part of this effect may be psychological; physical activity has been found to produce increased self-confidence, perceived self-efficacy, and increased energy in cancer patients, even during chemotherapy (21). Since both the psychological and physical dimensions of cancer fatigue have been established, activity is likely to result in at least the perception of greater energy and lower fatigue.

For individuals with cancer, the impact of a long-term (24 weeks or more) training program will vary considerably as a function of several key factors, including the stage of treatment, premorbid strength and overall conditioning, side effects and aftereffects of chemotherapy, the impact of aging on muscle function, and the possible impact of other medical conditions. These factors, either alone or in combination, can contribute to marked variations in training effects among individuals, confirming that resistance-training protocols should be highly individualized. The most comprehensive published source of information, and examples pertaining to the feasibility of progressive cancer exercise protocols, can be found in research by Schneider and colleagues (64).

The question might be raised as to the value, or even the feasibility, of planning a long-term resistance-training program, given the marked individual variability in progress and outcomes described above. After all, what is the point of laying out long-term goals for individuals whose progress at times may be slow, erratic, or even appear to be going in reverse? Individuals may be demoralized when their efforts may not seem to result in expected benefits despite persistent adherence to an exercise program. The counterargument is simple: Exercise planning enhances efficiency by providing a structured environment in which to assess changes in performance, whatever their nature. The success or failure of employing a structured approach depends largely on how the program is presented to the individual and the individual's interpretation. The impact of being physically active, irrespective of progress toward program goals, can be overwhelmingly positive for individuals for whom survival is of fundamental concern. The opportunity to engage in any form of physical activity can promote a sense of optimism and hope that from a motivational standpoint is potentially a unique byproduct of facing a life-threatening

illness. The key is to work with each individual on a session-by-session basis, taking into account the inevitable ebb and flow of energy, strength, stress level, and motivation.

In working with cancer survivors, keeping this perspective in mind is helpful when framing discussions of goals. When survival is the immediate goal, most other future-oriented events, such as becoming fit and being healthy, may tend to pale in comparison. Proceeding slowly and gradually is best; set manageable, short-term goals and use these to establish longer-term projections as appropriate. In fact, some individuals use language that speaks of "intention" rather than goal-oriented language. Individuals with cancer often literally do not know what the future holds for them, and as a result, emphasizing "living in the present moment" is an effective way to focus attention and make the most of every training session.

Training Program Components

The emphasis in resistance training for individuals with cancer should be on fostering improvements in functional capabilities. Retaining or improving strength in the trunk and extremities is of fundamental importance. Schwartz and colleagues (66) suggest an initial exercise dosage of 50 percent of 1RM two to three times per week, with 2 to 3 sets that may range from 3 to 12 repetitions. Reliably establishing 1RM in the initial stages of training is difficult, so the use of the Borg RPE scale at the light to somewhat hard level, 9 to 13 out of 20, is recommended (11). Courneya and colleagues (17) and others (64) have also provided recommended resistance-training guidelines for cancer survivors that can serve as a useful starting point in designing resistance-training programs, along with adaptations of resistance-training recommendations for older adults recommended by the ACSM (27, 47). A summary of principles derived from these sources is presented in Table 15-3.

Muscle groups that should be exercised include those of the upper and middle back (trapezius, latissimus dorsi), chest (pectorals), shoulders (deltoids), arms (biceps and triceps), abdominals,

Table 15-3 Recommended Resistance-Training Guidelines for Healthy Cancer Survivors

Parameter	Guidelines
Muscle group and exercise	Major muscle groups, as feasible
Frequency	Train three sessions per week with a minimum 24-hour rest between sessions. Adjust as needed depending on treatment status and fatigue.
Intensity	Begin with very light resistance, preceded by range-of-motion assessment without weights.
	Increase resistance gradually, doing the first set at the previous level, the second set at the new level.
	Use graduated reps, gradually increasing range of motion during a set as needed, especially at the outset.
	Adjust intensity based on pre-session fatigue level, effects of treatment, and risk of lymphedema (breast cancer).
Duration	Begin with 2 sets of 10 repetitions each, working up to 15 repetitions or volitional fatigue as tolerated
Progression	Maintain flexible approach toward progression, taking into account fatigue, effects of treatment, and other factors that may vary from session to session.
	Recommend increasing resistance after individual is capable of performing 3 sets for 15 repetitions; begin new resistance level at 2 sets and 10 repetitions

upper legs (quadriceps and hamstrings) and lower legs (gastrocnemius and soleus). The emphasis in such a program for most individuals is to enhance functional strength needed for day-to-day activities. Corresponding exercises for each of the major muscle groups are compiled in Table 15-4. This table is organized into three groups: 1) exercises on machines, 2) exercises on cable/pulley machines, and 3) free weights.

Of these exercise modalities, the cable/pulley machines are especially useful because of their flexible adaptation to individual differences in range of motion, often a significant limiting factor for resistance exercise for individuals with cancer. Several upper-body, free-weight exercises are included, although in general these are not recommended initially due to safety considerations.

Use of light free weights for initial instruction and early resistance training in the 1 to 5 pound range, or even no weight at all, may also be considered. Variable resistance bands offer another viable alternative as a strength-building stimulus for individuals with severe deconditioning or limited range of motion.

The ACSM has published a series of position papers outlining resistance-training guidelines for older adults. These guidelines provide an especially useful framework for working with individuals with cancer, who on average tend to be of relatively advanced age. Key recommendations include the following:

○ Keep intensity levels low (lighter weights, more repetitions) at the outset and progress slowly (27).

Table 15-4 Representative Machine and Free-Weight Exercises for Resistance Training

Primary Muscle(s)	Exercise Machine	Cable/Pulley Machine	Free Weights
Chest (pectorals)	Dual-axis chest press (basic motion)	Seated chest press/fly	Bench press using hand weights
Upper chest (upper pectorals)	Incline press	Cable cross	Incline bench press
Back (trapezius, latissimus dorsi, posterior deltoid)	Dual-axis row, rear deltoid (vertical handles)	Row (angled)	
Upper back (latissimus dorsi, teres major)	Lat pulldown	Lat (angled)	Life Fitness multi
Shoulders (anterior and medial deltoids)	Dual-axis overhead press (basic motion)	1- or 2-arm seated press	Shoulder press Front raise
Arms, biceps (biceps brachii, brachialis)	Arm curl	Basic/reverse curl	Biceps curl Hammer curl
Arms, triceps (triceps brachii)	Arm extension	Basic/reverse extension	Triceps extension
Legs (quadriceps, gluteals)	Seated leg press	Upright squat	
Legs (quadriceps, hamstrings, gluteals)	Leg curl	Hamstring/knee curl	
Legs (quadriceps)	Leg extension	Standing or seated leg extensions	
Abdominals (rectus abdominus, obliques)	Abdominal crunches (abdominal frame)	Abdominal machine	Abdominal crunches

○ Perform repetitions slowly through a full range of motion; sustain the eccentric (release) phase somewhat longer than the concentric (contraction) phase (25).

○ Adapt training protocols to novice, intermediate, and advanced levels (47).

Many persons with cancer begin resistance training for the first time as part of their rehabilitation program, often after years of inactivity. Others may be accustomed to being highly active and fit and are capable of more complex and challenging prescriptions. For most individuals, beginning with a single set of exercises is appropriate, adding additional sets as endurance increases. In terms of functional strength, increase the number of sets to at least 2 prior to increasing resistance. This format permits an initial light-weight set to be used as a warm-up prior to a second set performed at a target resistance. An additional adaptation that is often helpful is to limit range of motion at the beginning of a set then progressively increase it so that the final repetition is done using the full range of motion. This procedure can help detect "sticking points" or other anomalies that impact movement fluidity to give the individual more control over the repetition and encourage moment-by-moment attention.

Initial exercise training sessions should be closely supervised. Training should be conducted by exercise professionals familiar with the wide range of individual differences evident in cancer survivors, as well as marked variations in capabilities on a session-by-session basis for a given individual. Other useful recommendations based on clinical ACSM guidelines for resistance training with older adults include:

○ Begin with minimal resistance to allow for adaptation and to assess range of motion.

○ Teach correct form and breathing with minimal resistance (exhale during muscle contraction; inhale during release).

○ Control concentric and eccentric contractions to avoid bouncing

and promote smooth, deliberate movements.

○ Perform all movements in a pain-free manner, adjusting for range of motion, limits, and other medical factors.

These guidelines can increase the efficiency of a training session, an important consideration given the susceptibility to fatigue and possible adverse immune system effects of overly strenuous exercise. Encouraging relatively slow, smooth contractions and avoiding ballistic movements keeps the target muscles under sustained load, thereby optimizing the physiological benefit of each repetition. This effect can be further enhanced by encouraging proper breathing with each repetition cycle, which helps maintain an optimal pace. Collectively, these guidelines can help increase both the individual specificity and efficiency of a training session, an important consideration given the susceptibility to fatigue. The guidelines also foster a more attentive yet relaxed approach to resistance training, which is typically more foreign to most people than aerobic activity.

The recommendations discussed above, while generally appropriate, may need to be adjusted according to the needs, limitations, and capabilities of each individual. One way to accomplish this goal is to develop a set of whole-body exercises graduated by level, from beginner to advanced, as illustrated in Table 15-5. This approach offers several potential advantages, three of which are especially significant: 1) the assurance of success for individuals of almost any conditioning level; 2) the integration of resistance training with functional activities of daily living, and 3) the avoidance of specialized resistance-training equipment at the outset, which is frequently intimidating to novice lifters.

SAMPLE 24-WEEK PROGRAM

The following 24-week program incorporates the considerations described above and provides a template for program development for all individuals

Table 15-5 Sample Exercises Based on Training Level

Beginner	Intermediate	Advanced
Legs:		
Standing and sitting from chair	Body-weight wall squats with back against a stability ball to allow for squatting motion	Squats holding dumbbells at sides of the body
Body-weight lunge holding on≈to bench for stability	Body-weight lunge, hands on hips	Standing lunge holding dumbbells in hands
Chest:		
Standing wall push-up, body nearly parallel to wall at arm distance	Standing wall push-up at a 45-degree angle from the wall	Floor push-up, knees on the ground
Seated chest press	Supine barbell press	Supine dumbbell press
Back:		
Seated row	Dumbbell row	Lat pulldown
Superman back extensions on hands and knees	Prone back extensions	Back extension (machine)
Shoulders:		
Dumbbell lateral raise	Seated dumbbell military press	Standing military press
Arms:		
Seated dumbbell biceps curl	Standing dumbbell biceps curl	Barbell biceps curl
Triceps pushdown	Overhead dumbbell triceps extension	Seated dips

with cancer. Medical authorization is essential when working with individuals with cancer. Both an oncologist and an internist or general practitioner should be consulted about the suitability of a resistance-training program. This recommendation is important because of contraindications for resistance training related to noncancer concerns, such as unstable angina, uncontrolled hypertension, and other risk factors related to cardiac or other systemic functions. The cardiotoxic effects of many chemotherapy agents further underscores the need for close collaboration with the oncology and general medical team. An informed consent document that contains a detailed description of the proposed program, and an enumeration of possible benefits and risks, is also recommended.

Considering the given recommendations summarized in Table 15-4 and Table 15-5, a 24-week resistance-training program is outlined below. Weeks 1 and 2 are intended to provide participants with an orientation to the program and facilities and to conduct a baseline assessment.

Week 1: Baseline Health Assessment

- ○ Perform PAR-Q assessment.
- ○ Obtain health and cancer history.
- ○ Perform lifestyle assessment.
- ○ Determine body composition.

- ○ Obtain resting heart rate and blood pressure.
- ○ Obtain physician authorization (general practitioner, oncologist, others as needed).

Week 2: Testing and Education

- ○ Perform range-of-motion assessment (no weights).
- ○ Teaching session on mechanisms of resistance training. Although often highly motivated, individuals with cancer may not appreciate the mechanisms and processes involved in increasing strength. Providing a basic working knowledge of muscle activity related to strength gains is a good way to foster cooperation and beneficial training.
- ○ Practice technique, illustrating eccentric and concentric movement patterns and proper breathing.
- ○ Measure upper-extremity circumferences for breast cancer patients to provide a baseline for subsequent detection of lymphedema-related swelling.
  - ○ Midway between shoulder and elbow
  - ○ Midway between wrist and elbow
  - ○ Wrist

Weeks 3 through 6

- ○ Initiate resistance-training program: Stage I.
  - ○ Derive starting resistance levels for each exercise. This can be done through use of the Borg scale to determine a working range in the moderate

range (light to somewhat hard). During this stage, greater emphasis should be placed on proper form and breathing than on resistance level. Individuals often do best when given the opportunity to become gradually acclimated to resistance training, and there is no reason to start training at overly challenging levels.
  - ○ Begin a circuit-type program involving all primary muscle groups as tolerated, and take into account any mechanical limitations imposed by surgery or radiation.
  - ○ Gradually increase repetitions per set from 10 to 15 as tolerated, followed by increased resistance; return to 8 to 10 repetition sets.
  - ○ Focus on form and technique, emphasizing that 1 set per exercise performed correctly and with focused attention is of greater benefit than doing multiple sets too rapidly or with compromised form.

Weeks 7 through 12: Stage II

- ○ Reassessment: evaluate gains in initial neuromuscular adaptation.
- ○ Assess for physical changes in limb circumference for individuals at risk for lymphedema.
- ○ Review program goals and adjust accordingly.
- ○ Continue with progressive training.

Weeks 13 through 18: Stage III

- ○ Reassess and adjust as needed.
- ○ Continue with progressive increases in resistance as tolerated.

Weeks 19 through 24: Stage IV

○ Perform a final program review and develop a new periodized schedule.

CASE STUDY

Ms. D, age 49, began a combined resistance and aerobic conditioning program following bilateral mastectomies, the most recent of which occurred 3 months ago. Athletic and fit both before and after treatment, Ms. D played competitive tennis regularly and had run a half-marathon prior to her most recent surgery. Fitness program goals included developing additional strength and improving cardiovascular fitness. Her basic 12-week program began with aerobic training, primarily using an elliptical trainer to enhance lower-body endurance and to prepare for resistance training.

Following acclimation, a resistance-training program was progressively implemented following a range-of-motion assessment with a combination of lower- and upper-body exercises using cable/pulley machines and exercise machines. Upper-body training began with 5-pound weights in the low-intensity RPE range for bicep curls, triceps extensions, and chest presses; 10-pound weights were used for lat pulldowns. Proper form and breathing were continually emphasized as being of greater importance than resistance. Leg extensions using exercise machines were initiated at 30 pounds and leg curls at 17.5 pounds, rated as involving moderate RPE intensity. The initial training session consisted of a single set of 8 to 10 repetitions, subsequently progressing to a standard 2 sets of 10 to 12 repetitions as adaptation increased, with the first set treated as a warm-up. Additional exercises were gradually added over approximately a 6-week period to include abdominal and back exercises, along with leg and shoulder presses and eventually squats. Training consisted of two combined aerobic and resistance-training sessions per week, in addition to Ms. D's regular tennis regimen. Highly motivated and conscientious, she

made steady progress with the program, which was briefly interrupted at one point for outpatient surgery. By the time she completed the program, Ms. D was playing tennis with new-found strength and endurance as a result of her persistence and commitment to training on a regular basis.

Summary

Clinical research concerning the benefits of resistance training for individuals with cancer is currently in its infancy. In contrast, research on the benefits of aerobic training for individuals with cancer has been better established. Concerning the studies reviewed for this chapter, resistance training during cancer treatment has received somewhat less attention and documentation than post-treatment protocols. Results of these studies suggest the following conclusions:

○ Resistance training may help alleviate cancer-specific or treatment-specific symptoms, such as loss of muscle mass, and may also serve as one component of a more general strength and conditioning program in combination with aerobic fitness training.

○ Provided the program is implemented with adequate supervision and instruction, resistance training appears to be well tolerated, safe, and unlikely to have adverse consequences such as immune system impairment or lymphedema.

○ Resistance training is likely to be most effective when individualized with careful attention to needs and capabilities, including those related not only to cancer and treatment but to other health challenges especially common with advancing age, which holds a greater risk of cancer occurrence.

○ ACSM guidelines for resistance training described earlier provide a useful starting point in designing resistance-training interventions for individuals with cancer. Clinical guidelines published by Courneya and colleagues (17) and Schneider, Dennehy, and Carter (64) are also extremely helpful resources for program design and implementation.

Key Terms

Cancer
Carcinogen
Lymphedema
Metastasis
Staging
TNM staging system

Study Questions

1. What are the most common forms of cancer for males and females, and what general trend has been evident in recent years with respect to survival prospects?

2. Why is resistance training a potentially important aspect of cancer rehabilitation?

3. Cancer rehabilitation typically has to contend with treatment side effects, as well as effects of the disease itself. What are among the most important treatment-related effects of cancer that may impact resistance training?

4. What are some principles of resistance training used with healthy older adults that can be effectively adapted for use with people who have cancer?

5. Summarize general recommendations with respect to resistance-training modes, intensity, duration, and progression for people with cancer.

References

1. Adams, KJ, Salmon P. Acute adjustments for stress. *Strength and Conditioning Journal.* 2002;24(1):63–64.

2. Adamsen L, Midtgaard J, Rorth M, et al. Feasibility, physical capacity, and health benefits of a multidimensional exercise program for cancer patients undergoing chemotherapy. *Support Care Cancer.* 2003;11(11):707–716.

3. Adamsen L, Midtgaard J, Roerth M, Andersen C, Quist M, Moeller T. Transforming the nature of fatigue through exercise: qualitative findings from a multidimensional exercise programme in cancer patients undergoing chemotherapy. *Eur J Cancer Care.* 2004;13:362–370.

4. Akima H, Takahashi H, Kuno S, et al. Early phase adaptations of muscle use and strength to isokinetic training. *Med Sci Sports Exerc.* 1999;31(4):588–594.

5. American Cancer Society. *Cancer Facts and Figures 2005.* Atlanta, GA: American Cancer Society;2005.

6. American Cancer Society. *Cancer Facts and Figures 2008.* Atlanta, GA: American Cancer Society;2008.

7. American College of Sports Medicine. *ACSM Guidelines for Exercise Testing a Prescription.* 6th ed. Philadelphia, PA: Lippincott, Williams & Wilkins; 2000.

8. Berglund G, Bolund C, Gustavsson UL, Sjoden PO. Starting again: a comparison study of a group rehabilitation program for cancer patients. *Acta Oncol.* 1993;32(1):15–21.

9. Berglund G, Bolund C, Gustavsson UL, Sjoden PO. One-year follow-up of the "Starting Again" group rehabilitation programme for cancer patients. *Eur J Cancer.* 1994a;30A(12):1744–1751.

10. Berglund G, Bolund C, Gustavsson UL, Sjoden PO. A randomized study of a rehabilitating program for cancer patients: the "Starting Again" group. *Psychooncology.* 1994b;3:109–120.

11. Borg G. *Borg's Perceived Exertion and Pain Scales*. Champaign, IL: Human Kinetics;1998.

12. Brown ML, Lipscomb J, Snyder C. The burden of illness of cancer: economic cost and quality of life. *Annu Rev Public Health*. 2001;22;91–113.

13. Coleman E, Coon S, Hall-Barrow J, Richards K, Gaylor D, Stewart B. Feasibility of exercise during treatment for multiple myeloma. *Cancer Nurs*. 2003;26(5):410–419.

14. Comings DE. A general theory of carcinogenesis. *Proceedings of the National Academy of Science*, 1973. 70, 12 (Part 1):3324–3328.

15. Courneya KS. Exercise in cancer survivors: an overview of research. *Med Sci Sports Exerc*. 2003;35(11):1846–1852.

16. Courneya KS, Mackey JR, Jones LW. Coping with cancer: can exercise help? *Phys Sports Med*. 2000;28:49–73.

17. Courneya KS, Mackey JR, McKenzie DC. Exercise for breast cancer survivors: research evidence and clinical guidelines. *Phys Sports Med*. 2002;30(8):33–42.

18. Courneya KS, Jones LW, Fairey AS, et al. Physical activity in cancer survivors: implications for recurrence and mortality. *Cancer Ther*. 2004;2:1–12.

19. Cramp FDJ. Exercise for the management of cancer-related fatigue in adults. *Cochrane Database of Systematic Reviews*. DOI:10.1002/14651858.CD006145.pub2. Accessed June 19, 2008.

20. Cunningham B, Morris G, Cheney C, Buergel N, Aker S, Lenssen P. The effects of resistive exercise on skeletal muscle in marrow transplant recipients receiving total parenteral nutrition. *JPEN*. 1986;10(6):558–563.

21. Dimeo FC, Stieglitz RD, Novelli-Fischer U, Fetscher S, Keul, J. Effects of physical activity on the fatigue and psychologic status of cancer patients during chemotherapy. *Cancer*. 1999;85:2273–2277.

22. Doyne EJ, Ossip-Klein DJ, Bowman ED et al. Running versus weight lifting in the treatment of depression. *J Consult Clin Psychol*. 1987;55(5):748–754.

23. Durak EP, Lilly PC. The application of an exercise and wellness program for cancer patients: a preliminary outcome report. *J Strength Cond Res*. 1998;12:3–6.

24. Durak EP, Lilly PC, Hackworth JL. Physical and psychosocial responses to exercise in cancer patients: a two-year follow-up survey with prostate, leukemia, and general carcinoma. *J Exerc Physiol*$_{Online}$. 2. Available at: http://faculty.css.edu/tboone2/asep/fldr/fldr.htm. Accessed April 4,1999.

25. Evans WJ. Exercise training guidelines for the elderly. *Med Sci Sports Exerc*. 1999;31(1):12–17.

26. Feigenbaum MS, Pollock ML. Strength training: rationale for current guidelines for adult fitness programs. *Phys Sports Med*. 1997;25(2):44–64.

27. Feigenbaum MS, Pollock ML. Prescription of resistance training for health and disease. *Med Sci Sports Exerc*. 1999;31(1):38–45.

28. Fiatarone MA, Marks EC, Ryan ND, Meredith CN, Lipsitz LA, Evans WJ. High-intensity strength training in nonagenarians: effects on skeletal muscle. *JAMA*. 1990;263(22):3029–3034.

29. Fleck SJ, Kraemer WJ. Designing resistance-training programs. Champaign, IL:Human Kinetics;1997.

30. Ford MB, Mitchell MF. Cancer epidemiology. In: Boyers KL, Ford MB, Judkins AF, Levin B, eds. *Primary Care Oncology*. Philadelphia, PA: W. B. Saunders;1999.

31. Galvao DA, Newton RU. Review of exercise intervention studies in cancer patients. *J Clin Oncol*. 2005;23(4):899–909.

32. Greene FL, Page DL, Fleming ID, et al. and American Joint Committee on Cancer. *Cancer Staging Manual*. 6th ed. Philadelphia, PA: Springer; 2002.

33. Hanahan D, Weinberg RA. The hallmarks of cancer. *Cell.* 2000;100:57–70.

34. Harris SR, Niesen-Vertommen SL. Challenging the myth of exercise-induced lymphedema in breast cancer: a series of case reports. *J Surg Oncol.* 2000;74(2):95–98.

35. Hayes SC, Davies PS, Parker T, Bashford J. Total energy expenditure and body composition changes following peripheral blood stem cell transplantation and participation in an exercise programme. *Bone Marrow Transplant.* 2003;31(5):331–338.

36. Hayes SC, Rowbottom D, Davies PSW, Parker TW, Bashford J. Immunological changes after cancer treatment and participation in an exercise program. *Med Sci Sports Exerc.* 2003;35(1):2–9.

37. Heald SL, Riddle DL, Lamb RL. The shoulder pain and disability index: the construct validity and responsiveness of a region-specific disability measure. *Phys Ther.* 1998;77:1079–1089.

38. Hicks JE. Exercise for cancer patients. In: Basmajian JV, ed. *Therapeutic Exercise.* 5th ed. Baltimore, MD; Williams & Wilkins; 1990;351–369.

39. Holmes MD, Chen WY, Feskanish D, Kroenke CH, Colditz GA. Physical activity and survival after breast cancer. *JAMA.* 2005;293:2479–2486.

40. Howe HL, Wingo PA, Thun MJ, et al. Annual report to the nation on the status of cancer (1973 through 1998) featuring cancers with recent increasing trends. *J Natl Cancer Inst.* 2001;93:824–842.

41. Invergo JJ, Ball TE, Looney M. Relationship of push-ups and absolute muscular endurance to bench press strength. *J Appl Sport Sci Res.* 1991;5:121–125.

42. Kinakin K. Optimal muscle training: biomechanics of lifting for maximum growth and strength. Champaign, IL:Human Kinetics; 2004.

43. Knols R, Aaronson NK, Uebelhart D, Fransen J, Aufdemkampe G. Physical exercise in cancer patients during and after medical treatment: a systematic review of randomized and controlled clinical trials. *J Clin Oncol.* 2005;23(16):3830–3842.

44. Knudson AG. Mutation and cancer:statistical study of retinoblastoma. *Proceedings of the National Academy of Sciences, 1971.*

45. Knuttgen HG. What is exercise? *Phys Sports Med.* 2003;31(3):31–42.

46. Kolden GG, Strauman TJ, Ward A, et al. A pilot study of group exercise training (GET) for women with primary breast cancer: feasibility and health benefits. *Psychooncology.* 2002;11(5):447–456.

47. Kraemer WJ, Adams K, Cafarelli E, et al. Progression models in resistance training for healthy adults. *Med Sci Sports Exerc.* 2002;34(2):364–480.

48. Kraemer WJ. Strength training basics: designing workouts to meet patients' goals. *Phys Sports Med.* 2003;31(8):39–45.

49. Kung HC, Hoyert DL, Xu J, Murphy SL. Deaths: final data for 2005. *National Vital Statistics Reports.* 56(10). Hyattsville, MD: National Center for Health Statistics;2008.

50. McKenzie DC. Abreast in a boat: a race against breast cancer. *CMAJ.* 1998; 159(4):376–378.

51. McKenzie DC, Kalda AL. Effect of upper-extremity exercise on secondary lymphedema in breast cancer patients:a pilot study. *J Clin Oncol.* 2003;21(3):463–466.

52. McNeely MK, Parliament M, Courneya KS, et al. A pilot study of a randomized controlled trial to evaluate the effects of progressive resistance exercise training on shoulder dysfunction caused by spinal accessory neurapraxia/neuroectomy in head and neck cancer survivors. *Head and Neck.* 2004;26:518–530.

53. Mock V. The benefits of exercise in women with breast cancer. In: Dow KH, ed. *Contemporary Issues in Breast Cancer.* Boston, MA:Jones and Bartlett;1996:99–106.

54. National Cancer Institute. Cancer Trends Progress Report:2005 Update.

55. National Cancer Institute. Cancer Trends Progress Report:2007 Update. Available at: http://progressreport.cancer.gov. Accessed June 17, 2008.

56. Nieman DC, Cook VD, Henson DA, et al. Moderate exercise training and natural killer cell cytotoxic activity in breast cancer patients. *Int J Sports Med.* 1995;16(5):334–337.

57. Ornish D, Weidner G, Fair WR, et al. Intensive lifestyle changes may affect the progression of prostate cancer. *J Neurol.* 2005;174:1065–1070.

58. Peters J, Loud J, Dimond E, Jenkins J. Cancer genetics fundamentals. *Cancer Nurs.* 2001;24(6):446–461.

59. Plante TG, Lantis A, Checa G. The influence of perceived versus aerobic fitness on psychological health and physiological stress responsivity. *Int J Stress Management.* 1998;5(3):141–156.

60. Porter MM. The effects of strength training on sarcopenia. *Can J Appl Physiol.* 2001;26(1):123–141.

61. Ries LAG, Melbert D, Krapcho M, et al. eds. *SEER Cancer Statistics Review*:1975–2005. Bethesda, MD:National Cancer Institute. Available at: http://seer.cancer.gov/csr/ 1975–2005/. Accessed June 19, 2008.

62. Rosenberg, IH. Sarcopenia: origins and clinical relevance. *J Nutr.* 1997;127:990S–991S.

63. Salmon PG, Swank AM. Exercise-based disease management guidelines for individuals with cancer: potential applications in a high-risk mid-southern state. *J Exerc Physiol* [online]. 2002;5(4):1–10.

64. Schneider CM, Dennehy CA, Carter SD. *Exercise and Cancer Recovery.* Champaign, IL:Human Kinetics;2003.

65. Schmitz KH, Holtzman J, Courneya KS, Masse LC, Duval S, Sand Kane R. Controlled physical activity trials in cancer survivors: a systematic review and meta-analysis. *Cancer Epidemiol Biomarkers Prev.* 2005;14(7):1588–1595.

66. Schwartz AL. Cancer. In: Durstine LL, Moore G, eds. *ACSM's Exercise Management for Persons with Chronic Diseases and Disabilities.* Champaign, IL: Human Kinetics; 2003:166–172.

67. Segal RJ, Reid RD, Courneya KS, et al. Resistance exercise in men receiving androgen-deprivation therapy for prostate cancer. *J Clin Oncol.* 2003;21(9):1653–1659.

68. Sherwood NE, Jeffery RW. The behavioral determinants of exercise: implications for physical activity interventions. *Annu Rev Nutr.* 2000;20:21–44.

69. Spielholz NI. Scientific basis of exercise programs. In: Basmajian JV, Wolf SL, eds. *Therapeutic Exercise.* 5th ed. Baltimore, MD; Williams & Wilkins. 1990;49–76.

70. Turner J, Hayes S, Reul-Hirche H. Improving the physical status and quality of life of women treated for breast cancer: a pilot study of a structured exercise intervention. *J Surg Oncol.* 2004;86:141–146.

71. Visovsky C, Dvorak C. Exercise and cancer recovery. *J Issues Nurs.* [online] 10(2). Available at: http://nursingworld.org/ojin/ hirsh/topic3/tpc3_2.htm. 2005.

72. Yates JW. The role of exercise and weight control in breast cancer prevention and rehabilitation. In: Donegan WL, Spratt JS, eds. *Cancer of the Breast.* 5th ed. Philadelphia, PA:W. B. Saunders. 2002;225–247.

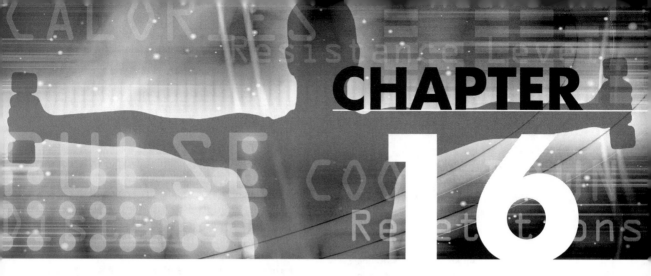

CHAPTER 16

RESISTANCE-TRAINING STRATEGIES FOR STROKE SURVIVORS

Objectives

Upon completion of this chapter, the reader should be able to:

- Discuss the health implications of stroke
- Describe the etiology of stroke
- Identify research supporting the safety and efficacy of resistance training for stroke survivors
- Describe different methods of resistance training and special considerations to enhance participant safety during exercise testing and training
- Describe program variables used to design resistance-training programs
- Explain the concept and application of periodization to the design of resistance-training programs for stroke survivors
- Design safe, effective, and progressive resistance-training programs for stroke survivors

INTRODUCTION

A **cerebral vascular accident,** commonly called a **stroke,** is the result of a reduction of blood supply to parts of the brain. When blood supply to a portion of the brain is diminished, oxygen delivery is also diminished, causing the affected brain cells to die and severely affecting neurologic function. Less than 30 percent of strokes are fatal, but the associated physical trauma can cause variable levels of impairment and loss of the ability to complete activities of daily living, which may result in loss of independence. The most common effects of stroke include hemiparesis, hemiplegia, aphasia or dysphagia, decreased field of vision and visual perception, and behavioral and cognitive changes. Of these effects, **hemiparesis,** weakness on one side of the body, and **hemiplegia,** paralysis on one side of the body, cause the majority of physical impairments that can be treated with a proper rehabilitation and training program.

Classically, physical rehabilitation for stroke survivors takes place within the first 30 days post-stroke and is completed on an inpatient basis with the assistance of physical and/or occupational therapists. During this period, acute recovery of motor function is the greatest, with smaller changes occurring during the next 3 to 6 months. After this time, recovery without the assistance of an external training program designed to teach the individual how to use the affected musculature is minimal. Resistance-training programs for stroke survivors will vary in complexity and intensity depending on the extent of physical impairment. This chapter will address some of the major resistance-training program components common to most stroke survivors.

PREVALENCE AND ECONOMIC IMPACT OF STROKE

Approximately 500,000 Americans experience their first stroke each year, and another 200,000 have recurrent strokes. On average, a stroke occurs every 45 seconds. While less than 30 percent of strokes are fatal, nearly 157,000 people a year die from strokes, making it number three among all causes of death (2). While stroke can occur at any age, the majority of incidents occur after age 55 in both men and women, and incidents increase with age. More men than women have strokes, but more women die from strokes. Stroke is also the leading cause of serious long-term disability in the United States (2). More than 1.1 million American adults reported having difficulty with functional limitations, activities of daily living, and so on resulting from stroke (2). The estimated direct and indirect cost of stroke nationwide for 2006 is $57.9 billion (2). The average cost per individual for inpatient care, rehabilitation, and follow-up care for lasting deficits following a stroke is estimated at $140,048 over a lifetime for a mild stroke, after which the individual was able to return to independent living again. Survivors who require nursing home care, in-home care, or have recurring strokes will incur much greater expenses.

ETIOLOGY OF A STROKE

Stroke is a general term that describes the cerebrovascular accident in the simplest terms. Classification of strokes by etiology is an ongoing process as the causes of stroke become more thoroughly understood with advances in medical technology. About 80 to 85 percent of strokes are **ischemic strokes** (2), which occur when an artery supplying the brain becomes clogged. There are several different types of ischemic stroke, each caused by a different mechanism. A **thrombotic stroke** is the result of arteriosclerosis that either completely blocks a blood vessel or narrows the vessel to the point that an insufficient supply of blood passes through. An **embolic stroke** occurs when an embolus, or wandering clot, becomes lodged in an artery leading to the brain. An embolus can originate from anywhere downstream of the vessel and is classified as either arterial or cardiac in origin. Cardiac sources of embolism include atrial fibrillation, sinoatrial disorder, acute myocardial infarction, cardiac tumors, valvular disorders, and bacterial endocarditis. A systemic hypoperfusion stroke occurs when circulatory failure caused by the heart results in insufficient delivery of blood to the brain. This mechanism is how 1 to 3 percent of all myocardial infarctions result in a stroke as well (11).

Hemorrhagic strokes caused by a ruptured blood vessel in the brain account for 15 to 20 percent of strokes (2). When a blood vessel is interrupted, blood flow is detoured from a normal path through the vessel into the extravascular space surrounding the vessel. A subarachnoid hemorrhage occurs when a blood vessel on the surface of the brain ruptures and bleeds into the space between the brain and the skull. An intracerebral hemorrhage is the result of a blood vessel bleeding into the tissue deep within the brain. In both types of hemorrhagic stroke, a ruptured aneurysm caused by high blood pressure is the most common cause.

For most individuals, a stroke may have more than one potential cause. The major risk factors that predispose a person to atherosclerosis—such as hypertension, cigarette smoking, and diabetes—promote plaque formation and occlusive disease in the coronary arteries, peripheral vasculature, and aorta, as well as the craniocervical arteries (2). The single most controllable risk factor for stroke is high blood pressure. Individuals with blood pressure less than 120/80 mm Hg have about half the lifetime risk of stroke compared to people with hypertension (24). Smoking doubles the risk of having a stroke at any age, and it takes 5 years after cessation of smoking for stroke risk to reach the level of a nonsmoker (31).

Transient ischemic attacks (TIAs) are "ministrokes" that produce stroke-like effects but no lasting effects. Recurring TIAs are a leading signal of impending stroke, because they are caused by clots that block an artery temporarily. Only about 15 percent of strokes are preceded by a TIA; but after a TIA, the risk of stroke within the next 90 days increases up to 17 percent and is highest within the first 30 days (14–16, 19).

PHYSIOLOGICAL EFFECTS OF STROKE

Although the survival rate for stroke is good, many survivors are affected by neurologic impairments due to brain cells damaged during the stroke. Despite intensive rehabilitation in the first few months after a stroke, survivors may be left with significant disability (7). The effects of the neurologic impairment varies among individuals and can include paresis, paralysis, spasticity, loss of balance, loss of sensation, trouble with visual perception or field of vision, and neuromuscular imbalances.

BENEFITS OF RESISTANCE TRAINING FOR STROKE SURVIVORS

A common physical impairment resulting from damage to the brain is muscle weakness combined with spasticity, an uncontrolled contraction that results in a shortened and stiffened joint that the individual is unable to release. This effect manifests as a combination of one or more of the following sustained changes in normal posture: wrist, elbow, and shoulder flexion; ankle plantar flexion; and knee and hip extension. One of the challenges for a stroke survivor with spasticity in the lower limbs is mastering the ability to walk. Rehabilitation is often centered on regaining mobility, with an improved gait and/or gait speed, because a survivor's ability to move about on their own is a major component of living independently (27). Walking with one leg in constant plantar flexion, with knee and hip extension, makes regular ambulation awkward and ungainly. Additionally, the inability to easily flex the hip and knee makes climbing stairs, stepping up on or down from a curb, or maneuvering into and out of a car difficult. Resistance training can improve both the gait speed and synchronization of arm and leg swing for stroke survivors, making daily errands less cumbersome (6, 25, 27, 29).

The limited range of motion caused by spasticity forces an individual to rely heavily on the nonaffected side to complete normal daily activities. This increased use of the nonaffected side further widens the imbalance in strength between the affected and nonaffected limb. Through the use of resistance training, this imbalance can be made smaller, and the increased strength in the affected limb can lead to increased regular use of that limb, which leads to increased ability to maneuver independently. This ability is often seen in a survivor's increased ability to balance while standing and rising from a sitting position, using both legs to propel them upward (8).

Muscle strength in affected limbs has been documented anywhere from 23 to 94 percent of the nonaffected limb (1), and that weakness is considered one of the most prominent consequences of stroke (17, 18). While muscle weakness resulting from disuse is a limiting factor in rehabilitation, the strength deficit may be furthered by reductions in muscle fiber firing and increased fatigability, decreased motor unit numbers, and altered recruitment order (5, 23, 32).

Resistance training has been shown to improve strength in both the affected and unaffected limbs of stroke survivors (3, 21, 25, 28–30). Although increased strength is a benefit to unaffected individuals, the benefit of increased strength to a stroke survivor has additional implications beyond being able to lift more weight. The stroke survivor has to contend with maneuvering throughout the day with only limited use of one of the arms or legs or both an arm and leg.

Literature Review of Research Supporting Resistance Training for Stroke Survivors

Until the mid 1990s, little research was available on the effects of resistance training for stroke survivors. As a result, many of the participants in research completed since that time are several years post-stroke, which allows us to see that resistance training has an effect even some time after a stroke, when the individual has settled into a regular pattern of use or disuse of the affected limbs. Table 16-1 lists relevant research on resistance training post-stroke.

Unfortunately, only eight studies have been completed thus far that specifically address the effect resistance training has on strength, and none of them addresses all the needs of a stroke survivor. Therefore none of them are applicable for implementation as a stand-alone resistance-training program. Very little of the available research utilized equipment normally found in health clubs and fitness centers. Half of the testing and training was done using isokinetic equipment, with results specified in increased torque rather than strength. The research that utilized conventional equipment (3, 21, 28, 30) found substantial increases in strength in as little as 4 weeks of training.

Research thus far has also failed to provide a full-body resistance-training program. In fact, the training programs used in research to date have focused on knee extension, knee flexion, ankle plantar flexion and dorsiflexion, and hip extension. The one study that included any component of upper-body musculature used a single exercise, the arm press, for elbow extension and shoulder horizontal adduction. While gait and mobility are important, a complete resistance-training program should include as many of the major muscle groups as possible in both the upper and lower body and should address movements other than gait that contribute to being able to complete activities of daily living. The resistance-training program detailed in this chapter will include the exercises found in the available literature, as well as exercises that work additional areas of the body, to provide a comprehensive training program.

DESIGNING RESISTANCE-TRAINING PROGRAMS FOR STROKE SURVIVORS

A growing number of stroke support groups include exercise training information for their members, and a growing number of exercise professionals are specializing in working with stroke survivors. Training this population requires an understanding of the varying ways in which neurological deficits can

Table 16-1 Summary of Research on Resistance Training Post-Stroke

Author	Design/n	Type of Training	Strength Gains
Weiss (30)	Pre/Post/7	12 wks, 2x/wk, 3 sets, 8 to 10 reps at 70% 1RM Weight-stack hip flexion, abduction, extension Pneumatic knee extension, leg press Also improved score on repeated Chair-stand test time.	68%
Ouellette (21)	Random/42	12wks, 3x/wk, 3 sets, 8 to 10 reps at 70% 1RM Pneumatic leg press, knee extension Weight-stack dorsiflexion, plantar flexion Also increased 6-minute walk distance, maximal gait velocity, and peak power	LP 16% KE 31% PF 36% DF 33%
LP = leg press; KE = knee extension; PF = plantar flexion			
Badics (3)	Pre/Post/56	4 wks, 3 to 5 sets. 20 reps at 30 to 50% 1RM	LP 31% AP 37%
LP = Leg press; AP = arm press			
Teixeira-Salmela (28)	Random/13	10 wks, 3x/week, 3 sets, 10 reps at 80% 1RM Isokinetic hip and knee flexion/extension Isokinetic ankle plantar flexion, dorsiflexion Increased torque 42%, gait speed 28%, and stair-climbing speed 37%	
Teixeira-Salmela (29)	Pre/Post/13	10wks, 3x/wk, 3 sets, 10 reps at 80% 1RM Hip flexion/extension/abduction, knee flexion/extension, ankle dorsiflexion and plantar flexion using bodyweight, Therabands, and sandbag weights. Increased power, gait speed (37%), stride length, and cadence	
Sharp (25)	Pre/Post/13	6wks, 3x/wk, 3 sets, 6 to 8 reps Isokinetic knee extension and flexion Increased torque and gait velocity	
Engardt (9)	Pre/Post/20	6wks, 2x/wk, 3 sets, 10 reps Isokinetic knee extension	25 to 30%
Cramp (6)	Pre/Post/10	12wks, 2x/wk Isometric/concentric knee extension	58%

manifest themselves. Not all stroke survivors present the same complications. Anecdotally, the older a stroke survivor is, the more symptoms will manifest, and the greater the neurological deficits will be. Likewise, the more time that has passed since the stroke, the more likely a survivor has established new motor patterns to help achieve a level of mobility. Without proper training, these new motor patterns are often the result of using the affected side as a brace while the unaffected side performs a majority of the required movements. For instance, a spastic leg that remains in plantar flexion with knee and hip extension will not be moved through the normal range of motion during walking, but will be held in this stiffened position and swung around like a crutch while the unaffected leg is used to step up on curbs or steps and propel the person forward. The spastic arm that is perpetually held with the fist clenched, wrist and elbow flexed, and arm held against the chest will be used to hold objects such as a purse or bag; the unaffected arm will be used for picking objects up, writing, and opening and closing doors. One of the difficulties of training a stroke survivor is untraining these new motor patterns and retraining the original patterns.

Exercise Testing Considerations

Exercise testing for this population is possible with some slight modifications to regular protocols. The standard one-repetition maximum (1RM) testing for strength (12) is applicable to this population if the testing is done unilaterally, one limb at a time. In a typically bilateral exercise such as the leg press, the unaffected leg will compensate for the affected leg, and the results will not indicate the difference between legs. This compensation causes difficulty in determining whether a resistance-training program is having an effect during retesting. To combat this problem, the same test can be done unilaterally, one limb at a time, so that differences between limbs can be measured and charted. Adapting the 1RM test protocol so that each limb is tested individually requires more time for testing and more rests between attempts. The test can be structured so that an attempt is completed on each limb before the weight is increased, or all attempts for a limb can be completed and then the opposite side can be tested.

When using 1RM testing for muscle strength, each exercise included in the training program should be tested. With the differences in neurological deficits a stroke survivor may exhibit, some areas of the body may adapt to the training program faster than others. For example, in some cases the strength of the upper body may improve before any changes in the lower body manifest; or the strength of the elbow flexors may increase before the strength of the elbow extensors. Always test each movement individually for changes in strength to obtain baseline values and a practical understanding of whether the resistance-training program is effective.

The range of motion of a joint is also a good indicator of the effects of the training program. In joints in which spasticity is present, range of motion is limited, and voluntary movement of that joint is reduced in comparison to the unaffected side. Measurement of voluntary range of motion and passive range of motion are both good measures of spasticity. **Passive range of motion** is the range within which the joint can be moved manually by the examiner without inducing either pain or movement in another joint. In areas of spasticity, the stroke survivor usually has very little ability to move the joint actively, although the joint can be moved quite a bit more passively. Measurements should be taken with a goniometer on both the affected and unaffected side to measure side-to-side differences and changes induced by the training program.

A stroke survivor's muscular endurance is typically very low, because their reduced mobility prevents them from completing repetitive tasks very easily. There are several tests of muscular endurance that are typically used with stroke survivors, and each one can be modified for the person's particular physical deficits. Common tests used in the research on stroke and resistance training include the chair-rise test (21, 30) and the stair-climb test (21, 25, 30). In the **chair-rise test,** a person attempts to rise to full standing height from a sitting position and then sit back down as many times as possible in 15 to 30 seconds; longer tests are used for those with more endurance. The length of the chair-rise test can be adjusted as the person gains more muscular endurance.

The **stair-climb test** evaluates how much time a person takes to climb a set number of steps. Tests typically use between 4 and 10 steps, depending on the ability of the person, the height of the available stairs, and the ability of the examiner to maintain a safe test as steps rise higher. Whereas the chair-rise test evaluates the number of repetitions in a given time frame, the stair-climb test evaluates the time to complete a given number of repetitions. Both tests thereby involve a component of speed and a component of power. Neither test has established standards or scores, so they can be used for pre- and post-testing to determine change. No specific tests are reported in the literature for determining upper-body muscular endurance of stroke survivors. Commonly used tests of 10- to 15-repetition maximums (10RM to 15RM) for a given upper-body exercise would be appropriate if they were performed unilaterally, with comparisons made between affected and unaffected sides and long-term comparisons made before and after training.

Balance is another area that is of great concern to stroke survivors. Along with the neurological deficits that cause weakness and spasticity, the loss of sensation in an affected foot can lead to trouble standing, walking, and climbing stairs, simply because the person does not feel how much pressure they are exerting on that foot. Combined with muscular weakness, the loss of sensation leads the person to rely more on the unaffected side, thus putting more pressure on that leg and removing as much stimulus as possible from the affected leg. This action in turn leads to more disuse and atrophy of the affected leg. Testing balance can be done with the **stork-stand test** (13). In this test, the person is required to stand on one leg as long as possible. Simple before and after comparisons can determine changes induced from the training program.

SPECIAL CONSIDERATIONS FOR EXERCISE TRAINING

Although the literature has reported strength gains in stroke survivors as high as 68 percent, these were gains made from a significantly atrophied state within the first 12 weeks of training. During the initial stages of a new training program, the majority of improvements are neurologically based (4), which is great for stroke survivors, because most of their deficiencies are neurologically based. The effects of a resistance-training program that continues beyond 12 weeks has not been reported, but based on research on normal subjects, improvement could continue as long as training continued.

Safety is a major issue that must be addressed with stroke survivors. Because of the possible loss of visual and sensory perception accompanying a stroke, care should be taken to maintain a training environment free from unnecessary obstacles, especially small objects on the floor that may cause a trip-and-fall situation. During balance training, and any resistance training in which a weight is held over the head or chest, appropriate spotting techniques should be employed (4). Resistance training with stroke survivors should always be monitored and supervised.

For stroke survivors with spasticity, range of motion may be limited in some joints. During the execution of resistance-training movements, encourage working through as much of the range of motion as possible. Allow a repetition to be considered complete when the individual moves through their maximum voluntary range of motion. Tracking range of motion over time will help show changes in range of motion, along with changes in strength. Additionally, assisting an individual to move through the remaining range of motion on an exercise is acceptable. Manually moving or "spotting" them through the rest of the exercise can assist in retraining the lost motor pattern.

Exercise Program Components

Because the muscular weakness found after a stroke is the result of both neural and muscular changes, in some ways the results of a stroke are similar to the results of normal aging, for which the benefits of resistance training have been clearly shown (10, 20, 26). Because research has shown that individuals can increase strength from a resistance-training program post-stroke, and that such a training program does not cause an increase in spasticity (3, 22), we can safely assume that a moderate training program will benefit most stroke survivors.

Given the limited information from investigations to date, some common themes can be used to form the basis of a resistance-training program. To improve strength, the literature recommends working at a minimum of 70 percent of 1RM with a maximum of 10 repetitions per set for 3 sets, performed 3 days per week for at least 10 weeks. The current recommendations for a program emphasizing improvements in strength recommends 2 sets of loads greater than 85 percent of 1RM and 6 or less repetitions (4). However, this type of program is primarily targeted toward athletes, and improvements in strength can be found with lighter loads combined with more repetitions, so the current literature is within the range of acceptable loads, repetitions, and sets for the given population.

The program outlined below is based on a circuit-training style of exercise, in which the individual performs a single set of a series of exercises in a row and then repeats the series for additional sets as required. Over the course of the 24-week program, the variable of load, sets, repetitions, and exercises is manipulated according to the principles of undulating periodization. **Undulating periodization** involves increasing the load and volume of exercise over the course of several training sessions, then decreasing the load and volume of exercise for a short time, then increasing both again to higher levels than before. Undulating periodization creates a cycling effect that allows a person to increase the workload and intensity of each exercise session slowly, allowing the body to rest completely before increasing the load again. Each time the load and volume of exercise are increased, they move beyond the previous cycle to higher levels of strength and performance.

In any given fitness center, there are an unlimited number of combinations of exercises that could be put together to achieve the same result. The program design must address the most common needs of stroke survivors by focusing on exercises that include major muscle groups, both multiple- and single-joint exercises, unilateral and bilateral movements, and a changing combination of exercises to ensure that the body is constantly required to learn new motor patterns. Because some exercises will require the prescribed number of sets to be completed on each limb individually, the number of exercises completed will constantly change. Rest between each set should be kept to less than 1 minute, unless the person is not able to keep up the pace, in which case additional rest is allowed.

SAMPLE 24-WEEK PROGRAM

To begin the program, baseline values of 1RM should be determined for each exercise in which an external resistance, such as a weight stack or dumbbell, is employed. Those exercises in which the resistance will consist of only the body weight or a small ankle weight need not be tested for 1RM. Retesting for 1RM should be completed at the end of each "light" cycle to determine how much the intensity is increased for the next "heavy" cycle. Over the course of a 24-week program, testing would be completed at the end of the first 3 weeks and again every 6 weeks thereafter.

The main exercises employed in the reviewed literature included the leg press, knee extension, knee flexion, plantar flexion, dorsiflexion, and arm press. A comprehensive resistance-training program should include exercises for each muscle group and joint, and it must include exercises that mimic the person's activities of daily living. Exercises should be done in a standing position if possible, so that side-to-side balance is trained while the exercise is being performed. Although other exercises could have been used for this program, the exercise choices here create a full range of strength, balance, coordination, and training for activities of daily living for the average stroke survivor. These exercises can be adapted to fit both beginner and advanced training levels.

Finally, the order of exercises has been set so that the person will rotate through every exercise over the course of several days, with every day having a different order and combination of exercises. The reason for this mixing up of the program is to challenge the individual to work the muscles in different combinations without getting set into a specific routine. Since life rarely takes the same course day after day, neither should training be the same every time. New motor patterns are learned with repetitive motion, but more complex motor patterns can be learned if the motion of each exercise is repetitive, but the order of exercises is different. Table 16-2 details a 24-week resistance-training program that includes specific exercises, sets, reps, percents of 1RM, and exercise order.

Table 16-2 Sample 24-Week Training Program for Stroke Survivors

Alternating 3-week cycles of light and heavy workloads and volume

Retesting 1RM after each light cycle

Light cycle 1

Week 1

2 sets, 5 reps, 70% 1RM

  Day 1: Test 1RM for each exercise
  Day 2: Leg presses, step-ups, squats, chest presses, upright rows, shoulder presses
  Day 3: Knee extensions, seated leg curls, knee raises, biceps curls, triceps presses, pulldowns

Week 2

2 sets, 7 reps, 70% 1RM

  Day 1: Standing leg curls, leg presses, squats, chest presses, rows, front raises
  Day 2: Step-ups, knee raises, knee extensions, triceps presses, shoulder presses, rows
  Day 3: Seated leg curls, leg presses, squats, pulldowns, biceps curls, upright rows

Week 3

2 sets, 9 reps, 70% 1RM

  Day 1: Standing leg curls, step-ups, knee extensions, front raises, shoulder presses, chest presses
  Day 2: Seated leg curls, knee raises, standing leg curls, biceps curls, triceps presses, upright rows
  Day 3: Retest 1RM

Heavy cycle 1

Week 4

3 sets, 5 reps, 74% 1RM

  Day 1: Squats, knee raises, step-ups, front raises, rows, pulldowns
  Day 2: Knee extensions, standing leg curls, leg presses, chest presses, biceps curls, pulldowns
  Day 3: Seated leg curls, squats, knee raises, upright rows, shoulder presses, front raises

(continued)

Table 16-2 Sample 24-Week Training Program for Stroke Survivors (continued)

Heavy cycle 1

Week 5

3 sets, 7 reps, 74% 1RM

Day 1: Step-ups, knee extensions, leg presses, rows, triceps presses, biceps curls

Day 2: Seated leg curls, knee raises, standing leg curls, chest presses, shoulder presses, pulldowns

Day 3: Leg presses, squats, knee extensions, front raises, upright rows, triceps presses

Week 6

3 sets, 9 reps, 74% 1RM

Day 1: Seated leg curls, step-ups, knee extensions, rows, chest presses, biceps curls

Day 2: Standing leg curls, knee raises, squats, pulldowns, front raises, chest presses

Day 3: Leg presses, knee extensions, seated leg curls, triceps presses, upright rows, shoulder presses

Light cycle 2

Week 7

2 sets, 8 reps, 72% 1RM

Day 1: Rows, chest presses, triceps presses, standing leg curls, squats, step-ups

Day 2: Pulldowns, chest presses, front raises, leg presses, step-ups, seated leg curls

Day 3: Biceps curls, upright rows, rows, knee raises, knee extensions, standing leg curls

Week 8

2 sets, 10 reps, 72% 1RM

Day 1: Shoulder presses, front raises, triceps presses, seated leg curls, squats, standing leg curls

Day 2: Rows, biceps curls, pulldowns, leg presses, step-ups, squats

Day 3: Upright rows, shoulder presses, rows, knee extensions, knee raises, seated leg curls

Week 9

2 sets, 10 reps, 72% 1RM

Day 1: Triceps presses, biceps curls, chest presses, standing leg curls, leg presses, step-ups

Day 2: Pulldowns, upright rows, shoulder presses, squats, seated leg curls, knee raises

Day 3: Retest 1RM

Heavy cycle 2

Week 10

3 sets, 5 reps, 76% 1RM

Day 1: Chest presses, rows, knee extensions, seated leg curls, biceps curls, triceps presses, squats

Table 16-2 Sample 24-Week Training Program for Stroke Survivors (continued)

Heavy cycle 2

Week 10 (continued)

Day 2: Leg presses, standing leg curls, front raises, upright rows, seated leg curls, step-ups, pulldowns

Day 3: Shoulder presses, biceps curls, step-ups, knee extensions, triceps presses, rows, chest presses

Week 11

3 sets, 7 reps, 76%1RM

Day 1: Upright rows, shoulder presses, standing leg curls, knee raises, pulldowns, front raises, step-ups

Day 2: Squats, seated leg curls, front raises, rows, leg presses, knee extensions, upright rows

Day 3: Shoulder presses, pulldowns, leg presses, standing leg curls, triceps presses, biceps curls, front raises

Week 12

3 sets, 9 reps, 76% 1RM

Day 1: Squats, knee raises, standing leg curls, upright rows, pulldowns, chest presses, shoulder presses

Day 2: Rows, biceps curls, knee extensions, knee raises, front raises, triceps presses, pulldowns

Day 3: Standing leg curls, step-ups, squats, biceps curls, chest presses, shoulder presses, knee extensions

Light cycle 3

Week 13

2 sets, 8 reps, 74% 1RM

Day 1: Upright rows, rows, pulldowns, knee raises, leg presses, step-ups

Day 2: Front raises, shoulder presses, chest presses, seated leg curls, leg presses, standing leg curls

Day 3: Front raises, biceps curls, triceps presses, squats, knee extensions, step-ups

Week 14

2 sets, 10 reps, 74% 1RM

Day 1: Seated leg curls, leg presses, knee raises, rows, upright rows, shoulder presses

Day 2: Squats, standing leg curls, knee extensions, triceps presses, rows, chest presses

Day 3: Step-ups, knee raises, leg presses, biceps curls, pulldowns, front raises

(continued)

Table 16-2 Sample 24-Week Training Program for Stroke Survivors (continued)

Light cycle 3

Week 15

2 sets, 10 reps, 74% 1RM

Day 1: Triceps presses, upright rows, pulldowns, seated leg curls, squats, knee raises

Day 2: Front raises, shoulder presses, rows, knee extensions, standing leg curls, step-ups

Day 3: Retest 1RM

Heavy cycle 3

Week 16

3 sets, 5 reps, 78% 1RM

Day 1: Biceps curls, leg presses, triceps presses, seated leg curls, upright rows, knee extensions, chest presses

Day 2: Rows, squats, shoulder presses, standing leg curls, front raises, knee raises, pulldowns

Day 3: Chest presses, seated leg curls, biceps curls, step-ups, upright rows, knee raises, shoulder presses

Week 17

3 sets, 7 reps, 78% 1RM

Day 1: Leg presses, triceps presses, squats, rows, knee raises, pulldowns, biceps curls

Day 2: Step-ups, chest presses, standing leg curls, front raises, knee extensions, pulldowns, upright rows

Day 3: Seated leg curls, triceps presses, leg presses, rows, knee extensions, shoulder presses, chest presses

Week 18

3 sets, 9 reps, 78% 1RM

Day 1: Upright rows, front raises, standing leg curls, knee raises, triceps presses, biceps curls, pulldowns

Day 2: Leg presses, seated leg curls, rows, chest presses, step-ups, knee extensions, standing leg curls

Day 3: Biceps curls, shoulder presses, squats, leg presses, triceps presses, pulldowns, front raises

Light cycle 4

Week 19

2 sets, 8 reps, 76% 1RM

Day 1: Rows, chest presses, triceps presses, standing leg curls, squats, step-ups

Day 2: Pulldowns, chest presses, front raises, leg presses, step-ups, seated leg curls

Day 3: Biceps curls, upright rows, rows, knee raises, knee extensions, standing leg curls

Table 16-2 Sample 24-Week Training Program for Stroke Survivors (continued)

Light cycle 4

Week 20

2 sets, 10 reps, 76% 1RM

Day 1: Shoulder presses, front raises, triceps presses, seated leg curls, squats, standing leg curls

Day 2: Rows, biceps curls, pulldowns, leg presses, step-ups, squats

Day 3: Upright rows, shoulder presses, rows, knee extensions, knee raises, seated leg curls

Week 21

2 sets, 10 reps, 76% 1RM

Day 1: Triceps presses, biceps curls, chest presses, standing leg curls, leg presses, step-ups

Day 2: Pulldowns, upright rows, shoulder presses, squats, seated leg curls, knee raises

Day 3: Retest 1RM

Heavy cycle 4

Week 22

3 sets, 5 reps, 80% 1RM

Day 1: Front raises, shoulder presses, knee extensions, squats, upright rows, biceps curls, leg presses, knee raises

Day 2: Pulldowns, chest presses, seated leg curls, step-ups, triceps presses, rows, standing leg curls, leg presses

Day 3: Upright rows, front raises, squats, seated leg curls, pulldowns, shoulder presses, knee extensions, knee raises

Week 23

3 sets, 7 reps, 80% 1RM

Day 1: Biceps curls, chest presses, pulldowns, front raises, step-ups, knee extensions, standing leg curls, upright rows

Day 2: Rows, triceps presses, shoulder presses, biceps curls, squats, leg presses, knee raises, pulldowns

Day 3: Chest presses, front raises, upright rows, seated leg curls, step-ups, knee extensions, biceps curls, rows

Week 24

3 sets, 9 reps, 80% 1RM

Day 1: Standing leg curls, squats, front raises, shoulder presses, step-ups, leg presses, chest presses, pulldowns

Day 2: Triceps presses, standing leg curls, upright rows, knee extensions, shoulder presses, knee raises, biceps curls, seated leg curls

Day 3: Rows, standing leg curls, triceps presses, knee extensions, front raises, step-ups, chest presses, pulldowns

CASE STUDY

This case study illustrates how the tests and training program presented in this chapter work in a one-on-one training situation. The subject, Mrs. V, is a 64-year-old woman who had a stroke 4 years ago. At that time, she was physically active, participating in water aerobics twice a week, walking 2 miles each day with her dog, and enjoying weekly ballroom dancing lessons. The most pronounced effects of the stroke were left-arm and left-leg spasticity.

Mrs. V received inpatient physical therapy for 3 weeks post-stroke, which taught her how to manipulate a self-standing cane so that she could walk. Since then, she has not participated in any type of rehabilitation, and she dropped out of the water aerobics class, dance lessons, and discontinued her daily walks. By all measures she became physically inactive and sedentary. As a result of this change in lifestyle, Mrs. V gained 30 pounds and lost the

ability to stand up from a sitting position without the aid of another person or something to hold on to for support and assistance. Mrs. V relies on a cane to assist her in walking, and when she encounters a step or curb, she always uses the unaffected leg to step up. Her left arm is practically useless, and the spasticity has increased in the years since her stroke. Her left hand is continually clenched into a fist, the wrist is flexed, the elbow is flexed and pronated, and the entire arm is held against the chest at all times.

After deciding to start a training program, we determined that Mrs. V's goals were to be able to get out of a chair unassisted, walk without a cane, reduce the spasticity of the left arm, and try to regain some useful voluntary movement. Measurements of joint range of motion were taken on both sides of the body (Table 16-3). Voluntary straightening of the left elbow was minimal; however when passively stretched, the arm would resume a fully extended position momentarily. Mrs. V had retained some range of

Table 16-3 Range of Motion for Each Joint Pre- and Post-Training

Measurements were taken from a standing position at rest				
	Pre	Post	Normal	% change
R-shoulder flexion	180°	180°	150–180°	none
L-shoulder flexion	45°	110°	150–180°	144%
R-shoulder abduction	180°	180°	180°	none
L-shoulder abduction	30°	90°	180°	200%
R-elbow flexion	130°	140°	140–150°	7%
R-elbow extension**	0°	0°	0°	none
L-elbow flexion*	10°	40°	140–150°	300%
L-elbow extension*	30°	60°	0°	100%
R-hip flexion	90°	110°	110–120°	22%
L-hip flexion	40°	90°	110–120°	125%
R-knee flexion	140°	150°	135–150°	7%
L-knee flexion	45°	85°	135–150°	88%

** Elbow extension is measured with the elbow at the side, already fully extended.

* The spastic left elbow was measured from the resting spastic position, which is partially flexed; so flexion was measured as additional voluntary flexion, and extension was measured as extension out of the spastic position.

motion in the left leg, because she continued to use it while walking. She was able to flex her hip and knee so that her left foot lifted off the ground approximately 5 inches (a normal step or curb is 8 inches).

Maximal one-repetition strength testing was completed on each exercise unilaterally (Table 16-4). In some cases during pretesting, the spastic arm was unable to move through the full range of motion required for one repetition. The chair-rise and stair-climb tests were also administered (Table 16-5). The chair-rise test was given for 20 seconds; however, since Mrs. V was unable to rise from a chair without assistance, a score of zero was given for the pretest. The stair-climb test measured the time required to climb five steps.

Resistance training was completed over the next 24 weeks according to the program outlined in Table 16-2. The equipment used included standard selectorized machines, dumbbells, and ankle weights

(5, 10, and 15 pounds). Because the weight stack on a selectorized machine typically graduates in 5-pound increments, small additional weights of 1 pound each were added to the weight stack as needed to make the small resistance increases needed after testing.

At the end of the 24-week program, Mrs. V saw an increase in muscular strength (Table 16-4) and endurance (Table 16-5) and range of motion for the affected limbs (Table 16-3). Additionally, she was able to rise from a chair without assistance and move about her home without the use of a cane. She reported feeling less spasticity in the arm and leg, although this was not measured. During times of rest, the arm and leg retained their pretraining spastic positions, but the subject was able to voluntarily move both the arm and leg through a greater range of motion post-training and therefore improved both her mobility and her ability to use those limbs during normal daily activities.

Table 16-4 1RM Measurements for Each Exercise Pre- and Post-Training

Measurements were taken in pounds			
	Pre	Post	Normal
Leg press L	50	90	80%
Leg press R	120	130	8%
Knee extension L	10	30	200%
Knee extension R	50	65	30%
Seated leg curl L	20	35	75%
Seated leg curl R	40	45	12%
Standing leg curl L	5	10	100%
Standing leg curl R	15	20	33%
Knee raises L*	5	15	200%
Knee raises R	25	30	20%
Step-ups L#	0	10	100%
Step-ups R	40	50	25%
Squats**	1	10	1000%

(continued)

Table 16-4 1RM Measurements for Each Exercise Pre- and Post-Training (continued)

	Pre	Post	Normal
Biceps curl L	5	15	200%
Biceps curl R	10	20	100%
Triceps press L##	0	10	100%
Triceps press R	10	15	50%
Chest press L	5	15	200%
Chest press R	30	40	33%
Upright row L	5	10	100%
Upright row R	15	20	33%
Pulldown L	20	30	50%
Pulldown R	40	50	25%
Row L	10	25	150%
Row R	30	50	67%
Shoulder press L##	0	10	100%
Shoulder press R	15	20	33%
Front raise L***	0	5	100%
Front raise R	10	15	50%

* Knee raises were measured for number of repetitions completed. Each repetition must be completed to the same height as the first repetition to count.

Step-ups were measured as the number of repetitions completed. Zero repetitions were completed for the left leg pretraining because the subject was not able to lift her leg to the top of the step.

** Squats were measured as the number of repetitions completed where the angle of the top of the thigh reached at least 45° (commonly called *a half-squat*).

Subject was unable to fully extend the elbow for a complete repetition.

*** Subject was unable to lift the dumbbell to shoulder level for a complete repetition.

Table 16-5 Chair-Rise and Stair-Climb Tests Pre- and Post-Training

	Pre	Post	% change
Chair rise: number of repetitions in 20 seconds	0	3	100%
Stair climb: time in seconds to climb five steps	20	13	54%

Summary

Although stroke can be a debilitating condition, resistance training has the potential to help stroke survivors regain some of the mobility and independence that can be lost. Every stroke survivor will present with different levels of physical deconditioning and possibly spasticity, so resistance-training programs must be individualized according to the needs of each person. Typical exercise equipment and movements can be utilized in the training program for a stroke survivor, but some exercises must be performed unilaterally, so that the affected side is made to work without compensation from the unaffected side. Overall, resistance-training programs for stroke survivors are fairly straightforward, and research has shown the effects to be very promising.

Key Terms

Cerebral vascular accident
Chair-rise test
Embolic stroke
Hemiparesis
Hemiplegia
Hemorrhagic stroke
Intracerebral hemorrhage
Ischemic stroke
Passive range of motion
Spasticity
Stair-climb test
Stork-stand test
Stroke
Subarachnoid hemorrhage
Systemic hypoperfusion stroke
Thrombotic stroke
Transient ischemic attack (TIA)
Undulating periodization

Study Questions

1. Explain the different types of stroke and the causes of each.

2. Describe the effect spasticity has on a stroke survivor's ability to perform activities of daily living.

3. What are the components (exercises, sets, repetitions, loads) of a resistance-training program for stroke survivors?

4. How is 1RM testing for a stroke survivor with spasticity different from testing other populations?

References

1. Adams RW, Gandevia SC, Skuse NF. The distribution of muscle weakness in upper motoneuron lesions affecting the lower limb. *Brain.* 1990;113:1459–1476.

2. American Heart Association. Heart disease and stroke statistics: 2006 update. *Circulation.* 2006;113:e85–e151.

3. Badics E, Wittman A, Rupp M, Stabauer B, Zifko UA. Systemic muscle-building exercises in the rehabilitation of stroke patients. *NeuroRehabilitation.* 2002;17(3):211–214.

4. Baechle T, Earle R, eds. *NSCA Essentials of Strength Training and Conditioning.* 2nd ed. Champaign, IL: Human Kinetics; 2000.

5. Bourbonnais D, Vanen Noven S. Weakness in patients with hemiparesis. *Am J Occup Ther.* 1989;43:313–319.

6. Cramp MC, Greenwood RJ, Gill M, Rothwell JC, Scott OM. Low-intensity strength training for ambulatory stroke patients. *Disabil Rehabil.* 2006;28(13):883–889.

7. Duncan PW. Stroke disability. *Phys Ther.* 1994;74:399–407.

8. Engardt M. Rising and sitting down in stroke patients: Auditory feedback and dynamic strength training to enhance symmetrical body-weight distribution. *Scand J Rehabil Med Suppl.* 1994;31:1–57.

9. Engardt M, Knutsson E, Jonsson M, Sternhag M. Dynamic muscle strength training in stroke patients: Effects on knee extension torque, electromyographic activity,

and motor function. *Arch Phys Med Rehabil.* 1995;76:419–425.

10. Fatouros IG, Kambas A, Katrabasas I, et al. Strength training and detraining effects on muscular strength, anaerobic power, and mobility of inactive older men are intensity dependent. *Br J Sports Med.* 2005;39(10): 776–780.

11. Fibrinolytic Therapy Trialists' (FTT) Collaborative Group. Indications for fibrinolytic therapy in suspected acute myocardial infarction: Collaborative overview of early mortality and major morbidity results from all randomized trials of more than 1,000 patients. *Lancet.* 1994;343:311–322.

12. Fleck SJ, Kraemer WJ. *Designing Resistance Training Programs.* 3rd ed. Champaign, IL: Human Kinetics; 2004.

13. Hagerman P. *Fitness Testing 101: A Guide for Personal Trainers and Coaches.* San Jose, CA: iUniverse Press; 2001.

14. Hankey GL. Treatment and secondary prevention of stroke: Evidence, costs, and effects on individuals and populations. *Lancet.* 1999;354(9188):1457–1463.

15. Hill MD, Yiannakoulias N, Jeerakathil T, Tu JV, Svenson LW, Schopflocher DP. The high risk of stroke immediately after transient ischemic attack: A population-based study. *Neurology.* 2004;62:2015–2020.

16. Johnston SC, Fayad PB, Gorelick PB, et al. Prevalence and knowledge of transient ischemic attack among US adults. *Neurology.* 2003;60:1429–1434.

17. Knutsson E, Martensson A. Dynamic motor capacity in spastic paresis and its relation to prime mover dysfunction, spastic reflexes and antagonist co-activation. *Scand J Rehab Med.* 1980;12:93–106.

18. Langton-Hewer R. Rehabilitation after stroke. *Quart J Med.* 1990;279:659–674.

19. Lisabeth LD, Ireland JK, Risser JM, et al. Stroke risk after transient ischemic attack in a population-based setting. *Stroke.* 2004;35:1842–1846.

20. Lopopolo RB, Greco M, Sullivan D, Craik RL, Manigione KK. Effect of therapeutic exercise on gait speed in community-dwelling elderly people: A meta-analysis. *Phys Ther.* 2006;86(4):520–540.

21. Ouellette MM, LeBrasseur NK, Bean JF, et al. High-intensity resistance training improves muscle strength, self-reported function, and disability in long-term stroke survivors. *Stroke.* 2004;35(6):1404–1409.

22. Riolo L, Fisher K. Is there evidence that strength training could help improve muscle function and other outcomes without reinforcing abnormal movement patterns or increasing reflex activity in a man who has had a stroke? *Phys Ther.* 2003;83(9):844–851.

23. Scelsi R, Lotta S, Lommi G, Poppi P, Marchetti C. Hemiplegic atrophy: Morphological findings in the anterior tibia muscle of patients with cerebral vascular accidents. *Acta Neuropathol.* 1984;62:324–331.

24. Seshadri S, Beiser A, Kelley-Hayes M, et al. Lifetime risk of stroke: Results from the Framingham study. *Stroke.* 2006;37(2): 345–350.

25. Sharp SA, Brouwer BJ. Isokinetic strength training of the hemiparetic knee: Effects on function and spasticity. *Arch Phys Med Rehabil.* 1997;78:1231–1236.

26. Sousa N, Sampaio J. Effects of progressive strength training on the performance of the functional reach test and the timed get-up-and-go test in an elderly population from the rural north of Portugal. *Am J Hum Biol.* 2005;17(6):746–751.

27. Teasell RW, Bhogal SK, Foley NC, Speechley MR. Gait retraining post stroke. *Top Stroke Rehabil.* 2003;10(2):34–65.

28. Teixeira-Salmela LF, Nadeau S, McBride I, Olney SJ. Effects of muscle strengthening and physical conditioning training on temporal, kinematic and kinetic variables during gait in chronic stroke survivors. *J Rehabil Med.* 2001;33(2):53–60.

29. Teixeira-Salmela LF, Olney SJ, Nadeau S, Brouwer B. Muscle strengthening and physical conditioning to reduce impairment and disability in chronic stroke survivors. *Arch Phys Med Rehabil.* 1999;80(10):1211–1218.

30. Weiss A, Suzuki T, Bean J, Fielding RA. High-intensity strength training improves strength and functional performance after stroke. *Am J Phys Med Rehabil.* 2000;79(4):369–376.

31. Wolf PA, D'Agostino RB, Kannel WB, Bonita R, Belanger AJ. Cigarette smoking as a risk factor for stroke: The Framingham study. *JAMA.* 1988;259:1025–1029.

32. Young J, Mayer R. Physiological alterations of motor units in hemiplegia. *J Neurol Sci.* 1982;54:401–412.

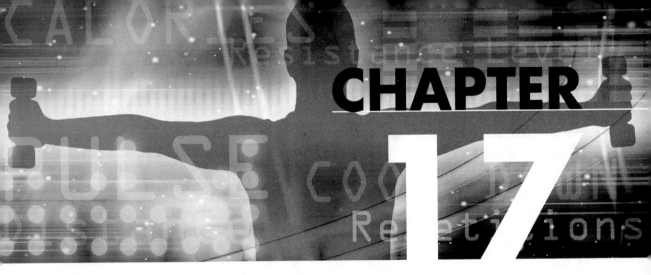

CHAPTER 17

RESISTANCE-TRAINING STRATEGIES DURING PREGNANCY

Objectives

Upon completion of this chapter, the reader should be able to:

- ○ Discuss the contraindications for exercise for pregnant women
- ○ Explain the safety precautions for resistance-training exercises
- ○ Describe resistance-training exercises for pregnant women
- ○ Design a safe resistance-training program for pregnant women

INTRODUCTION

Recent medical advice from the American College of Obstetricians and Gynecologists (ACOG) states that a woman with a low-risk pregnancy can participate in moderate exercise for 30 minutes or more a day on most if not all days of the week (1, 2, 3). Although the ACOG promotes exercise during pregnancy, concrete guidelines are not provided, because they do not distinguish between aerobic exercise and resistance-training activities. Conversely, the "PARmed-X for Pregnancy" includes a medical prescreening questionnaire to identify contraindications for exercise during pregnancy, a list of safety considerations, and aerobic and resistance-training guidelines and precautions (44). The "PARmed-X for Pregnancy" document, first published by the Canadian Society for Exercise Physiology (CSEP) in 1996 and revised in 2002, was endorsed by the Society of Obstetricians and Gynecologists of Canada (13, 14) and the American College of Sports Medicine (4).

The effects of resistance exercise performed during pregnancy have rarely been examined. Possible advantages to incorporating resistance-training activities into an exercise program may be improvement in overall strength, posture, and core muscle strength that may help in labor and delivery. By strengthening muscles of the body core, perhaps lower back pain and pelvic joint pain may be avoided as pregnancy progresses, and the body's center of gravity shifts forward (22). This chapter discusses resistance-training strategies during pregnancy.

BENEFITS OF EXERCISE DURING PREGNANCY

Very little scientific literature reports on resistance training for pregnant women, as most of the studies investigate the physiological effects of aerobic exercise. Conventional wisdom and traditional medical advice have suggested that pregnant women avoid heavy lifting or straining and especially those activities that have a static or isometric exercise component (5). Theoretical risks with resistance training during pregnancy have included changes in maternal blood pressure, especially if the Valsalva Maneuver is used (26); initiation of premature labor (15); and transient fetal hypoxia, a drop in fetal oxygen levels (21). Heavy resistance training, typically defined as training at more than 80 percent of the one-repetition maximum (1RM), may reduce blood flow and oxygen supply to the uterus, which could cause a mild, transient decrease in fetal oxygen concentrations (5) reflected by fetal heart rate decelerations or a drop in fetal heart rate, or *bradycardia* (33, 43).

However, increasing physical activity and leading an active lifestyle provides some benefit in the form of helping to prevent excessive weight gain during pregnancy, postpartum weight retention, gestational diabetes, and the associated risk of developing type 2 diabetes later in life (12). Other benefits of being active during pregnancy include improving heart and lung health, which may reduce the risk of hypertension and heart disease (35). Improved heart and lung health may increase stamina for labor and delivery and may assist in faster recovery from giving birth. Being active also improves self-esteem, moods, and sleep patterns; it promotes a healthy lifestyle and decreases state anxiety and depression following pregnancy (25, 43). Improvements associated with resistance training of specific muscle groups, such as the pelvic muscles or abdominal and core muscles, may improve or prevent urinary incontinence (28, 34) and back pain, respectively (20). Furthermore, developing upper-body strength will support the breasts and assist in carrying the infant after delivery (32).

Literature Review of Research Supporting Resistance Training During Pregnancy

Little research exists on the effects of resistance training on strength during pregnancy, possibly due in part to the unknown potential of what this type of exercise might do to maternal and fetal blood pressure, blood flow, or uterine contractions. Studies examining maternal response to exercise have found that healthy pregnant women have not exhibited a hypertensive response to resistance exercise (5, 7, 26, 41). A stable fetal heart rate pattern during isotonic and isometric exercise has been reported in some studies (5, 22, 27, 36, 41), and others revealed transient changes in fetal heart rate, especially during maternal exercise performed in a supine position, that is, lying on the back (21, 33). Thus, the literature would suggest that maternal resistance training does not compromise maternal or fetal well-being in healthy pregnancies, but exercises performed in the supine position should be avoided.

When leisure activity was examined during pregnancy, participation was shown to be lower among pregnant women compared to nonpregnant women of the same age; walking was the most popular activity for both groups, followed by aerobics, resistance training, and home exercises (19). When activity was assessed by trimester, pregnant women were shown to decrease their activity levels during the third trimester, with walking still the most popular activity (30). A study of strength using leg press, leg extension, bench press, and lat

pulldown tests conducted before pregnancy and 6 weeks postpartum found that strength decreased over the term of the pregnancy (40). These studies would suggest that maintaining muscular fitness should be emphasized as an important component of overall fitness, because many pregnant women may be at risk for deconditioning and diminishing physical activity levels during gestation.

Resistance training to improve overall strength may not be the most appropriate goal during pregnancy, but several studies highlight the importance of using resistance training to prevent muscle-related complications of pregnancy. For instance, strengthening the pelvic floor muscles during pregnancy has been shown to prevent urinary incontinence during gestation and 3 months after delivery (28). Meta-analyses revealed that postpartum exercise of the pelvic floor muscles using **Kegel exercises** also appeared to be effective in decreasing urinary incontinence (23). Table 17-1 outlines instructions on using Kegel exercises. Likewise, low back pain and pelvic pain are common complaints during pregnancy and may interfere with activities of daily living (29). The main factors associated with these complaints may be due to an alteration in posture required to support the increase in body mass (29).

Table 17-1 Kegel Exercises for Pelvic Floor Muscles

Kegel exercises contract the pelvic floor muscles (44). They can be done in a sitting or standing position. The "Wave" and "Elevator" exercises are the most common Kegel exercises used during pregnancy.

To perform the "Wave" exercise, squeeze the pelvic floor muscles starting from the posterior and working forward, with more of the muscles being squeezed while working forward. Hold for a count of three and then release. Repeat up to 10 times.

Perform the "Elevator" exercise by squeezing the pelvic floor muscles as if in an elevator ascending floors. Thus on the bottom floor, the pelvic muscles are relaxed, and as the elevator ascends each floor, the pelvic muscles are squeezed a little tighter, up to the tightest squeeze on level 5. The elevator then descends back to the bottom floor, where the muscles are then again relaxed. Repeat up to 10 times.

Standard treatment for low back and pelvic pain during pregnancy may consist of a pelvic belt, a home exercise program, stabilizing exercises (isometrics), and acupuncture (18). A recent study examined previous leisure-time physical activity prior to pregnancy in women with low back pain and pelvic pain and found that a higher number of previous leisure-time physical activities decreased the risk of low back and pelvic pain (29). Another trial showed that acupuncture and stabilizing exercises were important treatments for pelvic-pain management during pregnancy (18). Furthermore, treatment with specific stabilizing exercises appeared to be more effective than standard physical therapy alone for reducing pelvic-girdle pain (38, 39). One study found that specific back, abdominal, and hamstring muscle exercises during the second half of pregnancy significantly reduced the intensity of low back pain, had no detectable effect on lumbar curvature, and increased the flexibility of the spine (20). Others have found no change in back pain, functional limitations, or posture in those women who participated in resistance training during pregnancy (16, 17).

PRECAUTIONS FOR RESISTANCE TRAINING DURING PREGNANCY

Because of the small amount of evidence-based research pertaining to resistance training during pregnancy, medical prescreening is important to ensure that the pregnant woman has a low-risk pregnancy. The "PARmed-X for Pregnancy" document is a tool that a physician or health care provider can use to screen for contraindications to exercise (44). If no contraindications exist for exercise and the woman has a low-risk pregnancy, there are five important precautions for resistance training that must be addressed, as well as safety considerations during warm-ups and cooldowns.

Body Position

After 4 months (16 weeks) of pregnancy, the uterus may impinge on the major abdominal blood vessels while in the supine position. As shown in Figure 17-1, the inferior vena cava returns venous

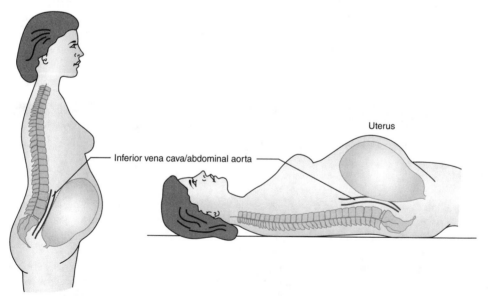

Figure 17-1 After 4 months (16 weeks) of pregnancy the uterus may impinge on the major blood vessels found in the abdomen while lying on the back (supine position). During standing the uterus does not impinge the inferior vena cava or abdominal aorta.

© Delmar/Cengage Learning.

blood from the lower body to the heart and may be obstructed while exercising in the supine position (3). If this is the case, the woman may experience symptoms of light-headedness or dizziness. The other major blood vessel along the posterior body cavity is the abdominal aorta, which provides the major blood supply to the uterus and developing fetus. During exercise in the supine position, the uterus may also impinge this vessel. There are no symptoms if this occurs, so caution is advised; beyond 4 months of pregnancy, exercises normally done in the supine position should be modified to be done in a sitting position (3, 44).

Joint Laxity

Ligaments may become more prone to injury during pregnancy because of a circulating hormone called **relaxin** (42). Relaxin loosens ligamentous connective tissue as the body prepares for delivery of the fetus through the birth canal (34). Relaxed ligaments may lead to joints that are more prone

to injury (8). As a result, some pregnant women may feel that they are more flexible in some joints. Rapid change of direction and bouncing ballistic movements should be avoided during pregnancy. In addition, stretching and flexibility movements should also be performed with caution to avoid ligament and joint injury (44).

Diastasis Recti

Diastasis recti, shown in Figure 17-2, is characterized by a bulging or rippling of connective tissue along the linea alba, the midline of the front of the abdomen when abdominal exercise is performed. The pregnant woman may also notice this bulging during a change in intra-abdominal pressure. If diastasis recti develops, abdominal exercises are contraindicated (10), because as the abdominal muscles are continuously strengthened, and the abdomen increases in size with the pregnancy, a tear may occur at the weakest point—in the connective tissue.

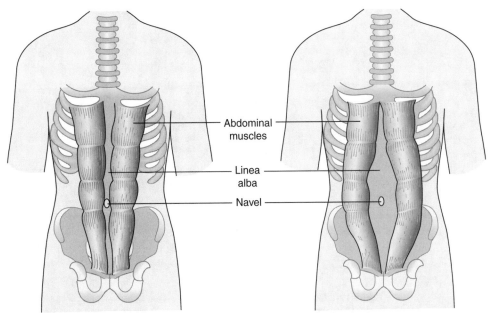

Figure 17-2 Strengthening the abdominal muscles may cause more tearing of the connective tissue (linea alba), as this tissue is the weakest point as the uterus continues to enlarge. Normal condition is pictured on the left and *diastasis recti* is pictured on the right.

© Delmar/Cengage Learning.

Breathing

During pregnancy, technique and proper breathing are extremely important to prevent injury and to ensure no change in blood pressure occurs with resistance training. Emphasis should be placed on continuous breathing during the activity, with exhalation upon exertion and inhalation upon relaxation. The Valsalva maneuver should be avoided during pregnancy, as this maneuver may cause an increase in blood pressure (44).

Posture

The enlarging uterus and breasts during pregnancy cause a forward shift in the center of gravity, which may cause the shoulders to slump forward (44) and increase lordosis of the lower back (24). Incorrect posture may lead to back and pelvic pain, thus correct posture and a neutral pelvic alignment is recommended (44). To find a neutral pelvic alignment, a pregnant woman should stand with her feet shoulder-width apart, knees slightly bent, with pelvic placement halfway between an accentuated lordosis and posterior pelvic-tilt position, pushing the pelvis as far forward as possible (Figure 17-3). These extreme positions are to be avoided during pregnancy; the neutral pelvic alignment is a comfortable position between the two extremes.

Warm-Ups and Cooldowns

Pregnant women may take a little longer to warm up before engaging in physical activity (44), therefore

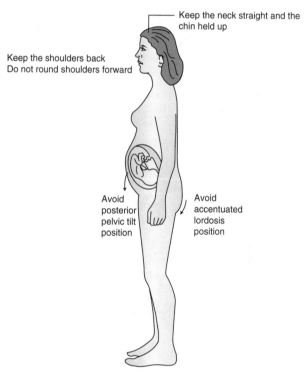

Figure 17-3 Correct posture is important for pregnant women who want to avoid lower back pain. Neutral pelvic alignment is recommended. To find the neutral pelvic alignment position, stand with feet shoulder-width apart, knees slightly bent, with pelvic placement halfway between an accentuated lordosis and posterior pelvic-tilt position.

© Delmar/Cengage Learning.

physical activity should be preceded by a 10- to 15-minute warm-up, followed by a 10- to 15-minute cooldown (44). Lower intensity calisthenics, stretching, and relaxation exercises should be included in all warm-up and cooldown sessions.

DESIGNING RESISTANCE-TRAINING PROGRAMS FOR PREGNANT WOMEN

The medical prescreening section of the "PARmed-X for Pregnancy" document includes absolute and relative contraindications to exercise and is in a checklist format for the health care professional to complete (44). Absolute contraindications to exercise include medical conditions such as ruptured membranes; preterm labor; uncontrolled type 1 or 2 diabetes; pregnancy-induced hypertension; incompetent cervix; intrauterine growth restriction; a high-order pregnancy, such as triplets; and vaginal bleeding (44). The relative contraindications are included because the risk to the pregnancy may exceed the benefits of being active. For example, iron deficiency or anemia (hemoglobin lower than 100 g/L) is listed as a relative contraindication. If this condition is corrected by iron supplements during pregnancy, and the hemoglobin concentrations are within the normal pregnancy range, the pregnant woman should be able to exercise (44).

Once medical approval has been given, a pregnant woman with a low-risk pregnancy can begin or continue an exercise program within the specified guidelines (44). Previous medical advice suggested that women who have not exercised should not start an exercise program during pregnancy. However, recent scientific literature and guidelines would suggest that if no contraindications to exercise exist, and if the pregnancy is low-risk, women may start an exercise program in the second trimester (32). Many women do not feel well, and some feel extreme fatigue in the first trimester, so they may be discouraged from exercise if the activity program

is started at that time (13). The best time to start an exercise program that may lead to a lifestyle change even after pregnancy is in the second trimester, around 12 to 13 weeks (32).

Pregnancy is not the time to initiate or continue athletic competition. Resistance training should be designed for maintaining strength and endurance, not for building muscle mass or increasing muscular strength. If a pregnant woman has not participated in any exercise previously, once she has medical approval, she can begin resistance training at the start of the second trimester, around 12 to 13 weeks, when pregnancy-related symptoms such as extreme fatigue, nausea, or vomiting are minimal. Pregnant women should also be advised of the safety precautions listed in Table 17-2 and the reasons to stop exercise and consult a physician listed in Table 17-3.

Table 17-2 Safety Considerations for Exercise During Pregnancy (44)

- Avoid exercise in warm, humid environments, especially in the first trimester.
- Avoid isometric exercise or straining while holding your breath (Valsalva maneuver).
- Maintain adequate nutrition and hydration; drink liquids before and after exercise.
- Avoid exercise while lying on your back (supine position) beyond the fourth month of pregnancy.
- Avoid activities that involve physical contact or danger of falling.
- Know your limits—pregnancy is not a good time to train for athletic competition.
- Know the reasons to stop exercise and consult a qualified health care provider immediately.
- It is important to monitor the temperature of heated pools. Maternal body temperature during exercise may be increased more by exercising in a warm environment.

Table 17-3 Reasons to Stop Exercise and Consult a Health Care Advisor (44)

- Persistent uterine contractions (more than 6 to 8 per hour)
- Bloody discharge from the vagina
- Any "gush" of fluid from the vagina suggesting premature rupture of the membranes
- Unexplained pain in the abdomen
- Sudden swelling of extremities: ankles, hands, face
- Swelling, pain, and redness in the calf of one leg suggesting phlebitis
- Persistent headaches or disturbance of vision
- Unexplained dizziness or faintness
- Marked fatigue, heart palpitations, or chest pain
- Failure to gain weight (less than 1 kg per month during last two trimesters)
- Absence of usual fetal movement

Each resistance-training session should begin with a warm-up that is low impact, starts with a small range of motion, and progresses to a larger range of motion for all major muscle groups. Static and/or dynamic stretches are to be performed with caution for all major muscle groups. Pregnant women are advised when stretching a muscle group to stretch until discomfort is felt and then release. The supine position is to be avoided.

Using a weight that allows 12 to 15 repetitions per set without fatigue is recommended (44). During the third trimester, at about 28 weeks gestation, the individual can decrease the load if fatigue is an issue, maintaining repetitions of 12 to 15 but at a lighter weight. Repetitions may also be decreased at this time to prevent fatigue. Resistance-training programs can be incorporated into an aerobic exercise routine, or they can be alternated with aerobic conditioning programs during the week. The frequency of structured exercise should not exceed five times per week, with the ideal number of exercise sessions in the range of three to four times per week (11).

One to two exercises should be used for each major muscle group for each side of the body, including the pelvic floor muscles. Table 17-4 lists specific exercises that can safely be included during pregnancy. Aerobic exercise to target heart-rate zones are provided in the "PARmed-X for Pregnancy" document for pregnant women based on age; however, these guidelines may be used for resistance-training programs as well:

○ 20 to 29 years of age, heart rate of 135 to 150 beats per minute (bpm)

○ 30 to 39 years of age, heart rate of 130 to 145 bpm

Intensity can also be monitored by the "Talk test," in which the intensity is sufficient if the pregnant woman can carry on a conversation while exercising (44). If the individual is out of breath while speaking, the intensity must be decreased.

Table 17-4 Exercises that can be Included During Pregnancy (37)

Standing trunk extension
Lat pulldown
Shoulder shrug
Seated row
Front raise
Lateral raise
Standing push-up against a wall
Dumbbell shoulder press
Dumbbell biceps curl
Dumbbell triceps press
Kickbacks
Cable lateral leg lift
Cable hip extension
Cable leg curl
Calf raises
Side-lying crunches
Side-lying oblique crunches
Kegel exercises

For a pregnant woman, the volume of exercise completed in each session is dictated by time rather than a prescribed number of sets. After a proper warm-up, begin with 15 minutes of exercise, increasing by 2 minutes each week until a maximum of 30 minutes is reached (37). This exercise-session length can then be maintained for the remainder of the pregnancy.

SAMPLE 24-WEEK PROGRAM

Once the individual is medically prescreened, she can begin exercise at about 12 to 13 weeks of gestation until delivery, which leaves approximately 27 to 28 weeks of activity before giving birth.

Week 1

Begin with three sessions per week with at least a day of rest in between. Each session will include a single set of 12 to 15 repetitions of the following seven exercises and should take approximately 15 minutes to complete: standing trunk extension, seated row, standing push-up, dumbbell biceps curl, side-lying crunches, dumbbell triceps press, and calf raises. In addition, Kegel exercises can be taught for at-home exercise.

Weeks 2 through 9

Continue a thrice-weekly schedule, adding an additional 2 minutes of exercise each week by including one additional exercise each week, alternating the addition of upper-body and lower-body exercises as follows:

Week 2: Front raise

Week 3: Cable leg curl

Week 4: Dumbbell biceps curl

Week 5: Cable hip extension

Week 6: Shoulder shrug

Week 7: Cable lateral leg lift

Week 8: Side-lying oblique crunches

Week 9: Kickbacks

Week 10 through 16

Continue with 30-minute exercise sessions, adding one additional day to change the exercise schedule to every other day.

Week 17 through Delivery

Continue with an every-other-day routine, but change exercise volume by decreasing to eight exercises and completing a second set of each. Use a combination of the following upper- and lower-body exercises: cable leg curl, dumbbell biceps curl, cable lateral leg lift, lateral raise, cable hip extension, dumbbell triceps press, calf raises, and seated row.

CASE STUDY

Mrs. M is 35 years old and a first-time mom with a low-risk pregnancy. She is about 16 weeks along in her pregnancy and has been complaining about lumbar back pain and would like specific exercises to help strengthen her back muscles. After taking her exercise history and assessing her posture, the exercise professional notes that she has an accentuated lordosis. The exercise professional educates Mrs. M about a neutral pelvic alignment and gives her an exercise program to strengthen her core muscles. She is instructed to follow the exercise program outlined in the 24-week template above and told to include an additional set of standing trunk extensions and side-lying abdominal crunches each session.

After 4 weeks of exercise, Mrs. M noted significant improvement in her back pain and an increase in her ability to complete her daily activities without fatigue. At the end of her pregnancy, she stated that she thought the exercise program made the pregnancy much easier for her, and she was interested in continuing to exercise postpartum.

Summary

Before starting or continuing a resistance-training program, every pregnant woman must be medically prescreened for contraindications to exercise. Once medical approval has been obtained, resistance training can be routinely added to an aerobic exercise program to enhance overall fitness levels. Possible advantages to incorporating resistance-training activities into an exercise program may be improvements in overall strength, posture, and core muscles that may help in labor and delivery. By strengthening muscles of the body core, perhaps lower back pain and pelvic joint pain may be avoided as pregnancy progresses and the center of gravity shifts forward. By strengthening the pelvic floor muscles, urinary incontinence may also be avoided.

Key Terms

Diastasis recti
Kegel exercises
Relaxin
Transient fetal hypoxia

Study Questions

1. What are the contraindications for exercise during pregnancy?

2. What are the safety precautions for resistance exercise during pregnancy?

3. What are the key resistance-training exercises for pregnancy?

4. How can you make sure that pregnant women exercise safely when they engage in resistance exercise?

5. What are the key signs and symptoms to stop exercise and seek medical help?

References

1. American College of Obstetricians and Gynecologists. Pregnancy and the postnatal period. *ACOG Home Exercise Programs.* Washington, DC: American College of Obstetricians and Gynecologists; 1985.

2. American College of Obstetricians and Gynecologists. Exercise during pregnancy and the postpartum period. *ACOG Technical Bulletin.* 1994;189(Feb):2–7.

3. American College of Obstetricians and Gynecologists. Opinion no. 267: Exercise during pregnancy and the postpartum period. *Obstet Gynecol.* 2002;99:171–173.

4. American College of Sports Medicine. Endorsements. *Sports Med Bull.* 2004;39(5): September/October, 2004.

5. Avery ND, Stocking KD, Tranmer JE, Davies G, Wolfe LA. Fetal responses to maternal strength conditioning exercises in late gestation. *Can J Appl Physiol.* 1999;24:362–376.

6. Barakat R, Sterling J, Lucia A. Does exercise training during pregnancy affect gestational age? A randomised, controlled trial. *Br J Sports Med.* 2008:42(8):674–678.

7. Barron W, Jujais S, Zinaman M, Brava E, Lindheimer MD. Plasma catecholamine responses to physiologic stimuli in normal human pregnancy. *Am J Obstet Gynecol.* 1986;154:80–84.

8. Borg-Stein J, Dugan S, Gruber J. Musculoskeletal aspects of pregnancy. *Am J Phys Med Rehabil.* 2005;84:180–182.

9. Brankston G, Mitchell B, Ryan E, Okun N. Resistance exercise decreases the need for insulin in overweight women with gestational diabetes mellitus. *Am J Obstet Gynecol.* 2004;190:188–193.

10. Bursch SG. Interrater reliability of diastasis recti abdominis measurement. *Phys Ther.* 1987;67:1077–1079.

11. Campbell MK, Mottola MF. Recreational exercise and occupational activity during pregnancy and birth weight: A case-control study. *Am J Obstet Gynecol.* 2001;184:403–408.

12. Charkoudian N, Joyner MJ. Physiologic considerations for exercise performance in women. *Clin Chest Med.* 2004;25(2):247–255.

13. Davies G, Wolfe LA, Mottola MF, MacKinnon C. Joint SOGC/CSEP clinical practice guideline: Exercise in pregnancy and the postpartum period. *J Obstet Gynecol Can.* 2003;25(6): 516–522.

14. Davies G, Wolfe LA, Mottola MF, MacKinnon C. Joint SOGC/CSEP clinical practice guideline: Exercise in pregnancy and the postpartum period. *Can J Appl Physiol.* 2003A;28(3): 329–341.

15. Durak E, Jovanovic-Peterson L, Peterson C. Comparative evaluation of uterine response to exercise on five aerobic machines. *Am J Obstet Gynecol.* 1990;162:754–756.

16. Dumas GA, Reid G, Wolfe LA, Griffin MP, McGrath M. Exercise, posture, and back pain during pregnancy, part 1: Exercise and posture. *Clin Biomech.* 1995;10:98–103.

17. Dumas GA, Reid G, Wolfe LA, Griffin MP, McGrath M. Exercise, posture, and back pain during pregnancy, part 2: Exercise and back pain. *Clin Biomech.* 1995A;10:104–109.

18. Elden H, Ladfors L, Olsen MF, Ostgaard H, Hagberg H. Effects of acupuncture and stabilizing exercises as adjunct to standard treatment in pregnant women with pelvic girdle pain: Randomized single blind controlled trial. *BMJ.* 2005;330:671–665.

19. Evanson KR, Savitz D, Huston S. Leisure-time physical activity among pregnant women in the US. *Paed Perinatal Epid.* 2004;18:400–407.

20. Garshasbi A, Zadeh SF. The effect of exercise on the intensity of low back pain in pregnant women. *Int J Gynecol Obstet.* 2005;88:271–275.

21. Green RC, Schneider K, MacLennan AH. The fetal heart rate response to static antenatal exercises in the supine position. *Aust J Physiotherapy.* 1988;34:3–7.

22. Hall DC, Kaufmann DA. Effects of aerobic and strength conditioning on pregnancy outcomes. *Am J Obstet Gynecol.* 1987;157:1199–1203.

23. Harvey MA. Pelvic floor exercises during and after pregnancy: A systematic review of their role in preventing pelvic floor dysfunction. *J Obstet Gynecol Can.* 2003;25:487–498.

24. Heckman JD, Sassard R. Current concepts review: Musculoskeletal considerations in pregnancy. *J Bone Joint Surg Am.* 1994;76:1720–1730.

25. Koltyn KF, Schultes SS. Psychological effects of an aerobic exercise session and a rest session following pregnancy. *J Sports Med Phys Fitness.* 1997;37(4):287–291.

26. Lotgering FK, van der Berg A, Struijk P, Wallenberg H. Arterial pressure response to maximal isometric exercise in pregnant women. *Obstet Gynecol.* 1992;166:538–542.

27. Marsal K, Gennser G, Lofgren O. Effects on fetal breathing movements of maternal challenges. Cross-over study on dynamic work, static work, passive movements, hyperventilation and hyperoxygenation. *Acta Obstet Gynecol Scand.* 1979;58:335–342.

28. Morkved SK, Schei B, Salvesen KA. Pelvic floor muscle training during pregnancy to prevent urinary incontinence: A single blind randomized controlled trial. *Obstet Gynecol.* 2003;101:313–319.

29. Mogren IM, Pohjanen A. Low back pain and pelvic pain during pregnancy. *Spine.* 2005;30:983–991.

30. Mottola MF, Campbell MK. Activity patterns during pregnancy. *Can J Appl Physiol.* 2003;28(4):642–653.

31. Mottola MF, Davenport M, Brun CR, Inglis SD, Charlesworth S, Sopper MM. VO_{2peak} prediction and exercise prescription for pregnant women. *Med Sci Sports Exerc.* 2006;38(8):1389–1395.

32. Mottola MF, Wolfe LA. Active living and pregnancy. In: *Toward Active Living. Proceedings of the International Conference on Physical Activity, Fitness & Health.* Quinney HA, Gauvin L, Wall AE, eds. Champaign, IL: Human Kinetics Publishers; 1994;131–140.

33. Nelser CL, Hassett S, Cary S, Brooke L. Effects of supine exercise on fetal heart rate in the second and third trimesters. *Am J Perinatol.* 1988;5:159–163.

34. Owens K, Pearson A, Mason G. Symphysis pubis dysfunction: A cause of significant obstetric morbidity. *Eur J Obstet Gynecol Reprod Biol.* 2002;105:143–146.

35. Pivarnik JM, Chambliss H, Clapp JF, et al. Impact of physical activity during pregnancy and postpartum on chronic disease risk: An ACSM roundtable consensus statement. *Med Sci Sports Exerc.* 2006;38(5):989–1005.

36. Ruissen C, Drongelen M, Hoogland H. The influence of maternal exercise on the pulsatility index of the umbilical artery blood velocity waveform. *Eur J Obstet Gynecol Reprod Biol.* 1990;37:1–6.

37. Sloboda DM, Weis CA, Mottola MF. *Prenatal muscle conditioning package.* The Exercise and Pregnancy Lab, Ontario, Canada: The University of Western Ontario; 1995.

38. Stuge B, Laerum E, Kirkesola G, Vollestad N. The efficacy of a treatment program focusing on specific stabilizing exercise for pelvic girdle pain after pregnancy: A randomised controlled trial. *Spine.* 2004;29:351–359.

39. Stuge B, Veierod M, Laerum E, Vollestad N. The efficacy of a treatment program focusing on specific stabilizing exercise for pelvic girdle pain after pregnancy. A two-year follow-up of a randomised controlled trial. *Spine.* 2004A;29:E197–E203.

40. Treuth MS, Butte N, Puyau M. Pregnancy-related changes in physical activity, fitness, and strength. *Med Sci Sports Exerc.* 2005;37:832–837.

41. Webb KA, Wolfe LA, Lowe-Wylde S, Monga M. A comparison of fetal heart rate (FHR) responses to maternal static and dynamic exercise. *Med Sci Sports Exerc.* 1991;23:S169.

42. Weiss M, Nagelschmidt M, Struck H. Relaxin and collagen metabolism. *Horm Metab Res.* 1979;11:408–410.

43. Wolfe LA, Brenner IKM, Mottola MF. Maternal exercise, fetal well-being and pregnancy outcome. *Exerc Sports Sci Rev.* 1994;22:145–194.

44. Wolfe LA, Mottola MF. *PARmed-X for Pregnancy.* Ottawa: Canadian Society for Exercise Physiology; 2002:1–4.

GLOSSARY

Absolute muscular endurance—the maximal number of repetitions performed with a specific pre-training load

Acute low back pain—is defined as activity intolerance due to pain in the low back of less than 3 months duration

Adolescence—refers to the period between childhood and adulthood and includes girls 12 to 18 years and boys 14 to 18 years

Allergens—triggers, such as air pollutants, pollen, tobacco smoke, chemical fumes, and exercise that trigger an allergic response in a hypersensitive individual

Alternating grip—hand position for gripping a weight which involves one hand pronated and one hand supinated

Android obesity—also known as central adiposity is described by individuals who carry excess amounts of body fat in the abdominal area and trunk

Angina—chest pain resulting from reduced blood flow through the coronary arteries

Ankle weights—small weights that are strapped to the ankle allowing for increased resistance

Apoptosis—is a "programmed" destruction of cells that occurs due to intracellular rather than extracellular processes

Arthritis—is an inflammatory condition of the joints, characterized by pain, swelling, heat, redness, and limitation of movement

Asthma—one of the three chronic, progressive diseases classified as COPD, characterized by airways that are hypersensitive to allergens or triggers, such as air pollutants, pollen, tobacco smoke, chemical fumes, and exercise

Atherosclerosis—build up of fatty material and plaque in the coronary arteries

Atlanto-axial instability—excessive mobility at the junction between the first and second cervical vertebrae due to either a bony or ligamentous abnormality

Autonomic neuropathy—diabetes-related damage to the central nervous system

Ballistic resistance exercise—exercise in which the load is maximally accelerated either by jumping (e.g., jump squats) or by releasing the weight using specialized equipment (e.g., Plyo Power System)

Barbell—made of a longer bar with weights on each end, meant to be held in both hands

Beta cells—insulin-producing cells

Beta-adrenergic receptor blockers—class of cardiac drug used to treat heart failure by reducing the work of the heart through a lowering of the heart rate

Body composition—the combination of fat mass and fat-free mass, can be an important tool for assessing fat distribution and health risk in the obese population

Body mass index (BMI)—ratio of weight to height used as an indicator of obesity

Bone mineral density—a measure of the structural integrity and strength of an area of bone

Bone modeling—the bone shape alterations which occur during puberty and young adulthood

Cable/pulley system—a form of exercise equipment that uses a stack of weights from which the user must insert a pin to select the desired resistance and a cable to which the user may attach a variety of handles depending on the exercise

Cancer—is a term that refers to a family of diseases marked by unregulated cell growth and proliferation that can affect virtually any bodily organ or system

Carcinogen—cancer-causing agents

Cardiac rehabilitation—systematic programming of exercise, nutrition, stress management, and risk factor education for individuals with heart conditions and their families

Central adiposity—is also known as android obesity and is described by individuals who carry excess amounts of body fat in the abdominal area and trunk

Cerebral vascular accident—commonly called a stroke, is the result of a reduction of blood supply to parts of the brain causing the affected brain cells to die, and severely affecting neurologic function

Chair-rise test—a test in which the individual attempts to rise to full standing height from a sitting position, and then sit back down as many times as possible in 15-30 seconds

Childhood—refers to a period of life before the development of secondary sex characteristics such as pubic hair and reproductive organs (approximately age 11 in girls and 13 in boys)

Chronic bronchitis—one of the three chronic, progressive diseases classified as COPD; characterized by a hypersecretion of mucus and chronic productive cough that continues for at least 3 months of the year for at least 2 consecutive years

Chronic heart failure—is a multi-system syndrome with a variety of pathological abnormalities that reduce exercise tolerance and contribute to the symptoms of functional disability

Chronic obstructive pulmonary disease (COPD)—chronic, progressive diseases characterized by gradual loss of lung function, airflow obstruction, dyspnea with exertion, weight loss associated with muscle wasting, recurrent bronchial infections, and chronic disability; includes asthma, chronic bronchitis, and emphysema

Closed-chain kinetic exercise—exercise where the distal segments are fixed such as the leg press, squat, and deadlift

Community-based exercise—exercise training that takes place in a setting such as a health or fitness center, is usually supervised, and allows several individuals to exercise together or at the same time

Compensatory acceleration—movement that requires the individual to accelerate the load maximally throughout the range of motion during the concentric muscle action to maximize bar velocity

Competitive training—training that involves resistance training to maximize muscle hypertrophy, strength, power, and/or local muscular endurance

Concentric—muscle shortening

Coronary heart disease—chronic condition caused by atherosclerosis (hardening of the arteries) that reduces blood flow through coronary arteries to the heart muscle typically resulting in chest pain and/or heart damage

Cortical bone—also known as compact bone, more dense than trabecular bone

C-peptide—is a protein marker used to detect the destruction of beta cells, and contributes to the diagnosis of type 1 diabetes

Deceleration phase—the phase that occurs near the end of the concentric range of motion where bar velocity decreases prior to completion of the repetition to bring the bar to a stop and to prevent injury

Deposition—rebuilding bone by osteoblasts

Development disabilities—a disability that develops pre or post natal and affects physical or mental development

Diabetic retinopathy—condition in which the eyes have weak, abnormal blood vessels in the retina that can break, tear, or bleed into the vitreous fluid in the center of the eye

Diastasis recti—is characterized by a bulging or rippling of connective tissue along the linea alba (midline of the front of the abdomen) when abdominal exercise is performed. If this condition develops then abdominal exercises are contraindicated during pregnancy

Diastolic dysfunction—cardiac dysfunction related to reduced filling of the ventricles

Diuretics—class of cardiac drug used to treat heart failure by reducing the volume load on the heart

Down syndrome—a condition characterized by an extra chromosome causing mental retardation and specific physical characteristics

Dumbbell—a short bar with weights on each end, meant to be held in one hand

Dynamic constant external resistance—formerly called isotonic training or training with a constant fixed resistance

Dyspnea—shortness of air, a common symptom for individuals with COPD; also a common symptom of heart failure

Eccentric—muscle lengthening

Embolic stroke—occurs when an embolus, or wandering clot, becomes lodged in an artery leading to the brain. An embolus can originate from anywhere downstream of the vessel, and is classified as either arterial or cardiac in origin

Emphysema—one of the three chronic, progressive diseases classified as COPD; characterized by the destruction of alveolar walls and the permanent enlargement of the airspaces distal to the terminal bronchioles

Energy balance—is achieved when the level of energy intake equals the level of energy expenditure

Environmental risk factors—include family dynamics (e.g., parental food choices and degree of parental adiposity), lack of safe places for physical activity, lack of consistent access to healthful food choices, increased consumption of energy-dense fried foods and carbonated beverages, changes in the availability of physical education, and increased access to television, videos, and computer games

Exercise intolerance—is the inability to sustain a submaximal level of exercise or activity

Exercise selection—refers to types of exercises chosen for inclusion in the program

Exercise sequencing—refers to the order exercises are placed within a training session

Exogenous insulin—insulin supplied from an injection or insulin pump

EZ-curl barbell—is bent or "wavy" to accommodate a more comfortable grip

Fetal alcohol syndrome—a permanent birth defect resulting from prenatal alcohol consumption

Forced expiratory volume in one second (FEV_1)—defined as the volume of air expired during the first second of expiration

Frailty—a condition in which mechanical weakening is compounded by concomitant issues of fatigue, diminished balance and coordination, reduced physical activity, slowed motor processing and performance, social withdrawal and cognitive decline

Frequency—refers to the number of times certain exercises or muscle groups are trained per week

Functional isometrics—involves performing isometric actions at specific weak points in a range of motion as a means of increasing strength at that particular point

Gastroparesis—a lesser ability to digest and absorb carbohydrates and food

Glycated hemoglobin—a measure of overall blood glucose levels over the previous 2-3 months; percentage of hemoglobin that is bound with glucose

Glycemic control—defined as a glycated hemoglobin of less than 7.0%

Gynoid obesity—characterized by excess amounts of body fat in the lower body region of the hips and thighs

Heart failure—is the pathological state in which an abnormality of cardiac function is responsible for failure of the heart to pump blood at a rate commensurate with the requirements of the metabolizing tissues, or to do so only from an elevated filling pressure

Hemiparesis—weakness on one side of the body

Hemiplegia—paralysis on one side of the body

Hemorrhagic stroke—caused by a ruptured blood vessel in the brain account for 15-20% of strokes

High pulley set up—set up that allows the individual to pull the handle up from the floor or below knee level

Home-based exercise—exercise that takes place in the individual's residence, is not supervised, and is often conducted alone

Hyperglycemia—is defined as fasting blood glucose above 125 mg/dl or a random glucose level of 200 mg/dl or greater

Hypoglycemia—defined as a blood glucose level of 65 mg/dl or below

Hypoxia—oxygen deficiency

Insulin—a hormone produced in the pancreas that facilitates the entrance of glucose into the cell and its conversion to energy or storage

Insulin receptors—a specialized site on a cell membrane where insulin acts

Intensity—describes the amount of weight lifted, or load

Intentional fast velocity–repetitions performed at a fast pace used with submaximal weights where the individual has greater control of the velocity

Intentional slow velocity–repetitions performed at a slow pace used with submaximal weights where the individual has greater control of the velocity

Ischemic stroke–occurs when an artery supplying the brain becomes blocked

Isometric–static actions with minimal change in length

Joint cartilage–cartilage which acts to cushion the ends of bones

Joint compression–occurs when two joints are pressed into one another, causing the anatomical space between them to decrease

Joint-angle specificity–a limitation of isometric resistance training in that strength gains are found only at the joint angle at which the training takes place

Kegel exercises–exercises used to strengthen the pelvic floor muscles

Ketoacidosis–the accumulation of excessive keto acids in the blood stream

Late-onset, post-exercise hypoglycemia–is defined by hypoglycemia that occurs 6–24 hours post-exercise or activity

Lifting belt–belt used to protect the back while performing resistance training exercises

Low back pain–non-specific chronic condition which is a complex and misunderstood interaction of physical, social, and psychological factors

Low pulley set up–set up that allows the individual to pull the handle down from above the head or shoulder level

Lymphedema–a condition involving swelling of the arm due to inadequate draining of lymphatic fluid that can be triggered by heavy upper body exertion or even partial occlusion of the arm due to tight-fitting jewelry or clothing

Maintenance training–involves resistance training to maintain the current level of muscular fitness rather than to develop further gains

Medicine balls–example of weighted implement

Mental retardation–an intellectual and developmental disorder characterized by substandard IQ and need of support

Metabolic syndrome–a clustering of traits that include hyperinsulinemia, obesity, hypertension, and hyperlipidemia

Metastasis–cancer cell migration

Minute ventilation–is the volume of air inhaled and exhaled in 60 seconds

Mobility disability–frail elderly person's capacity to complete purposeful movements at a required speed and maintain balance during these movements

Motivational readiness for change–refers to readiness to adopt and engage in regular, structured physical activity

Multiple-joint exercise–resistance training exercises that stress more than one joint or major muscle group

Muscle action–muscle movement classified as eccentric, concentric, or isometric

Muscle group split routine–involve performance of exercises for specific muscle groups during the same workout e.g. chest and triceps during one workout, biceps and back during another, then legs and shoulders during a third separate workout

Narrow grip–grip for holding a barbell that is narrower than normal or shoulder width

Needs analysis–consists of answering relevant questions based upon resistance training goals

Nephropathy–nerve damage

Neutral grip–used with dumbbells

Normal grip–defined as shoulder width distance of the individual and will differ according to the size of the individual

Obesity–is one of the most prevalent conditions among adults, and is commonly defined using body mass index which is a ratio of weight to height

OMNI RPE–scale similar to the Borg RPE scale, except that it is a 10 point scale

One repetition maximum (1RM)—the maximum amount of weight that can be lifted one time with proper technique

Opened-chain kinetic exercise—exercise that enables the distal segment to freely move against a resistance such as the leg curl

Orthostatic hypotension—fall in blood pressure that occurs in moving from a sitting/lying to a standing position which can result in light-headedness or fainting during activities

Osteoarthritis—is a chronic, degenerative joint disease that primarily affects lower extremity weight bearing joints such as the hips, knees, and spine

Osteocytes—cells located underneath the surface of bone in the mineralized matrix, function as strain transducers and communicate with the cells on the surface of bone where formation and resorption occur

Osteogenic—bone building

Osteopenia—term used to describe low bone density, or bone demineralization and weakening

Osteoporosis—brittle bone disease

Overtraining—training over the dosage that will typically result in positive changes

Oxygen saturation—oxygenation or aeration of blood expressed as a percentage

Passive range of motion—is the range that the joint can be moved manually by the examiner without inducing either movement in another joint or pain

Pediatric—broadly defined to include children and adolescents

Perceived barriers—are perceptions that an individual has that psychologically prevent them from exercising

Perceived exertion for children scale—contains verbal expressions along with a numerical response range of 0-10 and 5 pictorial descriptors that represent a child at varying levels of exertion while resistance training

Peripheral neuropathy—nerve damage in the periphery

Peripheral vascular disease (PVD)—a cardiovascular condition that limits blood flow to the lower extremities

Plate-loaded machine—exercise machine in which plates are loaded to provide the resistance

Pre-diabetes—a condition in which blood sugar levels are elevated but not high enough to be classified as diabetes

Primary osteoporosis—characterized by a marked acceleration of bone mass loss, categorized into three types, postmenopausal (also known as Type I osteoporosis), senile (also known as Type II osteoporosis), and idiopathic osteoporosis (where the cause of osteoporosis is of unknown origin)

Progression—the act of moving forward or advancing toward a specific resistance training goal

Progressive overload—entails increasing the stress placed on the body during the resistance training program

Pronated grip—grip for holding weights with the palms facing down

Proprioceptive acuity—awareness of body position

Pulmonary hypoplasia—incomplete development of lung tissue; reduced lung weight, volume, alveolar count, etc

Pulse oximeter—a non-invasive electronic device that selectively measures oxygen saturation of blood

Quality of life—defined as the gap between that which is desired in life and that which is achieved, is diminished

Recreational training—involves resistance training for moderate improvements in muscle strength, local muscular endurance, and hypertrophy for general fitness

Relative local muscular endurance—endurance assessed at a specific relative intensity, or %1RM

Relaxin—a hormone that loosens ligamentous connective tissue as the body prepares for delivery of the fetus through the birth canal

Repetition velocity—refers to the time it takes to perform a single repetition, and is usually divided into the concentric and eccentric portions of the movement

Resistance tubing—specialized tubing that can provide resistance during training

Resorption—dissolving of bone mineral by osteoclasts

Rule of 20—strategy that involves finding a weight that can be lifted safely and with proper form for 20 repetitions

Sarcopenia—a term used to describe age-related loss of skeletal muscle mass and strength; and entails progressive atrophy of skeletal tissue with reduced number and size of skeletal myocytes as well as intrinsic declines in their contractile performance

Secondary osteoporosis—a consequential condition resulting from another disease process and/or its treatment, such as corticosteroid treatment for asthma or rheumatoid arthritis

Selectorized machine—machine that uses a stack of weights from which the user must insert a pin to select the desired resistance

Shear force—found during the movement of joints, especially when bones move across each other in a sliding motion

Short physical performance battery (SPPB)—a convenient screening tool that can be administered in less than 10 minutes and is scored as a total of 12 points, 4 points each for timed tests that assess balance, walking speed, and chair rise time

Silent ischemia—is a reduction in blood flow to the heart muscle through the coronary blood vessels that is painless and symptom-free

Single-joint exercise—exercises that stress one joint or major muscle group

Skeletal muscle hypotonia—a diminution of muscle tone marked by a diminished resistance to passive stretching

Spasticity—is an uncontrolled contraction that results in a shortened and stiffened joint that the individual is unable to release

Specificity—refers to adaptations that take place that are specific to the training variables

Spondylolisthesis—shifting of the vertebral bodies

Spondylolysis—shifting of the vertebral bodies

Spotting—assistance provided by another individual used during exercises where a weight is held above the head or chest

Stability ball—ball used to modify resistance training exercises

Staging—is a procedure for assessing the range and severity of cancer progression

Stair-climb test—evaluates how much time a person takes to climb a set number of steps

Stork-stand test—a test of balance in which the individual is required to stand on one leg as long as possible

Strain—the deformation of bone tissue in response to mechanical loading resulting in bone hypertrophy

Stroke—the common name for a cerebral vascular accident

Supinated grip—grip for holding weights with the palms facing up

Systemic hypoperfusion stroke—occurs when circulatory failure caused by the heart fails to deliver enough blood to the brain

Systolic dysfunction—reduced cardiac function due to lowered ejection fraction and pumping ability

Thrombotic stroke—is the result of arteriosclerosis that either completely blocks a blood vessel, or narrowing the vessel to the point that an insufficient supply of blood passes through

TNM staging system—stands for Tumor, Lymph Node, and Metastasis and is among the most widely used and is endorsed by the National Cancer Institute and other regulatory groups. This system grades cancer according to: a) the size and scope of the primary tumor on a scale ranging from T1 (least extensive) to T4 (highly extensive); b) lymph node involvement, ranging from N0 (no involvement) to N3 (extensive involvement); and c) presence (M1) or absence (M0) of metastasis

Total body routine—involves performance of exercises stressing all major muscle groups (e.g., 1–2 exercises for each major muscle group)

Trabecular bone—cancellous, spongiosa bone, less dense than cortical bone

Training volume—is a summation of the total number of sets and repetitions performed during a workout, and can be manipulated by changing the number of repetitions performed per set, the number of sets performed per exercise, or the number of exercises performed per session

Transient fetal hypoxia—drop in oxygen levels in the fetal blood supply

Transient ischemic attack—are "mini strokes" that produce stroke-like effects but no lasting effects

Tubing door anchor—anchor that secures tubing during training

Type 1 diabetes—most often appears during childhood or adolescence and results from the autoimmune destruction of pancreatic beta cells which leaves the pancreas unable to make insulin

Type 2 diabetes—is characterized by the development of insulin resistance, which is a decreased ability to use the insulin the body produces, as well as a lesser production of insulin over time

Undertraining—training under the dosage that will typically result in positive changes

Undulating periodization—involves increasing the load and volume of exercise over the course of several training sessions, then decreasing the load and volume of exercise for a short time before increasing both again, but to higher levels than before

Unintentional slow velocity—velocities used during high-intensity repetitions in which either the loading and/or fatigue are responsible for the slow velocity of movement

Upper/lower split body routine—involve performance of upper-body exercises during one workout and lower-body exercises during another

Valsalva maneuver—holding the breath with a closed epiglottis

Variation—refers to consistently altering the stimuli related to the resistance training variables

Vasodilators—class of cardiac drug used to treat heart failure by reducing the afterload on the heart

Weight history—the history of average body weight including weight gains and losses during adulthood

Wide grip—gripping weighted implements with a wider than normal (shoulder) grip

Youth—broadly defined to include children and adolescents

INDEX

D

deadlift, 59, *60*

deceleration phase, 9, 14

deposition, 117, 118

depression, 208–209, 276, 281

description, 53

developmental disabilities, 290

diabesity, 229

diabetes, 230. *see also* type 1
   diabetes (T1D); type 2 diabetes
   (T1D)
   and autonomic neuropathy, 253
   as cause of blindness, 229, 244
   as cause of death, 229, 244
   as cause of kidney failure, 244
   as cause of pregnancy complica-
      tions, 244
   as cause of vascular damage,
      244
   and COPD, 276
   description, 228
   determinants of, 228
   diabetic nephropathy, 254
   diabetic retinopathy, 253
   economic impact, 244
   and elevated glucose/fats, 244
   eye complications, 253
   and heart failure, 244
   individual medical costs, 229
   and loss of central nerve
      function, 244
   and lower-extremity
      amputation, 244
   onset of angina during
      resistance training, 252
   peripheral neuropathy,
      252–253
   and prevascular disease, 252
   total medical costs of, 229

diabetes, gestational, 244

diabetes mellitus. *see* diabetes

diabetes mellitus type 1. *see* type 1
   diabetes (T1D)

diabetes mellitus, type 2. *see* type 2
   diabetes (T2D)

diabetes type 1. *see* type 1 diabetes
   (T1D)

diabetes type 2. *see* type 2 diabetes
   (T2D)

diabetic nephropathy, 254

diabetic retinopathy, 253

diastolic dysfunction, 170

digoxin, 175

diuretics, 175

Down Syndrome (DS)
   comparative levels, muscle
      strength, 292
   congenital heart problems, 297
   hypothyroidism with, 297
   physiological/physical charac-
      teristics, 291
   resistance training for people
      with, 299
   strength gains from training
      intervention, 301
   susceptibility to physical disor-
      ders, 291–292

dumbbell biceps curl, 49

dumbbell chest press, *54*, 54, *54*

dumbbell deadlift, 60, *61*

dumbbell fly, 57–58

dumbbell front raise, 48

dumbbell incline fly, 59

dumbbell incline press, 55

dumbbell lateral raise, 47, 48

dumbbell lunge, *79*

dumbbell prone fly, 58

dumbbell row/bent over row, *66*

dumbbell row/bent-over row, 65

dumbbell shoulder press, 55, *56*

dumbbell shrug, 67

dumbbell squat, 63

dumbbell triceps extension, 64

dumbbell triceps press, 64

dumbbell upright row, *66*

dynamic constant external
   resistance training, 13, 15

dynamic flexibility training, 156

dynamic resistance training
   vs. isometric muscle actions
      (ISOM), 5
   and isometric strength, 158
   low back pain, 155
   for pelvic stabilization, 158
   for spinal stability, 158
   studies of, 157
   for trunk rotators, 158

dynamic strength, and ISOM
   training, 5

dynamic warm-up activity, 213

dyslipidemia, 97

dyspnea, 172, 176, 276,
   277, 281

E

ECC force production, 14

ECC portions of movement, 13

eccentric exercises, 145

eccentric muscle action (ECC), 5,
   9, 144

echocardiogram, 175–176

ejection fraction, 171

electrocardiograph (ECG), 264

emphysema
   case study, 283–284
   causes, 277
   characteristics of, 277
   as COPD, 276
   prevalence of, in population,
      277
   progression of, 277

endothelial function, 232

endurance training, 9

energy balance, 186–187, 207

energy system utilization,
   targeted, 12

energy systems, 12

energy utilization, 16

enterovirus, 230

and rest intervals, 13
training strategies to improve, 15
training to increase, 13
velocity, 15

muscular endurance training, 156
ACSM recommendations, 8
loading strategies, 9
set duration, 15
velocity/repetitions, 15

muscular performance, and velocity, 14

muscular strength
age-related decreases, 124
and exercise sequencing, 7
and multiple-joint exercises, 6
neuromuscular contributions, 14
at novice level, 8

musculo-skeletal impairment, 103

musculoskeletal injuries, 211, 212

N

narrow grip, 24, *25*, 50

National Cancer Institute, 307, 310

National Health and Nutrition Examination Survey (NHANES III, 1988-1994), 116

National Institute on Aging, 105

National Strength and Conditioning Association Guidelines, 215

National Strength and Conditioning Association (NSCA), 4

Naughton protocol, modified, 175-176, 180

needs analysis, program design, 4

nephropathy, 231

nerve damage, and T1D, 229

neural adaptation, in novices, 16

neural conditioning, 189-190

neural responses, and training load, 8

neuromuscular adaptations, 145

neuromuscular contributions, movement pattern/skill coordination, 14

neuropathy, 229, 233, 234, 236, 237

neutral grip, 25
assisted dips, 39
dumbbell deadlift, 60
dumbbell fly, 57
dumbbell incline fly, 59
dumbbell lateral raise, 47
dumbbell prone fly, 57
dumbbell shrug, 67
dumbbell squat, 63
dumbbell triceps extension, 64
dumbbell triceps press, 64
dumbbell/bent-over row, 65
for dumbbells, 24, *25*
hammer curl, 52
kickbacks, 65
lat pulldown, 67, *68*

New England Journal of Medicine, 277

New York Heart Association (NYHA) classification system, 175

normal grip, 24, *25*
definition, 24
lat pulldown, 67
preacher curl, 50
width, *25*

normoglycemia, 228

novices
and frequency of exercises, 15
and resistance training, 10
and strength improvement, 16

nutrition, and aging, 99

O

obese adults
definition, 186
vs. overweight, 206

obese youths, 206
and cardiovascular problems, 208

consequences for adults with, 206
definition, 198
economic impact, 206–207
and energy balance equation, 207
and energy expenditure, 207
environmental factors, 207
epidemic of, 209
etiology, 207
genetic disposition, 207
impact on welfare of military, 207
and life expectancy, 208
medical concerns, 208
metabolic syndrome, 208
vs. normal-weight youths, 215
parental perception of, 207
and physical activity, 208
prevalence of, in population, 198, 206
and psychiatric disorders, 208
as public health threat, 206
resistance training and, 232
strength testing, 213
vs. juveniles of normal weight, 215
weight-related health problems, 206

obese youths, resistance training for, 206, 212–213
24-week sample program, 217
assessment for, 212–213
benefits, 208–209
choice/order of exercises, 214
as cornerstone of treatment, 208–209
designing programs for, 210
effects of, on weight, 211
effects of, on body composition, 211
and epiphyseal plate/growth cartilage, 212
exercise testing considerations, 212–213
goals, 212, 217
guidelines, 214
lower body, 215

R

range of motion, 14
  ballistic resistance exercise
    and, 14
  and compensatory
    acceleration, 14
  and exercise, 137
  exercises at weak points of, 5
  in obese adults, 193, 197
  in older adults, 101, 102, 103,
    106, 108
  in people with cancer, 311, 312,
    313, 315, 317, 319, 320
  in people with diabetes, 197
  in people with lower back pain,
    147, 161, 163
  in people with osteoarthritis,
    137, 139, 143, 144, 145, 147
  power development throughout,
    9, 14
  and repetitions with free
    weights, 14

recreational training, 5

relative local muscular
  endurance, 13

repetition maximum (RM), 7

repetition velocity, 13

repetitions
  deceleration phase, 14
  high-velocity, 14
  in intensity/volume program, 11
  intentionally slow, 14
  vs. load, 10
  for muscular hypertrophy
    training, 7
  an osteoarthritic adults, 145
  and set duration, 15
  an training to failure, 11
  and training volume, 10
  and velocity, 15, 216
  vs. weight lifted, 8–9

resistance training. *see also* under
  specific diagnoses
  benefits, 4, 5, 209, 232
  and bone fractures, 124
  early phase, 11

and high blood pressure, 252
higher velocity regimes, 101
lo g-term, 11
and load/repetition increases, 10
and muscular endurance, 13
optimal, 12
primary goal, 16
progression, rate of, 16
representative free-weight
  exercises, 316
representative machine
  exercises, 316
and resting metabolic rate, 189
studies of, for low back pain,
  158
and "traditional" weight lifting,
  124
and velocity, 14
and very low calorie diet, 189
and weight loss, 189

resistance training, people with
T2D
  diabetic retinopathy, 253
  rest/recovery, 254
  sample 24-week program, 255
  training components, 254–255

resistance training programs
  load components, 145
  multiple-set, 10
  neuromuscular adaptations
    from, 145
  and novices, 10
  periodized progressive, 178
  single-set, 10
  and untrained older adults, 10
  variables affecting, 10
  volume components, 145

resistance training, traditional
  description, 11
  and hypertrophy, 11

resistance training, types, 12
  competitive training, 5
  maintenance training, 5
  recreational training, 5
  traditional, 9, 11

resistance tubing, 24
  door anchor, *40*

exercise progression with, 27
for home, travel training, 40
for resistance training for obese
  adults, 197
safety of, 26
sizes, *27*

resistance-tubing exercises, 40

resorption, 117, 118, 121, 122

rest intervals
  choosing length of, 12
  description, 12
  effects of, 12
  and energy systems contribu-
    tions, 12
  impact on local muscular endur-
    ance, 13
  for youths, 215–216

retinopathy, 233

rheumatoid arthritis, and resistance
  training, 138

RM
  and overtraining, 9
  and training plateaux, 9
  zones and repetitions, 10

RM loading
  in intensity/volume program, 11
  in resistance training for obese
    youths, 214–215

Robinson et al, 12

rotavirus, 230

rows
  dumbbell/bent-over, 65–66
  standing, for older adults, 107
  upright, 66

rubella, 230, 291

Rule of 20, 160

S

sarcopenia
  and aging, 97
  atrophy of skeletal muscle, 101
  and body fat, 97
  causal theories, 98–99
  definition, 96–97

macro/microvascular complications, 230–231
mortality, 230
optimal medical/lifestyle management, 234
prevalence of, in population, 229
and self-care, 233
susceptibility, 230
symptoms, 229
vs. T2D, 230–231, 244

type 2 diabetes mellitus (T2D). *see also* type 2 diabetes (T2D)
exercise vs. weight loss, 246
risks of higher intensity exercise with, 250

type 2 diabetes, resistance training for people with, 243–261
and aerobic training, 246
assessments for, 247, 248–249
benefits, 245–247
and blood glucose control, 245
and carbohydrates, 252
case study, 255–256
designing, 247, 249
exercise testing considerations, 250
exercise-induced angina from, 256
GLUT4 increase, 245
glycemic control, 245
glycemic control during, 256
goals, 248
home-based training, 247
and hypoglycemia, 251
and increasing muscle mass, 245
and insulin action, 245–246, 251
and insulin resistance, 245–246
and insulin sensitivity, 245–246
and lean body mass, 246
metabolic control, 245
and muscle mass, 247
physician approval for, 250
precautions, 251
preexercise, 250–251
research supporting, 245–247
special concerns, 250
studies for, 248–249

vs. T1D, 244
visceral fat loss, 246

type 2 diabetes (T2D)
arthritis and, 254
benefits of resistance training for, 230–231
care of, 244
characteristics of, 244
description, 228
economic impact, 244
etiology, 245
glucose/fats and, 244
heart disease and, 244
and hypertension, 252
lifetime risk for, 244
macro/microvascular complications, 230–231
as medical condition precursor, 244
mortality attributed to, 244
and obesity, 229
and obesity in youths, 208
prevalence of, 229, 244
vs. T1D, 230–231
undiagnosed, 244
vascular damage from, 244

U

unintentional low velocities, 13
United kingdom, osteoporosis in, 116
upper-/lower-body split routines, 6–7, 15

V

Valsalvan maneuver, 26
valvular heart disease, 170
Vasalva maneuver, 126
vascular dysfunction, and resistance training for youths, 209
vasculature, and resistance training, 99

vasoconstriction, 280
vasodilators, 175
velocity, 7
and hypertrophy training, 15
intentional high velocities, 14
intentional low velocities, 13–14
lifting, 13, 14
low/ medium/high compared, 14
of movement/power, 101
and muscle power training, 9
and muscular endurance training, local, 15
repetition, impact of fatigue on, 13
repetition, impact of loading on, 13
and repetitions, 15
ventricular function, 312
visceral adipose tissue, 232
volume
components of, 145
description, 11
and hypertrophy, 9
vs. intensity, 11

W

walking programs, 138
wall push-up, 85
wall squats, 77, *78*
warm-up exercises, 7, 213
weakness prioritization, 7
Wechsler Adult Intelligence Scale, 290
weight lifting, 124
protocols, impact on bone mineral densities, 123
protocols, impact on strength, 123
vs. repetitions, 8–9
weight training, 124
weight-bearing, 124
wide grip, 24, *26*, 67

women
  Asian and osteoporosis, 116
  bone density and resistance
    training, 122
  bone loss in, vs. men, 116, 118
  Caucasian and osteoporosis, 116
  Hispanic, lifetime risk
    for T2D, 244
  Hispanic and osteoporosis, 116
  older, frequency and training
    effectiveness for, 15
  older, impact of weight lifting
    protocols on, 123
  older adults, 246
  osteoporosis, 116
  postmenopausal and resistance
    training, 99

with T2D, and resistance
  training, 247
with T2D and resistance
  training, 247
untrained, 15
young, bone density and
  resistance training
  for, 122

World Health Organization, 244

World Health Organization report
  (May 2006), 116

X

Xenical (orlistat), 193

Y

youths, definition, 206

youths, resistance training for
  and musculoskeletal overuse
    injury, 209
  research supporting, 210

youths, resistance training for
  people with
  vs. aerobic exercise, 209
  behavioral aspects, 209
  benefits, 210

IMPORTANT! READ CAREFULLY: This End User License Agreement ("Agreement") sets forth the conditions by which Delmar Cengage Learning will make electronic access to the Delmar Cengage Learning-owned licensed content and associated media, software, documentation, printed materials, and electronic documentation contained in this package and/or made available to you via this product (the "Licensed Content"), available to you (the "End User"). BY CLICKING THE "I ACCEPT" BUTTON AND/OR OPENING THIS PACKAGE, YOU ACKNOWLEDGE THAT YOU HAVE READ ALL OF THE TERMS AND CONDITIONS, AND THAT YOU AGREE TO BE BOUND BY ITS TERMS, CONDITIONS, AND ALL APPLICABLE LAWS AND REGULATIONS GOVERNING THE USE OF THE LICENSED CONTENT.

1.0 SCOPE OF LICENSE

1.1 Licensed Content. The Licensed Content may contain portions of modifiable content ("Modifiable Content") and content which may not be modified or otherwise altered by the End User ("Non-Modifiable Content"). For purposes of this Agreement, Modifiable Content and Non-Modifiable Content may be collectively referred to herein as the "Licensed Content." All Licensed Content shall be considered Non-Modifiable Content, unless such Licensed Content is presented to the End User in a modifiable format and it is clearly indicated that modification of the Licensed Content is permitted.

1.2 Subject to the End User's compliance with the terms and conditions of this Agreement, Delmar Cengage Learning hereby grants the End User, a nontransferable, nonexclusive, limited right to access and view a single copy of the Licensed Content on a single personal computer system for noncommercial, internal, personal use only. The End User shall not (i) reproduce, copy, modify (except in the case of Modifiable Content), distribute, display, transfer, sublicense, prepare derivative work(s) based on, sell, exchange, barter or transfer, rent, lease, loan, resell, or in any other manner exploit the Licensed Content; (ii) remove, obscure, or alter any notice of Delmar Cengage Learning's intellectual property rights present on or in the Licensed Content, including, but not limited to, copyright, trademark, and/or patent notices; or (iii) disassemble, decompile, translate, reverse engineer, or otherwise reduce the Licensed Content.

2.0 TERMINATION

2.1 Delmar Cengage Learning may at any time (without prejudice to its other rights or remedies) immediately terminate this Agreement and/or suspend access to some or all of the Licensed Content, in the event that the End User does not comply with any of the terms and conditions of this Agreement. In the event of such termination by Delmar Cengage Learning, the End User shall immediately return any and all copies of the Licensed Content to Delmar Cengage Learning.

3.0 PROPRIETARY RIGHTS

3.1 The End User acknowledges that Delmar Cengage Learning owns all rights, title and interest, including, but not limited to all copyright rights therein, in and to the Licensed Content, and that the End User shall not take any action inconsistent with such ownership. The Licensed Content is protected by U.S., Canadian and other applicable copyright laws and by international treaties, including the Berne Convention and the Universal Copyright Convention. Nothing contained in this Agreement shall be construed as granting the End User any ownership rights in or to the Licensed Content.

3.2 Delmar Cengage Learning reserves the right at any time to withdraw from the Licensed Content any item or part of an item for which it no longer retains the right to publish, or which it has reasonable grounds to believe infringes copyright or is defamatory, unlawful, or otherwise objectionable.

4.0 PROTECTION AND SECURITY

4.1 The End User shall use its best efforts and take all reasonable steps to safeguard its copy of the Licensed Content to ensure that no unauthorized reproduction, publication, disclosure, modification, or distribution of the Licensed Content, in whole or in part, is made. To the extent that the End User becomes aware of any such unauthorized use of the Licensed Content, the End User shall immediately notify Delmar Cengage Learning. Notification of such violations may be made by sending an e-mail to delmarhelp@cengage.com.

5.0 MISUSE OF THE LICENSED PRODUCT

5.1 In the event that the End User uses the Licensed Content in violation of this Agreement, Delmar Cengage Learning shall have the option of electing liquidated damages, which shall include all profits generated by the End User's use of the Licensed Content plus interest computed at the maximum rate permitted by law and all legal fees and other expenses incurred by Delmar Cengage Learning in enforcing its rights, plus penalties.

6.0 FEDERAL GOVERNMENT CLIENTS

6.1 Except as expressly authorized by Delmar Cengage Learning, Federal Government clients obtain only the rights specified in this Agreement and no other rights. The Government acknowledges that (i) all software and related documentation incorporated in the Licensed Content is existing commercial computer software within the meaning of FAR 27.405(b)(2); and (2) all other data delivered in whatever form, is limited rights data within the meaning of FAR 27.401. The restrictions in this section are acceptable as consistent with the Government's need for software and other data under this Agreement.

7.0 DISCLAIMER OF WARRANTIES AND LIABILITIES

7.1 Although Delmar Cengage Learning believes the Licensed Content to be reliable, Delmar Cengage Learning does not guarantee or warrant (i) any information or materials contained in or produced by the Licensed Content, (ii) the accuracy, completeness or reliability of the Licensed Content, or (iii) that the Licensed Content is free from errors or other material defects. THE LICENSED PRODUCT IS PROVIDED "AS IS," WITHOUT ANY WARRANTY OF ANY KIND AND DELMAR CENGAGE LEARNING DISCLAIMS ANY AND ALL WARRANTIES, EXPRESSED OR IMPLIED, INCLUDING, WITHOUT LIMITATION, WARRANTIES OF MERCHANTABILITY OR FITNESS FOR A PARTICULAR PURPOSE. IN NO EVENT SHALL DELMAR CENGAGE LEARNING BE LIABLE FOR: INDIRECT, SPECIAL, PUNITIVE OR CONSEQUENTIAL DAMAGES INCLUDING FOR LOST PROFITS, LOST DATA, OR OTHERWISE. IN NO EVENT SHALL DELMAR CENGAGE LEARNING'S AGGREGATE LIABILITY HEREUNDER, WHETHER ARISING IN CONTRACT, TORT, STRICT LIABILITY OR OTHERWISE, EXCEED THE AMOUNT OF FEES PAID BY THE END USER HEREUNDER FOR THE LICENSE OF THE LICENSED CONTENT.

8.0 GENERAL

8.1 <u>Entire Agreement.</u> This Agreement shall constitute the entire Agreement between the Parties and supercedes all prior Agreements and understandings oral or written relating to the subject matter hereof.

8.2 <u>Enhancements/Modifications of Licensed Content.</u> From time to time, and in Delmar Cengage Learning's sole discretion, Delmar Cengage Learning may advise the End User of updates, upgrades, enhancements and/or improvements to the Licensed Content, and may permit the End User to access and use, subject to the terms and conditions of this Agreement, such modifications, upon payment of prices as may be established by Delmar Cengage Learning.

8.3 <u>No Export.</u> The End User shall use the Licensed Content solely in the United States and shall not transfer or export, directly or indirectly, the Licensed Content outside the United States.

8.4 <u>Severability.</u> If any provision of this Agreement is invalid, illegal, or unenforceable under any applicable statute or rule of law, the provision shall be deemed omitted to the extent that it is invalid, illegal, or unenforceable. In such a case, the remainder of the Agreement shall be construed in a manner as to give greatest effect to the original intention of the parties hereto.

8.5 <u>Waiver.</u> The waiver of any right or failure of either party to exercise in any respect any right provided in this Agreement in any instance shall not be deemed to be a waiver of such right in the future or a waiver of any other right under this Agreement.